DAN MARSHALL

Home is Burning

HODDER

First published in Great Britain in 2015 by
Hodder & Stoughton
An Hachette UK company
First published in paperback in 2018

1

A CIP catalogue record for this title
is available from the British Library

ISBN 978 1 473 62431 3

Printed and bound by Clays Ltd, St Ives plc

Hodder & Stoughton policy is to use papers that are natural,
renewable and recyclable products and made from wood grown in
sustainable forests. The logging and manufacturing processes are
expected to conform to the environmental regulations of the
country of origin.

Hodder & Stoughton Ltd
Carmelite House
50 Victoria Embankment
London EC4Y 0DZ

www.hodder.co.uk

Dedicated to anyone who has lost
a loved one to cancer or ALS

PREFACE

Hello. I was once told that the best way to make new friends is to compliment them, and I want you to be my new friend, so let's start with a couple of compliments.

First, you have nice eyes with which you read these words. Or, if you're blind and doing the whole Braille deal, then you have silky smooth fingers made from a thousand angels' wings.

Second, you're the best thing that's ever happened to me. I love you already. Without you, dear reader, these words would just sit on my computer next to a folder called "Graduation Plans" where I hide some porno clips, and by *some*, I mean a lot.

Okay, now that we're already best friends and you love and trust me like a brother, let me quickly go over a few other things before we launch into the crazy, crude, sad, intense, and slightly inspirational story found on these pages.

As you know, this book is a supernatural memoir set in the year 3928—shortly after the first robot ghost was elected president, but before volcano monsters took over earth and added its second moon.

Just kidding.

Just a little goof up top. Sorry to stall. It's just that the subject matter of this book is pretty heavy, but fuck it. Here goes. This is the story of what happened to my family over the course of two years when my mom, Debi, was battling terminal non-Hodgkin's lymphoma and my dad, Bob, was diagnosed with amyotrophic lateral sclerosis (ALS), a terminal neurological disorder more commonly referred to as Lou Gehrig's disease.

Boom, there it is. Two terminally ill parents slammed with misfortune at the same time. Sort of an extreme situation, I know. That's why I started with that bullshit about the robot ghost.

My four siblings and I had no idea what we were doing. No one really does when dealing with life-altering tragedy, but we did the best we could, which wasn't great.

Before you decide whether to take the plunge and dive into our family tragedy, you might want to know a touch more about me. I'm Daniel Joseph Marshall. I have also gone by Danny, Dano, Danny Boy, Big Dick Dan (self-applied and untrue), Dickhead Dan, Mellow Yellow, Marshmellow, Marsh Marsh, D-Marsh, and Turtle Fucker, for reasons I'd rather not get into right now. Oh, and DJ. My dad called me DJ, short for Daniel Joseph. This nickname was fine until *Full House* rolled around and created a female character named DJ Tanner. I then had to request that I stop being called DJ in public so mean kids wouldn't tease me so much. Though I went by Danny for most of my life, I made a switch to Dan recently, because I think it's a little cooler and doesn't sound as childish as Danny.

Physically, I'm five foot nine, though at a recent doctor's visit, I was told I'm closer to five foot seven. It's pretty shocking when you spend your whole life thinking you're one height and then find out you're another. I still consider myself to be five nine. That doctor and his stupid science measuring stuff were full of shit. I was born weighing six pounds, twelve ounces, on September 17, 1982, in Pekin, Illinois, though I've gained a significant amount of weight since then. I currently weigh in around 175 pounds. With my semishort height and my weight, I'm a little dumpy. One friend described me as being a sad little cannonball. I feel that's accurate.

My favorite foods are pretzels, beef jerky, gummy bears, sunflower seeds, and Hot Tamales, which might explain why I've gained so much weight since birth.

Though I was born in Pekin, Illinois—where the high school teams were called the Chinks from 1930 to 1980, before being changed to the much less racist Dragons—I grew up in Salt Lake City, Utah. My family and I are not Mormon. Like most non-Mormons in Utah, I got out of there as soon as I could. Don't get me wrong, I love Utah. It's a hidden gem in this generally ugly world. Most people don't give it a chance because they view Mormonism to be a weird religion. Mormonism is certainly a weird religion, but aren't all religions a little strange? And who really cares what other people believe, so long as they don't believe in rape or kiddie porn? Like Catholics. But no one should live in Utah his or her whole life. It's too much of a warped reality.

So I left Utah for college. I was looking for a place that was at the opposite end of the cultural spectrum, so I decided to attend UC Berkeley. Berkeley is a strange mixture of academics and homeless people, and a refreshing place to live—the type of town where you can be as kooky as you like but also go completely unnoticed.

From Berkeley, I got a job working at a strategic communications and public relations firm in beautiful and scenic Los Angeles. I love traffic and pollution and assholes speeding around in BMWs, so Los Angeles was a great fit for me. I had started a pretty nice little life in Los Angeles. I lived in an apartment off Sunset Boulevard, had a job and a girlfriend I loved, and owned couches with built-in recliners—sort of the American dream in action. I was following that path we're told to follow: go to college, get a job, start instantly planning for retirement, find a significant other you enjoy being around who makes you feel like the world is bright instead of dark, be fun and happy and successful enough to have said significant other fall in love with you and see you as a long-term-provider-type figure, get married, buy a home, start a family, stay away from drugs and alcohol so you can raise that family in a functional way and thus give them a shot at following a similarly safe and happy path and pass along your genes, be proud of your children for doing well with the opportunities you gave them, retire, watch yourself wither away while reminding young people to live it up and have as much sex as possible while they can, etc.

The whole dying-parents mess interrupted that path. I was pulled from what I thought was the real world into a situation that made the real world seem fake.

Full disclosure: there is a lot of bad language in the book. Best to explain that up-front so you're not completely shocked when you see words like *fuck, shit, fart, hell, son of a bitch, asshole,* and *motherfucker* next to words like *dying, death, cancer,* and *Lou Gehrig's disease.* It's very difficult for me to write a sentence without using a bad word. That last sentence, for example, was fucking impossible for me to write.

My family has a very crude sense of humor. Our swear jar was always filled to the brim. When times were stressful, we'd take breaks where we were allowed to yell any obscenities we wanted at each other—sort of a venting mechanism. I'm sure some concerned neighbors would walk by our house and hear a burst of profanity-laced yelling flying out our front door. It was our way of dealing with the world and reducing some grief and depression.

And if I'm really being honest, we just like to offend Mormon people. I know this sounds stupid and petty, but growing up in the Mormon-dominated state that is Utah, we were often made to feel like outsiders, "The Other," which is an unusual thing for a prosperous white family in America to feel. When you are The Other, you begin to resent the majority and look for ways to piss them off. Swearing did that for us.

My mom and I, in particular, have very foul mouths. I always thought it was hilarious when she swore, so I mimicked her behavior. When I was about ten years old, I was lying on the couch reading—undetected by my parents—and I overheard my dad and mom having a little discussion about one of my dad's co-workers. My dad was complaining that the co-worker was a bit of a jerk, and my mom said, "Bob, here's what you do. You look him in the eye and tell him to shut the fuck up." I thought it was hilarious. After that, I decided that, like my mom, I'd swear all the time.

When my dad got sick, we all really amped it up. Increase the pain input, increase the swearing output. Makes sense. And because of the stress, we became increasingly blunt with each other.

I wrote this book because I'm just a sad dude with a big heart who really loves his dad. This book, in many ways, is a love letter to him. Jesus, that sounded sappy. But whatever, loving your dad isn't a crime. I owe him a lot.

My dream is that our story will give people who are currently caring for a loved one—no matter the age, ailment, or situation—some comfort in knowing that another family of shitheads has ungracefully gone through something similar. You're not alone. Tragedy has company, as someone aside from me probably said at some point.

I also hope this book paints me as a tragic hero (of sorts) and makes more people like me, or even love me. That's what life is all about, right? Being loved, loving others, and feeling good about yourself? I've also heard it's about collecting a bunch of material possessions to fill the void. Maybe I'll try that one day.

* * *

Okay, enough bullshitting. Let's get this show on the road. As you read, please keep in mind what great friends we are, and remember, through all this intense nonsense, that I'm just a slightly dumpy dude who loves pretzels and his dad.

HOME IS BURNING

THE BOMB

I fucking love it here," I said like a spoiled white asshole as I looked up at the cloudless sky, seeing only palm trees against the perfect blue.

"I know. I could stay here forever," said my girlfriend, Abby.

Abby and I were celebrating her twenty-fourth birthday at the JW Marriott pool in Palm Desert. She had flown into Los Angeles from Berkeley the night before, and then we had driven out to the desert in my shitty Subaru. We were drinking frozen tropical smoothies full of alcohol, the endless sun beating down on us as we read pointless books with entertaining storylines. The pool band played "Don't Worry, Be Happy" and various Beach Boys songs on a loop. We had incredibly important conversations about incredibly important topics, like where we should eat dinner and how much post-dinner sex we should have. Shit, maybe we'd even hit up a late-night hot tub session if we had the energy after all the eating and fucking. The world was ours.

My parents owned a time-share at this Palm Desert Marriott, and I had grown up vacationing there. It was our family spot. We were from Salt Lake City, Utah, so Palm Desert was one of the closest warm destinations. We liked coming here to get away from our problems and from all the Mormons who lived around us. My mom hated Mormons with a passion. When we first moved to Salt Lake from Pekin, Illinois, our beloved family dog, Basquo, was running around the neighborhood. An evil Mormon kid started throwing rocks at him and pulling his tail, so Basquo bit him. Our Mormon neighbors ganged up on my mom and dad and demanded that we put Basquo under. My mom had disliked Mormons ever since, blaming them for the death of our dog. She trained us to distrust them as well, and made sure we knew there was a normal world outside of Utah. So, as kids, when we'd land at the Palm Springs Airport, my mom was always sure to point out the glowing neon COCKTAILS sign in the terminal bar.

"See, this is what normal places are like that aren't run by a Nazi religion," she would say. "They have bars everywhere."

"Okay, great," we'd say back, not really sure what all that meant.

We spent several Thanksgivings and Easters in Palm Desert. Fuck, we were so comfortable with the place that my gay brother, Greg, came out of the closet here on a family vacation.

I brought Abby to Palm Desert to let her in on the Marshall family tradition of relaxing in the sun and getting away from all of our troubles.

At the time, I didn't have many troubles to get away from. Things were going great. I was living in Los Angeles working my first real job at a strategic communications and PR firm called Abernathy Mac-Gregor, making my own money for the first time in my life. Though the job was occasionally difficult and consuming, I was still very much in that post-college dicking-around phase. I lived in an apartment right off the Sunset Strip, where my roommate Gabe and I would sit on our balcony cracking jokes while watching beautiful struggling actresses walk by on their way toward chasing their Hollywood dreams.

Abby was getting her Ph.D. at Berkeley in materials science. We had met sophomore year of college at Berkeley and had been together since—four years now. She was way smarter than most attractive blondes and was amused by my offbeat sense of humor instead of repelled by it. We were madly in love. Even though we were in a long-distance relationship, marriage seemed inevitable.

Everything with my family was going pretty well, too. Sure, my mom still had non-Hodgkin's lymphoma. She had first been diagnosed in 1992, when she was only thirty-seven years old. I remember the day. She left for the doctor's one morning thinking she had a stomach bug and returned a cancer patient. My four siblings and I were all under eleven. We didn't know what cancer meant. My little sister Chelsea couldn't even pronounce the word. "What is can-sore?" she asked upon hearing the news.

"It's not good," I said, not really sure what it was myself.

Terrifying words accompanied my mother's diagnosis—words like *terminal, inoperable, untreatable,* and *advanced.* It was deemed stage four, or "end-stage," cancer, and she was given only a couple months to live. But, looking her kids in their watery eyes, she vowed to not let cancer leave her children without a mom. She decided to fight it with all her will and strength, no matter how many chemotherapy treatments and surgeries it took. She wasn't going to let cancer beat her.

And it didn't. After nearly seventy rounds of chemotherapy and several surgeries, at age fifty-one she was still standing. The cancer wasn't gone, but it was under control. She and her trusted oncologist, Dr. Saundra Buys, would keep a watchful eye on it. When her immune system or white blood count would begin to drop, she'd start chemo back up. It was a big part of her life and a constant battle. But right now she was feeling good and wasn't receiving any chemo. In fact, she had a full head of hair down to her shoulders.

My dad was doing better than ever. He was fifty-three and cruising along toward retirement. Sure his hair was graying and he was slowly going bald, but life was good. He owned and ran a few weekly newspapers in a variety of small towns across northern Utah, Idaho, and the Pacific Northwest. His business did well and he was financially secure. Plus, he worked for himself, so he was able to manage his hours in a way that allowed for him to have free time to spend with his dipshit family. He'd start every day with a cup of coffee and a dump, and end it with a glass of wine. He was living the dream.

Things were coasting along so nicely that he had recently picked up a new hobby: marathon running. His best friend, Sam Larkin, had gotten him into it a couple years back. I personally think you have to have some sort of mental disorder to want to torture your body via a marathon, but my dad seemed to love it. He had always been an active person—skiing every weekend in the winter—so I guess it made sense that he got addicted to another form of exercise. He was running at least fifteen miles most days of the week. He had to run no matter where we were. It was his meth, his life. It was how we all knew him now—our dad, the marathon-running health nut.

He had just finished running the Chicago Marathon on October 20, 2006. It had been his second marathon of the month. The first was St. George, in southern Utah. My dad was working on qualifying for the Boston Marathon, which is like the Super Bowl of marathons for these runner nuts. He needed to finish the St. George race in under three hours and thirty-five minutes to qualify for his age bracket. The obsessive training paid off. He qualified for Boston by only a few seconds.

My older sister, Tiffany, was working at Fidelity Investments in downtown Salt Lake. She had just finished undergrad at the University of Utah, where she majored in international studies. She had ambitions of going to law school next and was taking a class to help her study for the LSAT. She had just bought a house in a trendy Salt Lake neighborhood. She was a snowboarding fanatic, and even though her studies and work didn't leave her much free time, she'd get up to the mountains a few times a week during the winter season. She was seven years into dating her boyfriend, Derek. Derek was a Park City townie who worked at the Rocky Mountain Chocolate Factory and loved mountain biking. He had a tattoo of a naked lady running along his right arm that he'd let me look at when I was bored at family dinners, so I liked him. He had a giant heart and fit in perfectly with our family. My sister was still trying to figure out all of her career aspirations, but she was happy, settling into a very nice life in Salt Lake close to her beloved mountains.

My gay brother, Greg, was in his last year at Northwestern, in Evanston, Illinois. He was majoring in journalism and fine-tuning his incredible writing skills. He was busy enjoying the freedom that being out and proud brought about, especially now that he lived in a more liberal city than Salt Lake. Greg is a tall, wickedly smart blond, so he had his pick of cock. He was born with cerebral palsy, but after several leg surgeries, he was left with only a slight limp. Oh, and he was uncircumcised. He said that he had a "gimmicky cock that every guy on campus wanted to try out." If life is about fucking as much as possible, then Greg certainly seemed to be nailing it. After college, he planned on getting a journalism job at a newspaper or radio station in Chicago and living in the city with friends.

My little sisters, Jessica and Chelsea—who we always called "The Little Girls"—were in high school. My adopted Native American sister, Jessica, was a popular tenth grader who didn't give two fucks about school or anything. She spent most of her time flirting with boys and hanging with friends. In her early teens, one of the people she had been hanging around was her much older Mormon lacrosse coach. Because of the age difference we thought the relationship was just a bit creepy, so we started calling her coach Creepy Todd. But that appeared to finally be over. She had a couple more years of school, then hopefully she'd be off to college.

Chelsea was almost sixteen. She wasn't popular, so she focused on school. She was a little off socially. We always thought she was just immature, but we had recently begun to suspect that she actually had Asperger's, a mild form of autism. My parents had started looking into getting her some help for it. But Chelsea was a straight-A student and smart as a whip at anything she put her mind to. People with Asperger's often obsess over something, and her obsession was dancing. She was able to masterfully steer any conversation right back to ballet. Oh, and she was absolutely terrific at making fart and ass jokes—a trait I admired and one that had always made us close. A sense of humor is all you really need to get through life.

All in all, my siblings and I were lucky, living with the proverbial silver spoon jammed firmly up our asses. Having two loving parents who were financially stable gave us every advantage to succeed in this mostly unfair world. We always had a nice big roof over our heads, were able to pick whichever college we wanted to attend, and knew that, no matter our failures, our parents were there to help guide us toward success and happiness. I hate when a person uses the word *blessed* like some pious asshole, but we were so blessed—the genetic lottery playing out in our favor. Things had been good, were currently good, and were expected to continue to be good. The future was bright for the Marshall clan.

"Would you like another drink?" the poolside waitress asked Abby and me.

"Oh, fuck, yeah. I'll have another strawberry daiquiri with an extra shot of rum, and whatever she wants," I said back.

"Piña colada," said Abby.

"You got it," said the waitress.

"I love you, babe," said Abby as she looked over at me and smiled her beautiful, radiant smile.

"I love you, too," I said back.

We leaned over and did one of those obnoxious kisses assholes in love sometimes do in public. If I had been watching this display of affection instead of partaking in it, I would've shaken my head and muttered "dickheads" under my breath.

"Aruba, Jamaica, ooh I wanna take you to Bermuda, Bahama, come on pretty mama," sang the poolside band.

When we got back to our room, which looked out on the impeccably manicured golf course, we popped open a bottle of wine, because why the fuck not? I had left my phone charging in the wall socket as to not be distracted from the drinking and sitting around at the pool.

"Holy shit," I said as I picked it up.

I had six missed calls from my mom, three from Greg, and two text messages from Jessica, who primarily communicated via text message, unless she was shit-faced drunk—then she might offer up a drunk dial. The texts just read "Danny?" and "Where are you?"

I instantly knew something was up.

I initially thought, Oh fuck, something happened to one of our dogs. We had two golden retrievers, Berkeley and Mazie, who my parents loved and were always calling to talk about. A thousand hypothetical scenarios ran through my head. Maybe Berkeley had been hit by a car. Or maybe he had swallowed and choked on one of the two tennis balls he usually carried in his mouth. Shit, maybe one of the cruel Mormon neighborhood boys had beaten him to death and carved FUCK THE MARSHALLS into his heart. The Mormons had written FUCK THE MARSHALLS on our mailbox in chalk once. Had they taken it to the next level? Was this the next Basquo situation?

I called my mom back. She answered. "Where the fuck have you been?"

"At the pool. What the fuck is up?" I responded, wanting to match her swear word for swear word—one of our secret games.

"It's your fucking dad," she said back, her voice now trembling.

"Fuck, what happened to Dad?" I responded, suddenly concerned. My dad was beyond healthy, having only missed a couple days of work due to illness his whole life. He won attendance awards at Pocatello High School for never missing a class. He had recently choked on a chicken bone while eating some soup our Polish cleaning lady, Stana (pronounced *Stah*-nuh), had made. Maybe it was related to that? Or maybe it was something else. He had gone to the doctor recently because he had started to experience strange muscle twitches in his upper chest over the summer. We figured it was probably caused by all the running he was doing, and that he just wasn't drinking enough water, so we didn't think anything of it. But his doctor hadn't been sure, so he sent my dad up to see a neurologist, Dr. Mark Bromberg, up at the University of Utah. My dad went to the appointment with a this-is-pointless-but-I'll-go-along-with-it attitude. It certainly wasn't going to be anything serious. In fact, I had forgotten that he had even gone to get it checked out.

"Dad has . . ." My mom was crying too much to even get the words out.

"Dad has . . ." She tried again. "Here, talk to your dad." She shoveled the phone off to him, continuing to cry in the background.

"Hey, DJ. How was the pool?" he asked, as if the phone hadn't been passed to him by a frantic, crying person.

"It was fine. Dad, what's up? Is it the dogs? Did the neighbors carve 'Fuck the Marshalls' into Berkeley's heart?"

"What? No. It's not the dogs," he said.

"Oh, thank God," I said. "Well, what is it then? The fucking chicken bone? Fucking Stana."

"Well, I have—Well, they think I have—Well, they think I might have ALS, Lou Gehrig's disease," he managed.

"Really? That sucks." I paused for a few seconds, not knowing which of the many diseases Lou Gehrig's was. "Wait. Which one is Lou Gehrig's disease again?" I asked, while sipping my glass of wine and thinking about what positions Abby and I were going to try during our post-dinner fuck festival.

"It's a neurological disorder where your spinal cord loses its ability to communicate with the muscles. It's sort of a dying off of your motor neurons that can lead to paralysis," he said, sounding like he was just repeating the words his doctor told him without really processing them. "Those fasciculations in my chest, I guess those were the first signs of it."

"Shit, but you're going to be all right, right?" I asked, clearly not really contemplating the magnitude of this news. "It isn't too serious?"

"I'll be fine." I heard my mom crying in the background and muttering about how he wasn't going to be fine, about how he was going to die. "I can live a long, long time with this. Stephen Hawking has had the disease for forty years or something, so don't worry about me," he said with optimism in his voice.

"But isn't Stephen Hawking, like, crippled, and in a wheelchair, and unable to talk, and always about to die?" I asked.

After a long pause, my dad said, "Well, the point is, I can live a very long time."

"Well, shit, Dad. This can officially be placed in the 'shitty news' file. Are you getting a second opinion?" I asked while polishing off my glass of wine.

"Yeah, we're looking into it. There are a lot of things this could be instead of Lou Gehrig's. It could be Lyme disease," he said back.

"Fuck. Really? Lyme disease?" I had heard of that one.

"Hope I didn't ruin your trip. Is the weather nice?"

"Yes, it's always sunny and hot here."

"Well, you should go back to the pool, or to a nice dinner," he suggested.

"Yeah, might need to. Can I talk to Mom? I love you," I said.

My mom got on the phone, still crying—a stark contrast to my dad's relaxed tone. She seemed convinced my dad was going to die any minute. I told her to settle down and wait for the second opinion before we shit the bed and went into crisis mode.

But this was major news. Our dad was the rock of our family. The stable one. The healthy one. The parent who wasn't going anywhere. We thought if we were going to lose a parent, that it would be our mom. This was wildly off script.

Part of why my mom was able to fight cancer so successfully over the years was because of my dad's willingness to be the solid figure who kept our lives running smoothly. My mom was a terrific parent, but for a lot of my childhood, my dad had to take over parenting duties while my mom was undergoing chemo. There had been no hesitation on his part. His wife had cancer. He needed to step up, so he did. He was Mr. Mom. He built an amazing home and life for us all. It was very close to perfect, minus the whole bit about my mom having cancer.

When my mom was sick and busy with her cancer fight, we looked to our dad for homework help, rides around town, advice on life, allowance money, etc. He partook in all of our stupid hobbies: skiing with Tiffany, watching and playing basketball with me, playing tennis and talking politics with Greg, eating expensive Chinese food with Jessica, and aimlessly chatting about dance with Chelsea—all with patience and genuine interest. He never raised his voice. He was a kind, peaceful soul who was impossible to not like. The perfect dad for a bunch of imperfect children.

I wasn't expecting him to go anywhere. I was expecting for us to always have our rock. But this news—well, it could change all of that.

* * *

Once I got off the phone with my parents, we called Abby's mom—who always seemed to be near a computer—to find out more about Lou Gehrig's disease. This was before I owned an amazing iPhone, so Abby's mom was always our 411 whenever we were lost, needed a restaurant suggestion, or wanted to know more about a terminal illness killing my father. She pulled Lou Gehrig's disease up on Wikipedia.

I started to take the whole thing more seriously when she said things like, "lives for an average of two to three years," and "is considered terminal," and "may require a wheelchair after it leads to paralysis," and "many patients are on a respirator"—all of which I heard as: "Danny, your father and pal and road map to life is going to undoubtedly die soon and leave you a lonely bastard with a drinking and motivation problem."

Just so we're all clear, Lou Gehrig's disease—named after New York Yankees great Lou Gehrig—is a neurodegenerative disease that slowly kills off motor neurons. Without these neurons, the brain can't communicate with voluntary muscles. So say, for example, that someone with advanced Lou Gehrig's disease wants to move their arm or leg: their brain would tell their muscles to move, but they wouldn't be able to actually move their limb because the message can't get through. It also affects the diaphragm, which helps draw air into the lungs. The disease progresses rapidly and leads to muscle atrophy, fasciculations, spasticity, dysarthria, dysphagia, and a bunch of other words I can't pronounce. Its more technical medical name is amyotrophic lateral sclerosis, or ALS.

A person with Lou Gehrig's disease can still feel everything, and their brain functions normally. They essentially become a prisoner of their own body. Some go on a respirator to extend their lives, but the respirator, on average, only adds a couple more years. Doctors are still not sure what causes it, and very little progress has been made in slowing its progression once it's diagnosed.

In other words, Lou Gehrig's disease is a real ugly motherfucker, and is pretty much a death sentence.

After hanging up the phone, I gave Abby a big, sad kiss and ran my hand through her perfect blond hair to help make me forget the tragic news about my dad, my buddy, my pal.

Abby wanted to take a shower before dinner, so I decided to reach out to my siblings in the meantime. I was the last to hear the news because I had been busy letting my brain turn to mush at the pool. I was closest with Greg, so I decided to give him a call first. I went out to our balcony with a glass of wine and dialed.

"'Sup, Gregor?" I said. I was expecting him to be relaxed. He is a calm, levelheaded person, having more of my dad in him than my mom. It was rare to ever see him worked up about anything. Though he does hate bugs.

But instead of exuding his usual composure, he started bawling. Shit is serious if Greg is crying. "Can you believe this shit? Why can't things ever stay good with this fucking family? I mean, isn't Mom having cancer enough for us to deal with?"

"Yeah, I know. It's fucked up. Dad thinks he'll be okay, though," I said.

"Danny, get fucking real for a second. I looked it up on Wikipedia. This disease is a death sentence. We're going to have to take care of him. Mom can't do it."

"I know, I read the Wikipedia page, too. But you never know. That kook Stephen Hawking has had this fucker for like a million years," I said.

"This family, I swear we're cursed. I mean. Dad. Dad. This is happening to DAD. Not Mom. DAD."

"I know. Well, let's wait for a second opinion," I said.

"What's the point? He has it. And now we have TWO terminally ill parents. One hundred percent of our parents are terminally ill," he said.

I didn't want to think about all this. I wanted to go back to vacation mode. "Guess where I am?" I said, changing the subject as I watched some shitbag golfer duff his approach shot.

"Where?"

"At the birthplace of your coming out," I said.

"Oh, I love Palm Desert," he said. We were silent for a second. "God, Dad's going to fucking die."

After I got off the phone with Greg, I called Tiffany. She and I always hated each other: the old first/second child rivalry in full effect. She's a very serious person who doesn't like to joke around. She is prim and proper, and thinks we should all be the same. I'm less serious. Conversations between us would usually go like this: She'd say something. I'd make a horrible joke. She'd say something bitchy in response. I'd say something mean back to her. Then it would end. Maybe things would be different now.

"Hey, Tiff," I said.

"Hey, Dan, you hear about Dad?" she said. She was crying, too. Really bawling her head off. Fuck, should I be crying, too?

"What? No. What happened to Dad?" I said as if I hadn't heard the news.

"He has Lou Gehrig's disease. He's going to be paralyzed and we're going to have to take care of him on a respirator. He's going to die before Mom," she said.

"I was just kidding. I talked to Dad a bit ago. I already knew," I said nonchalantly.

"God, can you not be an unfunny asshole for two seconds?" she said.

"As soon as you pull the stick out of your ass for two seconds," I said back.

"I'm late for my LSAT class. I'm gonna go."

"All right, great catching up," I said. God, I was a fucking asshole.

I sent Jessica a text and asked her if she was okay. She texted back that she was okay and said that Mom was crying and freaking out. I told her that it was going to be okay, that things would calm down. Chelsea didn't have a cell phone at the time. This was before every dickhead over five was carrying one around. I figured that she was just focusing on dance, and possibly making a fart joke or two.

Abby got out of the shower, looking like a wet angel against the Palm Desert sunset. She put her arms around me. She seemed even more beautiful and perfect next to this horrible news.

"You okay?" she asked in her sweet voice.

"Yeah, I think so. I mean, this can't be for real, right? My dad can't have Lou Gehrig's disease," I said.

"Yeah, maybe he doesn't. He's so healthy. He runs all the time," Abby said and forced a smile, trying to play along with my denial.

"Yeah, I'm sure he'll be fine," I managed.

We went to a steak dinner at a nice restaurant and loaded up on wine. I tried to put on a happy face, but I was mainly trying to comprehend what this news meant. It seemed so unreal that our family rock would go down like this. We had expected and even planned for my mom's death at some point. My mom always joked that she was busy picking out my dad's next wife. But for my dad to go? That wasn't possible. I figured the healthy bastard would outlive me and run a marathon on the day of my funeral.

He had always been there for us, and because we were all very spoiled, we were still dependent on him to help with our finances, fix any of our little problems, and just generally give us very grounded and sane advice about how to function in this complex world. He was good at life, and, with his support, so were we. This news meant we might lose the guy who had made our lives as awesome as they were. It might mean no more time-shares in Palm Desert. It was a scary thought.

And what would all this mean for my mom? Would she still be able to fight off cancer without my healthy father at her side? Or would the disease gain momentum and finally make its game-winning attack? And if my dad died before my mom, how would she function? She, even more than the rest of us, was reliant on my dad to keep her life up and running. Fuck, were both my parents going to die soon? Was I going to be an orphan? Little orphan Danny.

And what would happen to all my siblings? Tiffany, Greg, and I were in our twenties and could sort of look after ourselves. But what about Jessica and Chelsea? They still needed parents to guide them into college and adulthood. Would Jessica be able to hang on and get through high school? My dad always helped Chelsea with her math homework. Was she now going to suck at math?

And what would happen to me? My plan was to keep working at Abernathy MacGregor, then try to find something in the Bay Area so I could be close to Abby. I would move in with her, and then propose. Then we'd spend the rest of our lives together completely in love without a care in the world, and then probably get burial plots right next to each other so that we'd always be at each other's side. I know people get married when they're in their late twenties or early thirties these days, but I didn't think I was ever going to find anyone I loved as much as Abby, so why the fuck not get married sooner rather than later? Was this plan now fucked? Would I have to move home and take care of my parents?

What about my poor, kind, loving dad? He was such a sweet, gentle guy to have such a horrific diagnosis. How would he handle all of this? He was supposed to fade to old while still running and skiing and traveling and drinking his nightly glass of wine, all while doing his best to keep his wife alive. Fuck, he was planning on running a couple marathons a year for the next ten years. How would he handle losing his favorite hobby? How would he manage slowly losing control of his trusted body one muscle at a time? He had figured that he'd have twenty-five to thirty more years to cram the rest of his life in. But Wikipedia said he had only two to three? Fuck that. How dare this asshole disease pop up and ruin him? I already hated it. Fuck Lou Gehrig's disease.

I didn't want to think about any of this. I just wanted to drink and eat steak, and go back to being a spoiled white asshole on vacation in Palm Desert.

"What are you thinking about?" asked Abby. Her eyes were a little puffy. She had been crying off and on; it seemed I was the only person who hadn't cried yet.

"Oh, nothing. Just my terminally ill parents and how my life might totally be fucked now . . . Let's get drunk," I said.

I ordered another bottle of wine and filled our glasses to the brim.

PREPARING FOR
THE SHITSTORM

Second and third opinions from Stanford and Johns Hopkins Universities confirmed the diagnosis. My dad officially had Lou Gehrig's disease.

Fuck. Shit. Goddamnit. Murder. Fart. Cock.

The ALS storm was brewing in the distance with ambitions of taking everything from my dad and ruining our perfect little lives. We now needed to figure out what to do about it.

My solution was to go back to Los Angeles and just ignore the whole thing. I was in denial mode. So I continued rocking my sunglasses and a shit-eating grin while living my silly L.A. life. What am I going to do, cure Lou Gehrig's disease? I thought. I can hardly do my own laundry. I assumed that the whole thing would work itself out, and that I wouldn't have to think about it for several years. This wasn't real. My dad was going to be fine. He was invincible. Nothing bad could *actually* happen to him.

"That's a real bummer about your dad," said my roommate Gabe as we were out drinking our dicks off at the Lava Lounge on La Brea, our local watering hole. "Man, life is so fucked up." Gabe had lost his dad to that soulless shit muncher leukemia when he was only fifteen, so he knew what it was like to have a sick father.

"Yeah, well, life goes on. Nothing I can do right now," I said, gulping down a gin and tonic and ordering another.

"What does ALS even stand for?" he asked.

"Ass-a-morph Latter Something-or-other. I don't fucking know. I just call it Lou Gehrig's disease," I said. I hadn't even taken the time to learn how to pronounce the disease that was killing my father.

I was probably so relaxed about the diagnosis because of my dad's calm demeanor. It was one of his talents, but also one of his flaws—to make tragic events seem totally okay. After Michael Jordan nailed that infamous jumper over Bryon Russell in the 1998 NBA Finals to win his sixth championship, a game we attended at the Delta Center in Salt Lake, my dad said, "Well, the Jazz lost this year, but they'll be good again next year." "Fuck off, Dad," I'd responded to his cheery observation as we walked away from the arena in defeat.

Following confirmation of his diagnosis, I'd call him every few days to check in. We'd chat a little about the disease, but then he'd change the subject to something about me. He didn't like talking about himself. When we did talk about the disease, he was in incredibly high spirits. It was as if nothing had changed. I guess he had the right to be optimistic. He wasn't showing many serious signs yet. The fasciculations in his chest were getting a little worse, but the rest of him was still strong. He was still running every day with Sam. His breathing was fine. Everything appeared to be close to normal.

"I can live a long, long time with this disease," he explained over and over again.

"Okay, that's great," I'd reply, kicking my feet up and relaxing in the California sun. I believed that if anyone could live with this thing, it was my sturdy, healthy dad.

"So how's work?" he'd ask, steering the conversation away from his terminal illness. "And when will you see Abby again?"

My mom was a different story. She was in full panic mode. For the first time in her life, she had to picture things without her loving, caring husband at her side. She had started calling me a lot, sometimes in the middle of the night.

"Danny, what the fuck are we going to do?" she'd ask.

"It's four in the morning, Mom. Can I call you tomorrow?" I'd say back.

"Yeah. But seriously, what the fuck are we going to do?" she'd say.

"I'm going to go back to sleep. So should you." I'd hang up, then instantly get a text message from her. "What are we going to do if Dad dies?" it'd read. I'd readjust in bed and try to get some more sleep before having to wake for work.

My siblings weren't quite as aloof as I was. Tiffany, in particular, was terrified. Being the oldest of the five kids, she was always under a lot of pressure to help out with family emergencies. If it wasn't my dad driving my mom to chemo or helping out with the little girls, it was

Tiffany. She had chosen to stay in Salt Lake while Greg and I went off to college to drink and fuck around. Since she was only a phone call away, a lot of the family burden fell on her.

By the time she reached her mid-twenties, she was burned out on dealing with family issues and wanted to get on with her life. She thought it was unfair that nothing ever fell on Greg and me. She resented our selfish asses. And now that my dad was getting sick, she had one more sack of shit to help manage. Separating her life from the family's life seemed to be getting harder and harder.

When the news broke about my dad, Tiffany's boyfriend Derek had been off visiting family and mountain biking in Vernal, some shit-kick town in Utah. Tiffany had asked him to come home because she was freaking out and she didn't know what to do. He said he would come home immediately, but he ended up staying for an additional week while feeding Tiffany lies and excuses. Tiffany took it as a sign that he wasn't going to be supportive when things got really bad, so she decided to cut it off right then and there.

"Dad getting sick made me realize life is short. I need to be with someone who is a little more serious," she explained to me when I came home for Thanksgiving. I was thinking about giving her some shit about it and saying something ruthlessly mean, as was our tradition, but breakups aren't easy, so I left her alone on this one.

Derek had been a part of the family—attending just about every important event all the way down to funerals—so we were upset by his exit. It seemed as though we had already started losing things because of this shit disease.

Tiffany started dating a guy she met in her LSAT class, Brian. Brian had loftier career goals and dreamed of traveling the world and owning a fancy house full of golden retriever puppies. He seemed like a good match for my sister. And on top of all that, Tiffany had accidentally told my mom that Brian had a large penis. My mom can't keep a secret, so she told the rest of us. I thought it was hilarious and started calling him BCB, standing for "Big Cock Brian."

My dad had always done a great job of looking after Tiffany. My mom stressed her out, while he calmed her down. They were ski pals, and got along beautifully. She was facing the possibility of losing that now, so it made sense that she'd want to date someone who could look after her and care for her. The big cock was just a bonus.

Greg decided that once he was done with his senior year at Northwestern he would move back home to help take care of our parents. He already had a job offer from a media company called Gannett. Living in Chicago near gay bars and nice restaurants with friends sounded nice, but that shit would have to wait. Maybe guys in Utah would also be interested in his gimmicky, uncircumcised penis.

Jessica was really confused by our dad's diagnosis. She had no idea what Lou Gehrig's disease was or what it would mean for our dad. She hadn't read the Wikipedia page like the rest of us. My mom had been getting chemo throughout most of Jessica's life, so she figured that our dad would be given similar treatment and would be okay. Jessica had always been introverted and shy around the family. She was a lot closer to my dad than she was to my mom. He had always been the one to drive her around to lacrosse practice and to friends' houses. She was also good at talking him into buying her things: clothes, DVDs, phones, new electronics, etc. Even if she wasn't outwardly saying she was affected by my dad's diagnosis, she definitely was.

Shortly after the bomb, my parents began occasionally finding Jessica drunk in our basement, sometimes passed out and covered in vomit. She had also charged thousands of dollars' worth of clothes and shit for her and her friends onto my mom's credit card without her permission. I guess we all cope in different ways.

At Thanksgiving dinner, which we spent at the Larkins'—my dad's running partner Sam's family—my parents asked me to talk to Jessica about the drinking. They had talked to her about it and notified the school counselors, but they thought she should hear it from me. I was the cool brother who she looked up to.

"So Jess, why the fuck are you drinking?" I asked, a little tipsy myself. I was holding a tall glass of wine filled to the brim. Sam's daughter, Becca, loved drinking as much as I did, so she kept pouring. It was my third or fourth of the night. I was losing track.

"I'm not," she said, always keeping her responses short and sweet.

"Mom and Dad said they've found you drunk a couple of times," I said.

"Well, you drink," she said, eyeing the glass of wine in my hand.

"But I'm an adult. I'm allowed to drink. I'm supposed to drink. You're a kid. Your brain is still developing. You're dumb to drink," I said, then gulped down the wine.

"K. Whatever." She walked off to sit alone in some other part of the house.

Chelsea also had no idea what was going on. Anytime I brought up the Lou Gehrig's, she'd crack a stupid joke and then change the subject.

"What do you think about this whole ALS thing?" I asked her.

"It's fine. Dad will be fine," she said. "Hey, so I was thinking that they should call it A-S-S instead of A-L-S." She giggled uncontrollably.

"I like that," I said back.

"Oh, our dad? He has A-S-S. It's nothing," she said back.

"But seriously, are you dealing with this okay? It's pretty big news," I said, trying my best to be a good brother.

She looked at me and smiled. "God, can you believe Tiffany is dating Big Cock Brian?" Chelsea would often repeat things she heard me say and was always trying to mimic my sense of humor, so she was already calling Brian by his new nickname.

There was no getting around the fact that my dad's disease meant Chelsea's life was going to change immensely. My parents did everything for her. My dad helped her with all her homework every night. They drove her to and from school and then to dance class. She was going to have to learn to be more independent. My parents were just beginning to seek help for some of her social issues, but therapy for Chelsea had been pushed to the back burner now that there were more serious issues at hand.

"That big cock must be really great to leave Derek for it," she giggled, not really having any idea what she was saying.

By Christmas, my mom had started to calm down a little bit. She realized that panicking wasn't productive. We needed to face this fucking disease head-on and try our best to remain positive. When she had been diagnosed with terminal cancer, like, a million years ago, and survived, she credited her hopeful attitude for getting her through it. She wasn't just going to roll over and let cancer fuck her to death. She was going to fight, and fight hard, and suggested that we all do the same, no matter what it was we were battling.

Over the years, hope became a part of her whole persona. She had branded herself as a survivor fueled by hope and the commitment to never give up. Her side of the bedroom was plastered with inspirational, hope-related words of wisdom and quotes. She had hope-themed T-shirts, greeting cards, and bracelets. She had a rock engraved with the word *Hope* that she'd bring to chemotherapy and rub as the cancer-fighting chemicals were blasted into her. For a while, she also wrote a column called "Silver Linings" that ran in some of my dad's weekly newspapers. The column detailed stories of hope and triumph, mainly from her personal life. Fuck, she even went as far as changing her e-mail address to nvrgvupdeb@frontier.com, the nvrgvup short for "Never give up." It was as though she was the self-proclaimed spokesperson for hope, because hope had worked for her.

Lou Gehrig's disease isn't cancer, but she wanted my dad to be around as long as possible. She wanted him to battle as hard as she had and to "never give up." So she stopped acting like a crazy person, and she and my dad started to formulate a plan for how we were going to manage this thing if and when it started to get bad.

I flew into snowy Salt Lake City with Abby for Christmas. Coming home for Christmas was always one of the best events of the year. It was a cozy time full of my favorite activity: acting like a spoiled white asshole. Friends were in town. Snow was on the ground. There was always a lot of drinking. Our living room had high ceilings, so we'd always get a tree in the fifteen-to-twenty-foot range, beneath which my mom would pack a seemingly endless supply of presents. We'd sit around watching Christmas movies with a light buzz, feeling that warm feeling you get around the holidays, that feeling like nothing bad is ever going to happen.

On Christmas Eve, we'd all crowd around the towering Christmas tree in goofy pajamas. My dad would toss on a Santa hat and read "'Twas the Night Before Christmas," even though we were all getting way too old for that shit. Tradition was tradition. Then we'd select someone to open the first present of Christmas. It was usually one of the little girls, since they were younger and Christmas meant more to them, but sometimes it would be whoever was having a hard year and needed a present the most. It had never been my dad.

But that Christmas, there was a certain intensity in the air. This trip wasn't all about watching *Elf*, getting too many presents, and letting alcohol slowly numb our brains. There were some serious issues to talk through.

On Christmas Eve, my mom called us all around the Christmas tree for our first post-diagnosis family meeting. We all still wore our silly pajamas, the Santa hat on my dad's head, our happy golden retriever dogs smiling at our feet. The ornaments danced and sparkled on the tree as if nothing were wrong. Outside, snow fell lightly, adding to the ambiance. I snuggled up on one of the living room sofas with Abby. We both had eggnog in our mugs, with an extra shot of whiskey, because why the fuck not?

"I know it's Christmas, but I don't know when we'll all be together again," my mom said as we all diverted our attention from the presents to her. Her inane pajamas had reindeer all over them. "We've got a shitstorm heading our way and we've got to figure out what to do."

"Maybe Dad should just go in a nursing home," suggested Greg, who was working on a hot cocoa and wearing Batman pajamas.

"Have you ever been to a nursing home? They're full of a bunch of old fuckers shitting their pants and watching *The Price Is Right* all day," I said, scratching an eggnog stain off my Grinch bottoms.

"Well, Dad will get that way eventually," he said.

"I won't get that way for a long, long time," my dad said while looking down at his Superman PJs.

"Maybe we should sell the house and just travel until you're dead," suggested Tiffany. She wore red pajamas covered in hearts.

"Maybe Dad should just take a dance class, and everything will be fine," giggled Chelsea from her Hello Kitty getup.

"God, you're dumb, Chelsea," said Jessica. Jessica wore her usual baggy jeans and a pullover sweater, apparently too cool to partake in tradition.

"When can we open the first present of Christmas?" asked Chelsea.

Poor Abby sat there stunned, wondering why she hadn't just gone home to spend the holidays with her family instead of coming to Utah to be with us morons.

"EVERYONE SHUT THE FUCK UP!" my mom yelled, slamming down her little red notepad. She was a list maker, and had apparently made a list of everything she wanted to discuss and plan for. We all shut the fuck up as my mom took the floor. She opened the notebook as if she was reading an alternative version of " 'Twas the Night Before Christmas" called " 'Twas the Night Before the Shitstorm."

"Shit is going to get bad, but we've all got to buck up and deal with it," she explained. "I didn't survive cancer by sitting around on my fat ass. And we're not going to sit around on our fat asses while your dad dies. He's going to live a long time, but we've got to be ready."

"Yep, I'm going to live a long, long time," confirmed my dad.

We all nodded in agreement. Lou Gehrig's disease is very unpredictable, so it's hard to know exactly how fast and hard it's going to hit. But my mom was right. It would be best to prepare for everything so we weren't surprised when it started to get bad. We didn't want to be the idiots who didn't take the necessary precautions.

"Your dad and I have talked, and here's the plan . . ."

The first order of business was what to do with the family house. We had moved into the house in 1991, a few months after we adopted Jessica and a year before my mom got cancer. The house was the gem of a predominately Mormon neighborhood called the Corn Patch, which we'd sometimes call the Porn Patch, just to offend our neighbors. We were the only non-Mormon family in the neighborhood, besides our across-the-street neighbor Ralph. It was a seven-bedroom, five-bathroom, three-story redbrick mansion surrounded by pine, aspen, and cottonwood trees. It boasted a tennis court, a swimming pool, a trampoline, a drinking fountain, three pinball machines, a hot tub, and a gazebo. And it was a giant middle finger to all our Mormon neighbors. "Ha ha. We don't even believe in God and we still have a bigger house than all of you," we'd think. They would then probably cite the cancer and Lou Gehrig's disease as signs that there was a God and remind us that God punished nonbelievers.

My mom said we could either keep the house and make it wheelchair accessible, or find a new house that was already wheelchair accessible. Renovations would include adding an elevator from the garage up to my parents' bedroom, making a couple of bathrooms wheelchair accessible, building a few ramps, replacing the carpet with thinner material that would allow the wheelchair to roll with ease, and widening some of the doorways.

Ultimately, my mom and dad decided that it would be easiest to stay in the house—that moving would be too much unnecessary work.

"We're keeping the house, and we're going to make it as comfortable and nice as ever," my mom said. "We're not moving into some dump because of this fucking disease. It's not getting everything."

My parents were going to meet with architects and contractors to get the renovations going. I was happy we weren't selling the family house. We had been through a lot in it; it was like an eighth family member. I'm sure some of our Mormon neighbors were hoping we'd get out and take our porn jokes with us, but the foulmouthed Marshalls were staying put.

"I know it sucks that Dad's dying and all, but it's pretty fucking sweet that we're going to have an elevator in the house," I said as I sipped on my eggnog. Greg nodded in agreement, while Tiffany gave me a bitchy look. Add "elevator" to the list of our house's awesome amenities.

The next order of business on my mom's list was how we were going to manage the disease once it started to get bad.

"Your dad has taken care of me over the years, so now it's my turn to take care of him. We're going to do everything we can for as long as we can," my mom said with some of her patented hope.

There isn't a cure for Lou Gehrig's disease, but there are ways to deal with it. With my dad, the disease had started its attack in his upper body. That's not good because it can go after the diaphragm, which in turn affects breathing. That's how most ALS patients go: their lungs weaken so they can't get the almighty oxygen to the rest of their bodies. But my mom made it clear that once an issue came up, we'd toss a solution at it. So, if my dad couldn't chew, he'd go on a feeding tube. If he couldn't stand in the shower, he'd get a shower chair. If he couldn't walk, he'd go in a wheelchair. If he couldn't breathe, he'd go on a respirator. If he couldn't talk, he'd use a communication device. If he couldn't make it to the toilet for a shit or piss, he'd use diapers and a urinal. It didn't matter how much any of this cost. My parents were willing to spend everything they had. A lot of ALS patients choose to do nothing and just let the disease take them. Or some will do the feeding tube and wheelchair grind. Only a small percentage elect to go on a respirator. But it sounded like my dad was going full bore. It was the full Marshall Never-Give-Up Package.

"I don't mind spending the rest of my life taking care of him," my mom said as she took my dad's Lou Gehrig's disease hand into her cancer hand and smiled a supportive smile.

But the thought of seeing my crippled dad in a wheelchair, shitting into a diaper while some robot replaced his gentle voice and some clunky machine breathed for him, sounded like a nightmare to me. I took a sip of my eggnog and looked at Abby's sweet face, trying to push the image out of my mind.

The next item on the list was what to do with my dad's newspapers.

My siblings and I were too busy pursuing our own interests to give a fuck about the family business. My dad had a partner, Kris, but Kris was looking to retire. So my dad figured that he'd sell the papers to make things easier when he got sick. He certainly couldn't run a newspaper from a wheelchair while hooked to a breathing machine.

Next on the list was the Boston Marathon. My dad had run his skinny little ass off to qualify for it, and he still wanted to do it. We weren't sure if he should be running now that he was terminally ill. But Dr. Bromberg seemed to think it would be okay, as long as he stayed hydrated and continued to eat well.

"He's still going to run it," my mom proclaimed.

"Really?" I said. "I mean, that's really inspiring and all, but is it really okay?"

"I'll be fine. I'm going to keep running," my dad explained.

On the one hand, I thought it was a complete mistake. By this point, I had read a lot more about ALS. I read that though they don't know what causes Lou Gehrig's disease, it seems to occur with greater frequency in those people who push their bodies to the max. Lou Gehrig himself was famous for setting the record for most consecutive baseball games played, 2,130—a record that stood for fifty-six years before Cal Ripken Jr. finally broke it. I thought all the running was a contributing factor to my dad's diagnosis. It certainly couldn't be good for the muscles, and it probably drained my dad of all the nutrients that had kept him so healthy and strong over the years.

But on the other hand, my dad loved running. It was his escape, his therapy, his release. Whether he ran or not, he still had Lou Gehrig's disease, so he might as well die doing something he loved.

My mom was a little uncertain about the marathon, but she knew how much he loved it, so she decided to fully support it. Sam and my dad's other running pals, Donna and Paula, said they'd run it with him to make sure he made it through.

Next up was managing our own mental health as things got bad. Dr. Bromberg had advised that my mom and dad both go on an antidepressant, because apparently slowly losing functioning in your body and no longer being able to do the things you love is quite a bummer.

"I actually really love these antidepressants. I should've been on this shit for years," my mom said, as she smiled as big as I'd ever seen her smile. "You guys should really try them."

They had also started seeing a therapist, Robin. Robin suggested that they try to cherish the time they had together and not fixate too much on the future. She said to focus on what my dad could do, instead of what he couldn't. She also suggested that my dad come up with a few activities he wanted to do with each of us before he turned into a crippled mess—sort of a bucket-list-type thing.

"We'll go to a Jazz game together," I said.

"I'm going to take him helicopter skiing in January," said Tiffany.

"We'll play a lot of tennis when I move back home," said Greg.

"You can take me to dance," said Chelsea.

"You can buy me a new digital camera," suggested Jessica.

"We're also trying to figure out a big family vacation to take this summer," said my mom.

"That all sounds great," my optimistic dad said.

Then finally, there was the issue of us all helping out. My parents were a little divided on this topic. My mom thought we all should move home instantly to lend a hand and spend time with our dad, but my dad didn't want to burden us. He knew our adult lives were starting and didn't want the disease to get in the way of that. He liked being the giver of attention, not the receiver. He wanted to just hire an aide when it got bad, but my mom thought we should be the ones to care for him.

"We're his fucking family, so you little shits really need to step it up now, especially you older kids," my mom said.

"Well, I'm already moving home this summer," bragged Greg.

"I might be at law school, and I have work, and Brian and I might take a vacation to Costa Rica next year, but I'll do all I can," said Tiffany in a panic.

"I already live here, remember?" Chelsea giggled.

"Listen, I don't want everyone sitting around feeling sorry for me and waiting for me to die. You have lives, too," my dad said.

"Oh, get over your denial, Bobby Boy," said my mom. "We had all these shithead kids for a reason."

Looking back, I should've called up my work right then and there and quit. I should've weaseled out of my apartment lease. I should've tossed everything I owned in boxes and raced out of Los Angeles and back home as quickly as I possibly could. I should've jumped at the opportunity to spend as much time as possible with my still relatively healthy dad. But I didn't know. I didn't know how serious this horrible disease actually is. I figured I'd start visiting more frequently, maybe

I'd even move back eventually, but for now I had a new career to worry about, a girlfriend, an apartment, a life—albeit a selfish, stupid one.

"And that's it for now, troopers," my mom said, closing her notebook.

We were all as silent as the falling snow as we looked over the wrapped presents, not really wanting to open them anymore. I glanced over at my dad, his Santa hat drooping on his head. I couldn't believe all this was happening. He looked so healthy, so alive. His usual self. Was he really going to slowly become paralyzed while his family ran around trying to put the fires out? It didn't seem real. I loved the man more than anything. He had done such a great job of taking care of all of us over the years, and it was weird that the roles would potentially be reversing—that we'd be taking care of him—and this early in life. Everyone expects to tend to their parents eventually, usually when they're in their eighties and have dementia and are writing their names in shit on the wall. But my dad was in his early fifties. Were my siblings and I going to have to derail our lives to try to help him manage this unlucky turn of events?

I took a big swig of my eggnog and cuddled up even closer to Abby's warm body. My dad was in for a long year, so I figured he finally deserved the first present of Christmas.

"Dad, you got the first present this year," I said as I grabbed a gift for him and tossed it his way. He caught it with his still-strong hands.

"Thanks, DJ," he said. He paused and looked over his family, then ripped it open.

THE YEAR BEFORE
THE WORST YEAR
OF OUR LIVES

My dad and I always had a great relationship. He was my pal. My buddy. My friend. It was never like, "Oh, fuck! I've *got* to hang with my dad." It was always more like, "Oh, fuck yeah! I *get* to hang with my dad."

We were guys who liked guy things. We didn't get too emotional about anything. I had only seen him sort of cry once—when his dad died. Even then, he cried for only a few seconds, and then he said, "It's part of life, and he was suffering. Let's get packed for his funeral." My dad trooped through life hardly ever showing grief or sadness. To him, life was short, so he thought we should enjoy it without unnecessary stress.

Our relationship was built on these laid-back, easygoing principles. We were in this mess together—a couple of goofballs who liked sex jokes, basketball, and trying to make sense of the complexities of our existence.

Over the years, he didn't get much of a break from caring for his children and his sick wife, but occasionally we'd sneak up to the mountains to ski—leaving all our problems back in the Salt Lake Valley. Some of our best conversations took place on the chairlifts heading up the mountain. He'd always start off the day by saying something incredibly blissful, like "There's no place I'd rather be right now," and "Boy, it's so beautiful up here," and "God, being up here makes me forget all of life's worries." We'd then get chatting about the small stuff: the Utah Jazz, the stock market, *The Sopranos*, the *Sports Illustrated* Swimsuit Issue, or how crazy my mom could get.

But as the day progressed, we'd both open up in ways we wouldn't when we were back in that grimy, polluted civilization. He'd encourage me to talk about whatever was troubling me: school, planning for the future, dealing with my mom's cancer. When I was feeling especially courageous, I'd even ask him about girls.

"How do you get a girl to like you?" I'd ask while knocking the snow off my boots with a ski pole.

"Just be you. And if she doesn't like you, fuck her. Move on. It's her loss," he'd say with a smile and pass me hand warmers to stuff into my gloves.

I loved how things were between us. I loved our meaningful, open conversations. I loved knowing that he had my back. I wanted that to last forever. The thing that scared me the most about Lou Gehrig's disease was that it would change our relationship. I liked having my dependable dad looking after me no matter what.

"You went fucking helicopter skiing?" I asked over the phone as I drove through L.A. traffic on my way home after work.

"Yep, they took Tiff and me up around Snowbird, dropped us, and we skied completely fresh powder," my dad said. "We did seven runs."

"But you have Lou Gehrig's disease, remember?" I said as I thought about honking at some dickhead who'd cut me off.

"Yeah, I struggled a little with some of the deeper powder, but it was absolutely fantastic," my dad replied.

I was ecstatic that my dad was still able to go skiing. And not just skiing, but some of the most intense, beautiful backcountry skiing in the world. It meant that he was still healthy. It meant that his body was still working. It meant that he was still able to do all the things he loved. Plus, he got to spend time in the mountains, his getaway from the hectic world.

The year 2007 appeared to be off to a strong start.

The skiing was the first of his bucket list items for the year. But there were others on the way. He had put his business up for sale, so he was busy with that, but he had enough free time to enjoy life while he was still healthy. Soon after the helicopter skiing, he and his best buddies went on a ski trip to Sun Valley, one of his favorite spots. They skied, drank, and sat in hot tubs—a dream vacation away from their wives. My dad was staying exceptionally active. He and my mom walked Berkeley and Mazie every night through our neighborhood. Jesus Christ, those two just won't die, I bet the Mormon neighbors thought as they saw my energetic parents speed by. Then, of course, there was the Boston Marathon on the horizon. That was the big one.

My mom started to frame my dad's running of the marathon as the ultimate act of never giving up. He wasn't just a man running a marathon, but a terminally ill hero who was beating the odds and not letting his disease get in the way of his dreams. My mom thought the story was so inspiring that she reached out to all the local TV stations and newspapers to pitch it to them.

"My husband has Lou Gehrig's disease, but he's still running the Boston Marathon," she explained to them. "He's never giving up."

She then expanded the story to include her own fight with cancer. "We always thought I'd die first," my mom explained. "But now it might be him."

The story ran locally on a few TV stations, and then *CBS Evening News with Katie Couric* reached out and said they'd be doing a nationally televised report as well.

The Boston thing became major. Friends and family rallied around my dad in support. Some would even get teary eyed. "Your dad—no, your whole family—is so brave and strong," they'd cry.

"Really? I think we're a bunch of idiots," I'd say back.

My mom even made T-shirts that said HEAVEN CAN WAIT BECAUSE BOB'S RUNNING BOSTON, which I thought was pretty silly since we weren't religious and didn't believe in a heaven or hell. My mom loved all the attention. It provided a nice distraction so she and my dad could delay worrying about all the depressing things heading our way. In an e-mail to me, my dad wrote:

> I don't know if running has anything to do with me getting ALS (I sincerely don't believe that it has) but it has made a tremendous impact on my life after getting this goddamn disease. Training for the Boston Marathon has given me purpose and focus at a time it would have been so easy to sink into concern and depression.

During this stretch, I was back in Los Angeles working and being a piece of shit. Abby and I were stronger than ever. Any chance I had to leave town, I'd head up to Berkeley to eat great food, cuddle, and fuck. Things weren't serious enough with my dad for me to go home yet. I wouldn't have had anything to do, except watch my parents prepare for the trip to Boston. I was hoping, praying, that things would stay like they were, that the disease wouldn't move too fast. I did, however, provide my parents with a new nickname: Team Terminal.

"How's Team Terminal doing today?" I'd ask over the phone.

"Good, good. I went for a long run. Then we just walked the dogs. I'm going to BBQ up some steaks soon here, and we're going to eat dinner out in the gazebo," my dad would say as if nothing was wrong.

"Great. Well, I'm going to get back to cuddling with Abby and not caring about anything important," I'd say.

In February, I flew home for a Utah Jazz game because having a beer with me at a Jazz game was on my dad's bucket list. I hadn't seen him since our family meeting at Christmas. For the first time since his diagnosis, I could tell something was up. He was skinnier than usual, and not just from running. His arms weren't as mobile and his voice was softer. It was hard for him to lift the beer up to his mouth. He could do it, but not with the natural smoothness he had perfected over the years. We'd traditionally share a big bucket of popcorn. When I was a little guy, he'd scoop up a big handful and let me pick it from his paw. But now I noticed I was the only one eating it.

"You okay, Dad?" I asked. "Not into popcorn anymore?"

"I am, but it's just hard for me to grab it," he said. Picking up small objects had become something of a struggle. I thought about grabbing some popcorn and feeding it to him, but figured that we'd get some strange looks from the rabid Jazz fans cheering around us. So I just took a big sip of my stadium beer instead.

We met up with a high school friend at halftime who later texted me, "Is your dad okay? Looked weird."

I wanted to text back, "He's slowly dying of a motherfucking terminal illness that there's no fucking cure to, you dickless dick." Instead, I just wrote back, "Yep, he's just running a lot." I think it was just part of my denial, or maybe I just didn't understand the disease well enough to talk about it, but I was almost silent about it with friends. Most of them didn't even know he was sick.

The next day, our cleaning lady, Stana, stopped by the house with some chicken noodle soup and potato salad. I once lied to her and said I loved her cooking, so now every time I was in town, she'd make a massive pot of soup and a giant bowl of potato salad. She spoke in blunt, broken English with a thick Polish accent.

"Danny, you is believin' Daddy is sick, too?" she asked as I picked bones out of the chicken noodle soup, trying my best to act like I was enjoying it.

"Yeah, crazy, but who knows. He might last a while," I said with forced optimism.

Stana just shook her head. "Daddy is sick. He get way, way worse. Soon he be . . ." she pointed down to the ground to imply death, like six feet under.

"We'll see. He's still pretty strong," I said.

"Danny, Daddy is die before Mommy," she said.

It was starting to seem real. There was no denying that my pal was getting worse.

In mid-April, it was finally time for the marathon. I flew to Boston to meet up with the rest of the family. I was more excited that the Hyatt we were staying at had a steam room and hot tub than I was for the marathon. I was beginning to think my dad had put too much pressure on himself to run the race. His health was clearly waning, but with all the news stories and articles, it was impossible for him to back out. I wanted him to not run. I wanted him to say fuck it and quit.

But I showed up to support him. Throughout the weekend, it rained like I'd never seen before—the wind blew our umbrellas inside out and the downpour drenched us in seconds. Say what you will about L.A., at least we never have to deal with that bullshit. I was hoping they'd cancel the race due to the weather. But it cleared up by Monday and my dad was raring to go.

On race day, Greg, my mom, and I were loaded into a CBS News van to follow my dad around. They wanted ample footage for the report. Greg and I were awarded the privilege because Tiffany, Jessica, and Chelsea were interviewed for the news clip, and my mom wanted to be fair. We'd get out and see him at the ten-mile marker, then the fifteen, then at the finish line.

The driver and the cameraman didn't seem very interested in my dad's story. Anytime my mom would try to tell them what a horrific disease ALS is, they'd instantly change the subject.

"So they say people with Lou Gehrig's disease usually only last two to three years, but we're hoping Bob can make it longer," said my mom.

The cameraman nodded, then turned up the volume on the Red Sox game that was playing over the radio. They were up 6–1 in the first inning against the Angels.

"Wow, you believe that. Six–one in the first inning," said the cameraman. It was clear that they didn't like to talk about anything tragic. I sort of admired their ability to block out sadness, but I was also sort of sickened by it. Was that what my denial over my dad's illness looked like?

We got out of the van and stood on the sidelines sipping on our Dunkin' Donuts coffee as healthy people darted by us. Though I'd probably blow my brains out before running a marathon, I actually quite enjoy watching them. Marathons have a distinct energy and collective effervescence that I find exciting. The Boston Marathon is particularly thrilling because of all the cheering drunks, and everyone seems to be running for some cause. It really is a spectacular display of humanity.

Finally, my dad and his pals emerged in the distance. I'll admit, it was inspiring to see my old, kindhearted dad smiling and waving as he saw us cheering him on from the sidelines, even though he was hunched over and clinging onto his three friends for support. Running the thing might have been a medical mistake, but it made him as happy as I've ever seen him, so it was worth it. He ran to the sideline and hugged my mom. The two cried in each other's arms. "I love you, Bob. Never give up," she said.

"I love you so much," he said back, and then rejoined the race.

"Give 'em hell," my mom shouted after him.

"Think the Sox have a legit shot at the pennant?" asked the aloof cameraman.

My dying dad finished the race in six hours, twelve minutes, and fifty-seven seconds—roughly two hours and thirty-eight minutes slower than his time at the St. George Marathon, which he had run only seven months prior. If that didn't prove how fast the disease was progressing, I don't know what would. We all cried as he crossed the finish line, his arms linked with those of his devoted friends.

After the race, we all went back to the Hyatt and drank champagne while my dad wrapped himself in one of those shiny, post-marathon Mylar blankets.

My dad's younger sister, Sarah, his sister-in-law, Martha, and a couple of our cousins had surprised him by coming to watch the race. There was no love lost between my mom and my dad's family. She thought they were a bunch of rich-bitch, blowhard alcoholics who weren't supportive enough of her when she got cancer. In her opinion, they were only around for the good moments in life and not the bad. She was really upset that they had shown up.

"They can't just pop up when they want to," my mom said. "This is a special moment for OUR FAMILY. Fuck those blowhards."

But my dad wanted to see them. He loved them despite my mom's hatred, and this day was about him. I always loved my dad's family— maybe because I also loved drinking and acting like a rich bitch. So my dad tasked me with calling them and inviting them to come drink champagne with us.

They now stood at one end of the hotel room chatting with him and drinking, while my mom vented on the other. I hated that they didn't get along with my mom. Family should always be a good thing, not a bad.

"We're so proud of you, Bobby," my aunt Sarah said, rubbing one of her older brother's bony shoulders.

"Thanks. I'm excited to see the CBS report," said my dad.

"Us, too. I have Jerry recording it back home," she said. Jerry was her husband.

Eventually, my mom shooed everyone out. The party was over. It was just us.

"I can't believe those fuckers had the balls to show up," my mom said of my dad's family after they left.

My dad was so physically exhausted from the race that he couldn't lift up his arms. They hung to his side like broken tree branches. He was sweaty and salty from the run. He needed a shower, and there was no way he could wash himself.

"I'm not washing my dad's balls, Mom," I said when she suggested I help him shower.

Unless they're drunk or involved in an act of passion, most people are shy when it comes to someone else touching or even looking at the parts of their body they've been trained to tuck away from the world. My dad is a person. He was thus reluctant to have his privates handled by others. And he certainly didn't want me of all people to help him shower. That was not within the bounds of our relationship.

But my mom insisted. "Don't be an asshole, Danny. You're both guys. You both have dicks. Get over it," she said.

"No, DJ doesn't need to do that," my dad said.

"Bob, you can't even move your fucking arms," my mom reminded him.

"Yes I can," he said as he tried to lift his tired arms, but couldn't.

"See, you can't," said my mom. "You have to accept the help you need."

And she was right. My dad didn't like to bother or inconvenience other people. He didn't like asking for help. But, if we were going to manage this situation, he'd have to become comfortable receiving help from us, and I'd have to become comfortable giving it.

Although I was really enjoying listening to my passive dad and aggressive mom bicker back and forth, I said, "I don't mind. Let's wash those balls."

"It's really okay. I'll just rinse off," my dad tried one last time.

"No, Dan will help." My mom slapped the soap into my hand and slammed the hotel bathroom door, effectively locking us in there. "Don't forget to get his foreskin," she added through the door. Like Greg, my dad wasn't circumcised.

"Sorry, DJ," my embarrassed dad said as I began to undress him. I slipped off his running shorts, looking away from his junk, but noticing how skinny he was from head to toe. I hadn't spent a lot of time in my life looking at him naked (believe it or not), so I didn't have much to compare it to, but I could tell that the disease was ruining him. He was always a little plump—like a king who'd had too many steak dinners and bottles of wine. He had started to thin down with all his running. But now he looked like he'd been plucked straight out of a POW camp. Each rib was outlined through his sagging skin. His shoulder blades were as sharp as volcanic rocks. His face was so gaunt, he already looked like a corpse. "Jesus, you're skinny. We've got to get you a million hamburgers," I said.

"Or maybe I should just drink more beer," he joked.

"I'll join you there," I said, craving a thousand beers and thinking how being drunk would make all of this much easier.

The muscles in his chest were twitching, really going wild.

"Those are the muscle fasciculations," he explained, once he noticed me looking. "That's the Lou Gehrig's disease working on me."

I placed my hand on his chest and felt the muscles pulsate just above his big, beating heart. I wanted to grab those muscles and tell them to chill out, to stop destroying my dad and relax. But they continued to shake and pop. The disease was in control. My dad was under attack.

He was naked now. We didn't make any eye contact. I turned on the shower, checking to make sure the water was warm. It was. Hotel water never seems to struggle to get hot. I helped him step into the tub and grabbed the soap.

"Let's get the balls out of the way first," I joked as I slowly made my way down there. I had used a vacation day from work to come to Boston for the marathon. Weird to think I was using my vacation to wash my dad's dick. "How was your trip?" I imagined a co-worker asking. "It was great. Washed my dad's dirty dick," I would casually reply.

As soon as the soap touched his privates, he changed the subject to something we used to talk about before this mess. "So, you think the Jazz will make the playoffs this year?"

"It's looking good," I said, rubbing the soap over the place where my life had started with a triumphant orgasm some twenty-four years earlier. "Seems like the combination of Williams, Boozer, Okur, and Kirilenko is finally working out."

"Would be fun if you came back for a playoff game," he said. I had finished with the privates, but continued to look away as I soaped up his legs.

"Yeah, it'd be nice to get back for another game. I'll see about getting another day off work." His body was now covered in soap from head to toe, from balls to butthole. I aimed the showerhead at him and washed all the suds off his brittle body. They ran down the drain as if they, too, were trying to get away from this horrific situation.

As I wrapped him in towels, he said, "First ball wash. Not bad."

"Yeah, I didn't vomit or anything. I feel like I could be one of those ball-cleaning machines on a golf course if the whole PR thing doesn't work out."

"You should look into that," he said. "And seriously, thanks."

"It honestly wasn't bad at all." And it wasn't. It was just different. We got him dressed. He looked good as new. Well, he looked like shit because he had just run a marathon and he had Lou Gehrig's disease. But he looked clean and refreshed, the best he could be. It was the first taste of how intense shit was going to get, the first sign that our relationship wasn't going to just be talking about basketball.

We left the bathroom. My dad took a nap. I went to the hotel bar for a strong one.

* * *

As May rolled around, my dad was still in good spirits. He and my mom walked the dogs up Millcreek Canyon every day—a stretch of national forest a few minutes from our house. My mom thought if he stayed active and kept his legs strong that maybe that son of a bitch Lou Gehrig's disease would have a tougher time with him. My mom was doing her best to keep his spirits up. She'd pin an inspirational quote on his pillow every night so he could dream inspiring dreams about kicking Lou Gehrig's disease in the nuts. He was going to live a long, long time with this disease. Hell, maybe he'd be the first person to beat Lou Gehrig's disease. He'd be like Magic Johnson and HIV. Maybe he'd even be the first person to live forever.

During this stretch, my mom was feeling pretty good, so she provided most of the care for him. They spent every second together and looked more in love than I'd ever seen them. They were happily designing the renovations to the house like they were planning their second wedding. They were holding hands and kissing all the time. It was sort of disgusting, really—a couple of dying fucks making out and shit.

Mid-May, my dad was out in the Bay Area to run the Golden Gate Relay, which started in Calistoga and went to Santa Cruz—a span of 199 miles. He had two legs of the race, one through Napa and one over the Golden Gate Bridge. His team members gave him the coveted Golden Gate Bridge leg because he was dying of Lou Gehrig's disease and they would've been dicks if they hadn't.

I decided to fly up to visit Abby and run the legs with him. Abby and her mom ran with us. Though he had finished the Boston Marathon a month earlier, my dad was clearly in worse shape. He couldn't tie his own shoes. His hands were barely working. His breathing was more labored. He couldn't undo his pants, so I had to help him go to the bathroom. Good thing I already had some experience dealing with his dick. We'd do run/walks, where we'd run about a hundred yards, then walk, then run. Then eventually we just walked.

The Golden Gate Bridge leg took place at two in the morning. They normally close the bridge down to pedestrians after 9 p.m. (probably to prevent people from tossing themselves off it), so having access to it was unique. I ran alongside my dad, the love of my life and her mom running on the other side, the bay breeze cooling our faces as the city sparkled in the background. I looked over to my panting dad, barely able to stand up but still trying to run.

"You sure you're okay to do this?" I asked as we slowed to a walk.

"Yeah. God, the city is so beautiful," he said, not wanting to talk about his struggles. I started to weep as we walked. It was so hard to see him in decline, but I was thankful I got to spend this time with him. I knew this was the last run I'd take with him. I knew that we weren't going to have many more beautiful moments with each other before it got really bad. I wanted my poor dad to get better, not worse, but was finally starting to realize that that wasn't how Lou Gehrig's disease worked.

After our run, Abby and I went back to her place in Berkeley buzzing from the experience. "Your poor dad," she said. "I'm so proud of him."

"I am, too," I said.

We fucked and then slept in the next morning.

In June, I flew out to Chicago to watch Greg graduate from Northwestern. It was his last taste of the good life before moving back home to Utah. I still had no official plans to move home. I had just been promoted at my job, and things were going great. I didn't want to give that up until I absolutely had to. Greg and Tiffany were sure to make me feel like shit for not committing to moving back.

"It's okay, Danny. Have fun in Los Angeles while I spend all the time in the world with Dad and become his favorite son," Greg passive-aggressively joked.

"Yeah, we'll get him to write you out of the will," said Tiffany in a rare attempt at humor.

"Last week, they made us dance for an extra two hours to get ready for our recital," said Chelsea. "Two hours. Can you believe that?"

Jessica didn't say anything.

"Sorry if I'm the only successful sibling with a good job," I fired back.

We all went out to dinner at a fancy restaurant on Rush Street to celebrate Greg's graduation. As we waited for our large table (we always had to wait because there were seven of us), I played with my dad's hands. He could hardly move them at this point. I uncoiled and recoiled his fingers. I didn't know what to say. My grandma Barbie, my dad's mom, was eighty-four and had some kidney issues. She had been telling us she was ready to go.

"So, do you think you or Grandma will die first?" I asked for some reason.

My dad got a little teary eyed and said, "I don't know. I hope we both live a lot longer, but probably Grandma."

Greg overheard the conversation. He started to cry.

"Shit, sorry, I was just joking, making small talk," I said.

"I know, but still, it's just—all of this is so sad," cried Greg.

"Relax, Gregor. Dad's gonna live a long, long time, remember?" I said. "You haven't had that much liquid on your face since your last blowie." I smiled at him, trying to get him to laugh. He kept crying. I was attempting to fight Lou Gehrig's disease with humor, but no one had the patience for cum-on-the-face jokes. Things were getting really serious.

And Greg was right. It was all so sad. The thought that we might lose a parent before a grandparent would have seemed ludicrous only a few months earlier, but now it seemed like a possibility. I don't know why I asked my dad this morbid question—probably because I'm an asshole—but it was the first time I'd outwardly acknowledged that my pal was going to actually die at the hands of ALS. My denial was officially beginning to give way to reality.

In July, we all went on what was depressingly billed as being our "last family vacation"—a twelve-day Mediterranean cruise that started in Barcelona and went to Cannes, Pisa, Rome, Naples, Pompeii, Capri, Florence, Venice, Corfu, and Dubrovnik, before returning to Barcelona. It was one of those luxury cruises full of a bunch of rich, spoiled assholes. We fit right in. We picked the cruise because it was the easiest way to see Europe. We just had to board the boat, get off to see the sights, then get back on.

My dad was getting worse by the day. His legs were still strong, but his arms and hands were very weak. Watching him try to give me a hug was like watching a four-year-old child try to lift a hundred-pound weight. The disease had also started a fierce attack on his diaphragm and lungs. He now had to be hooked to a bilevel positive airway pressure (BiPAP) machine while he slept, which essentially helped push air into his lungs. He was having more and more trouble eating, so it was decided that he'd get a gastric feeding tube inserted in his stomach right after the trip. Once that happened, all of his food would be in liquid form. This trip was his last chance to eat and drink whatever he wanted.

To top it off, my mom's cancer had flared back up like a bad case of herpes. She had been taking great care of my dad and dumping all her energy into him. It burned her out and allowed the cancer to sneak back up on her. This time around, the cancer was deemed more aggressive than her previous bouts had been. She was going to start "big guns chemo" right after the cruise. I wasn't sure what she meant by "big guns chemo," but it didn't sound good.

The whole mess was starting to sink in for me in a big way. I had told my work about what was happening with my dad so I could try to get the time off for the cruise, even though I was out of vacation days. "It's our last family vacation," I told them. "Morbid, I know." They understood and gave me the time off, with pay. I still wasn't sure when I would need to come home to help out, but I knew the time was getting closer.

Thankfully, it was easy to drink on the cruise. They gave you this little plastic card that they'd swipe when you wanted anything. It didn't seem like real money. And they served a couple bottles of wine at dinner every night. I guess rich people like to be drunk most of the time. My dad and I ended up running up a booze bill of over three thousand dollars.

I tried to keep the mood light by cracking dark jokes as we saw all the European sights along the way. I thought if I could joke about this serious disease that maybe it wouldn't seem so serious.

"Don't get close to that thing or it'll fall on your unlucky ass," I said as we looked at the Leaning Tower of Pisa.

"It could have been worse. They could have had Lou Gehrig's disease," I quipped as we inspected the plaster-cast bodies of a couple of Pompeii victims.

"We should get someone to do a sculpture of you naked in a wheelchair," I said as we looked at the *David* in Florence. "Your dick is bigger than his, even with Lou Gehrig's disease," I added, reminding my dad that I had recently seen his dick.

We were all on edge. About two days into the trip Tiffany was acting like a know-it-all travel guru. She and BCB had been doing a lot of traveling since they started dating, so she thought of herself as an expert. She was bossing us all around, and I finally snapped.

"Hey, I've got a fun idea, Tiff: how about you stop acting like a bossy bitch for a few minutes and shut the fuck up?" I said.

"Fuck you. I'm just trying to help us see as much as we can," she said. "It's Dad's last trip." We didn't talk for the rest of the vacation.

Greg somehow contracted pubic lice about halfway through the trip. We shared a very small cabin, a twin-sized bed on each side. He said he hadn't slept with anyone on the cruise; he figured he must have gotten it from the sheets.

"How didn't you get it?" he asked.

"I don't know. Maybe the lice prefer your gimmicky, uncircumcised cock," I joked.

"I'm going to wash my pubes again," he said as he scratched his way to our little cabin bathroom.

My mom's hope campaign was starting to fade as things got worse and worse with my dad. She was still pinning an inspirational quote on my dad's pillow each night, and she was still preaching that things would be okay. She and my dad would walk laps around the giant ship's track to keep his legs strong. But there was no denying that the disease was working on my dad faster than my mom had thought it would, faster than we all had thought it would. Everything was being sped up. Her goal was to get chemo and hopefully start feeling better before my dad had to go on a respirator, so she could resume taking care of him.

During the last dinner my mom asked us all to hold hands as we sat around a circular table. I reluctantly put down my wineglass and took Tiff's hand as my mom started her short speech.

"Things are going to continue to get bad. But we all need to be there for your dad. We are a family and we can do this. If nothing else, we will always have each other," she said.

For some reason, Chelsea was hypercritical of my mom on the trip and was attacking her at her most vulnerable moments. She assumed everything was fine, that both my parents were faking as a ploy to get our attention. So, instead of linking hands with the rest of us, Chelsea sat at the table, giggling and digging her gangly fingers into her water cup to fish out ice cubes to throw at my mom.

But the rest of us nodded in agreement. At least we had each other. At least we were still a family.

"Sounds good, Mom," said Greg while folding up his napkin. "Now, if you'll excuse me, I've got to go back to the room to scratch my pubes." Tiffany and I separated our hands and scowled at each other. Jess didn't say anything. Chelsea was busy with her water glass. What a family.

After the cruise, my dad got a feeding tube implanted into his stomach, and my mom started big guns chemo. I returned to Los Angeles. I knew I had to talk to my boss about taking a leave of absence from work so I could help at home, but I was still trying to put it off for as long as possible.

Right as the chemo started up, my mom seemed to drop the never-give-up bullshit and go back into full panic mode. She was on my ass about moving home to help out. She started sending me three or four guilt-inducing text messages each day while I was at work or out drinking. I wanted to kick whoever taught her how to text in the teeth. It was probably Jessica. The texts started coming in at all hours of the day and night.

We really need your help. Dad is going to die soon.

I can't do this.

Come home.

It's not looking good out here. How's work?

Dad shit his pants today. We need your help.

I'm just getting home from chemo. Your dad is way worse. Wish you were here to help.

I've been vomiting all day and your dad can't move his arms. Your siblings are starting to resent you. I hope you are well.

We all have those "What the fuck am I doing?" moments. Mine came at a bar called the Derby in Los Feliz. I was probably five drinks into what was shaping up to be another shitshow of a night when I got this message from my mom:

Dan, we met with the architect, elevator guy, and contractor today. This could really push me over the edge, but I am going to do it. I have been in bed all day trying not to throw up from twelve hours of chemo and blood transfusions. It would probably be a zoo to move home right now with all the construction, although we could really use the help.

I closed my phone and ordered another drink, trying to ignore the message, but the guilt was starting to get to me. I caught a glimpse of my fat, smiling face in a wall mirror—sweating out alcohol, like a spoiled white asshole—and had the moment.

"What the fuck am I doing?" Here I was, drunk in everyone-has-their-head-up-their-ass L.A., while my mom was lying in bed next to my dying dad, recovering from a horrible day of being injected with awful drugs to keep her from dying so she could continue taking care of our diseased father.

I flew home to Salt Lake the following weekend to assess the situation.

Home was certainly different this time around, and not just because of the construction to make our house wheelchair accessible. My dad had gotten much worse in the couple of weeks since the cruise. He could hardly move his arms, he was having some trouble walking, he was now on the feeding tube, and his breathing had gotten so bad he had to be hooked to the BiPAP machine a couple of times a day.

My mom was on edge and sick from the chemo. Tiffany immediately reminded me how much more she was doing for the family than I was. Greg still had pubic lice from the cruise that he couldn't seem to shake, so he was even crankier than usual. Jessica was wandering in and out of the house, trying her best to hide from everyone. Chelsea had her head in the schoolbooks, ignoring the situation via math and science. When she wasn't studying, she was dancing, or talking about it.

The calm, soothing force that had always been my dad displayed more anger than usual. He was clearly frustrated by his misfortune. Before heading out for a family dinner, Chelsea was slowly buttoning up my dad's shirt because he couldn't lift up his arms to do it himself. As she buttoned, she noticed that Tiffany had removed all the pictures of herself and Derek from the dresser next to her old bed.

"How could she get rid of those pictures of her and Derek? And now she's dating Big Cock Brian? What a whore," said Chelsea.

"Don't talk like that," said my dad, growing less and less patient by the second.

"What? She shouldn't take down those pictures and get rid of those memories, all just because Brian has a bigger cock. It's bitchy," said Chelsea, smiling a little.

"Chelsea. What did I just say? Don't talk like that. I want to smack you in the face," said my dad.

"You can't move your arms," said Chelsea.

My dad looked down at his shirt, bursting with frustration, and said, "How long does it take to button up a fucking shirt?"

He also had an uncharacteristically low tolerance for our hyperactive golden retrievers, whose cheerful tail-wagging natures seemed out of place with all the dying taking place around us. Anytime they would try to charge out the front door so they could freely run around the Mormon neighborhood—shitting wherever their hearts and anuses desired—my dad would greet them with a swift kick to the rib cage, making great use of the little strength he had left in his legs.

"These fucking dogs," he said. I had never seen my dad mad. He just wasn't the angry type. Everything was not normal on the home front.

Before I left Salt Lake, my dad and I went up to Snowbird resort—a place where we had spent many days skiing the steep slopes and chatting about life on the chairlifts. Though it was only August, some of the leaves were starting to change, giving the mountain a colorful glow.

"Boy, it's so beautiful up here, isn't it?" my dad said, and for a moment, it was like all the other times we had been up there, just a couple of healthy pals there to ski. I think we both momentarily forgot about all the developing problems in our lives.

"Yeah, it's pretty great. Beats L.A. The endless sunshine is nice, but consistency can be boring," I said.

"Nice to see the leaves changing. Always marks the beginning of my favorite time of the year. Also means that ski season is on the way," he said, forgetting for a moment that he'd never be able to ski again.

We took the aerial tram to the top of Snowbird's Hidden Peak, some eleven thousand feet above sea level. We looked out at the world—all the peaks and valleys, all the dark clouds mixed with the patches of blue sky.

"DJ, sorry to get all serious here, but the mountains bring it out in me. My life is falling apart here. This damn disease. Didn't think it would hit me this hard," he said, taking a deep breath and letting the slight mountain breeze run through his graying hair.

He continued, "I know you got your life going in Los Angeles, and we're really proud of you for that. But we need you back home. I need you back home."

Fuck, there it was. My mom had been begging me to come home for a month, but finally the request was coming from my dad. In a strange reversal, he was now asking for my help. He'd always had my back, and now it was time for me to have his. I was hoping he would snap out of it and say, "Just kidding. Go on being a kid and fucking around in Los Angeles. You're too young to take care of your parents." But he didn't. He needed my help, and I had to give it.

I placed a hand on his bony shoulder. "I'll do everything I can, Dad. I'm a bit of a selfish asshole, but if you want me here, I'll be here."

It was time to finally accept that things couldn't stay good forever, that my relationship with my dad would have to change. It was time to accept that life isn't all about gin and tonics and sunsets, that it's about spending as much time as possible with the people you love, through the good and the bad.

I decided that when I returned to L.A. the following Monday, I would talk to my boss and try to take a leave of absence from work so I could go back to Utah to help take care of Team Terminal. It was time to put my selfish life on pause. It was time to come home. My dad needed me.

LEAVING LOS ANGELES

When I got back to Los Angeles, I drafted an e-mail to my boss asking for a leave of absence from work. I really didn't want to flat-out quit. I liked my job. I was just starting out in my career. I couldn't stand the thought of just giving it up completely. My crazy mom—all fucked up on chemo drugs—had called my boss, Ian, at his home at eleven o'clock one night to tell him that she needed me back in Utah, so he understood the situation. I'm still not sure how my mom got his number. I guess she's resourceful like that, chemo drugs or not.

The whole thing was awkward. I felt very exposed by the situation, which seemed like a bad way to launch my professional life. But fuck it. My parents were dying. They were now the most important thing that ever existed in the history of anything. Fuck the rest.

I sent Ian this desperate e-mail:

August 22, 2007

Ian,

As you know, I spent last weekend at home with my family. Unfortunately, my father's condition is much worse than I had anticipated. His weight is down to 140 pounds and his breathing is down to around 33 percent (meaning he is only able to inhale and exhale using 33 percent of his lungs' capacity). They have already surgically implanted a feeding tube and are going to be putting him on a breathing machine shortly, at which point he will no longer be able to talk. To top it off, my mom is undergoing intense chemotherapy and is emotionally unstable (as you witnessed firsthand when she called you at 11 p.m.).

My family and I are in a state of panic right now and I'm not sure what to do about the whole situation. I've been thinking about solutions all day long and was wondering if I could talk to you about potentially taking an unpaid leave of absence to help out at home and spend time with my family. I don't know how long it would last or if Abernathy even allows for these, but I do know that I really enjoy working here and would love to continue once things get better at home, assuming they will.

I know the timing for this request is awful, and that my temporary departure would place extra stress on everyone, but I would be willing to assist in finding some extra help and stay on until mid– to late September to ensure we have the bases covered.

I apologize for this request. I wish I didn't have to make it. I thank you for considering it and for being such an accommodating employer. Let me know if you are available to talk in greater detail tomorrow.

Thanks,

Daniel Marshall

Daniel is my grown-up, professional name.

Ian and I met a couple of days later to discuss the letter.

"I'm so sorry, Daniel. This is really unfortunate," Ian said, looking out at the dirty Los Angeles skyline, traffic helicopters buzzing by. We were on the thirty-ninth floor of the Aon Tower in the heart of downtown, so we had an almost endless view of the filthy city. L.A. is an ashtray. Ian sat down in his desk chair and looked me over. "Things were going so well for you."

"I know. It really sucks. And sorry again about my mom calling you," I said.

"Is she okay?" he asked.

"Well, she gets a little loopy with chemo. She's insane right now."

"Understandable. I would be, too," said Ian.

He shook his head. He didn't know what to say about any of this. I was finding that no one really did. He was around my parents' age. I'm sure he felt lucky that such tragedy wasn't hitting him and his family.

"Well, let me know if I can do anything else to help," he said. I wanted to say, "Hey, why don't you go ahead and cure Lou Gehrig's disease and cancer." But instead I nodded and said that I would let him know.

My leave was to be three months long, unpaid, but I would still get health insurance. My last day would be September 15, 2007.

Initially, I thought there was a good chance that I'd return. I thought

I would go out to Mormontown, wipe some ass, get my dad stabilized, wipe some more ass, maybe sit in on a couple of chemotherapy sessions, get drunk alone in the basement, show the world what a great, unselfish person I actually was, and wipe some more ass.

But, for now, I was leaving Los Angeles, the city I often describe as a giant toilet bowl full of dying dreams, to return to Salt Lake, a city I often describe as a wholesome Norman Rockwell painting, but one now full of dying parents.

Even though I was sure I'd be coming back to L.A., I decided that it would be best to move all my shit back to Utah, just in case I had to stay longer than three months. I guess there was a part of me that knew I'd be in Salt Lake for a while. This meant moving out of my apartment with Gabe.

"I wish I didn't have to, but I do," I told a disappointed Gabe over a beer.

"I understand, man," he said. "Sucks, though. Fucking life."

I was amazed by how fast things could change. Just fourteen months earlier, my dad had helped me move from San Francisco down to Los Angeles. He didn't have Lou Gehrig's disease then. He was still the man he was made to be, still the caring father he always was, still my road map through this bullshit life of mine. The move had been easy because of him. He knew how it all worked—the best ways to carry heavy shit, the angles to move oddly shaped objects so we could finish in time to sip a glass of wine and watch the sun set over Sunset Boulevard.

As my time in L.A. wound down, I started to open up more about what was happening at home. I had previously been pretty quiet about it—mainly because I was in denial—but I felt like there was no sense keeping things to myself anymore. Fuck it. Might as well tell the whole world. When people would ask me why I was leaving Los Angeles, I'd get really blunt with them.

"I'm going home to take care of my dying parents," I'd say. "Lou Gehrig's disease and cancer. They're dying like super fast."

"Sorry man. That's horrible," they'd say back, a little uncomfortable. "You're a good man for going."

"I know. I'm a hero of sorts," I'd joke back. I sort of loved how uncomfortable the whole thing made everyone. I was pretty desensitized to tragedy because my mom had been sick my whole life, but other people my age weren't.

"Man, my parents are going to be dead soon," I'd say.

"I'm so, so sorry," they'd say, getting more and more uneasy.

My last few days of work were easy. I was just wrapping up a couple of projects and tying some loose ends, as they say in the business world. I couldn't take on any new projects, so there wasn't a lot for me to do. One of my bosses jokingly called me a "lame duck account executive." I had worked really hard during my time there, so it was kind of nice to go on cruise control. Mostly I spent my last days at the office in the break room, twisting off caps of the free Snapples they provided and reading the Snapple Real Fact aloud to whoever would listen: "A bee has five eyelids."

I wasn't sleeping much. I'd lie in my bed at night, a slight L.A. breeze fanning through my balcony door, carrying with it the faint sound of a few wild drunks still searching for excitement. I'd stare at the cottage-cheese ceiling thinking about what I was in for.

I was nervous. I had never been any good at taking care of people. My dad and I used to go boating at Bear Lake on the Utah-Idaho border every summer. The last time we went, he asked me to put sunscreen on his back. I did a lazy, sloppy job of it and he got the worst sunburn of his life. You could actually see all the spots my dumpy, lazy little fingers had missed. Was this going to be another Bear Lake situation? Was I going to be really shitty at taking care of him?

I hadn't spent a lot of time around my dad since his condition had worsened and he needed more care—certainly no more than just a few moments here and there, like the Boston Marathon dick washing. I'd mainly watch my mom or Greg care for him, electing to just sit on the outside looking in, while making silly jokes. It wasn't a world I had entered yet, but here I was, finally on the precipice, about to jump in.

I started to wonder how I should approach this whole situation when I got home. Should I just be a sad jerk? A stubborn asshole about helping out? Or should I be really positive and willing? I wasn't going to be working, with the leave from Abernathy MacGregor and all. I wouldn't have anything else to distract me. This could just be what I focused on for a while. I could just get wrist-deep in this dying-parents shit. Feel everything. Do everything. Roll around in the mud. Really experience the horrible reality of death firsthand. That would make me a wiser and better person, right? That would help me grow up, right? That would give me life experience that would put everything else in perspective, right?

But if I was wiping my dad's ass every day, what would our relationship become? Could we still crack sex jokes and talk about the Jazz? Or would it be all about the Lou Gehrig's disease? And how much more time would I actually have with my pal? Was I going to go home and watch him die within a couple of months? It seemed unfathomable that he would go that fast, but he had an aggressive version of an already aggressive disease. He could easily die soon. Or could we get him stabilized so he could live a long, long time? That was the goal.

Should we even be fighting this disease? Was making our house wheelchair accessible and having him go on a respirator mean, causing unnecessary suffering for him and the rest of us? Would we be better off doing nothing and letting him go quietly and quickly? I didn't know the answers to any of these questions, and I wasn't too eager to discover them.

Abby came to town from Berkeley to spend my last weekend in Los Angeles with me. It was also my birthday weekend. Big twenty-five. I had made a little L.A. bucket list of things to do before I left, so we went to a beach in Malibu, saw a concert at the Hollywood Bowl, and walked around the La Brea Tar Pits. Pretty lame bucket list, I know. But my parents were dying. Life wasn't just about fucking around anymore.

Abby had been incredibly supportive up until now, but as my departure back to Salt Lake approached, she seemed to get a little more distant. While we were sitting at Zuma Beach in Malibu, watching the endless California waves roll to the shore, I noticed that she was acting off—quiet, not her usual cheery, smiley self.

"What's the matter?" I asked.

"Nothing," she said as she intensified the speed at which she flipped through her *US Weekly*, a sign that something was definitely wrong. When you spend so much time with someone, even a slight change in behavior is obvious.

"Come on. What's up? Do you want me to put my shirt back on? Is my whiteness hurting your eyes or something?" I joked.

"It's just, you're taking time off work, and I was hoping you'd come spend a couple weeks with me up in Berkeley before moving back," she explained. That didn't really make sense to me. Things were bad at home. I wasn't going back for vacation. I was returning to deal with some real-life shit. I had put off going home for as long as I could.

"I'd love to go up to Berkeley, but I have to go back now. We're in crisis mode," I explained.

"I know, but . . . I love you and I don't want you to have to do this." She began to cry. I pulled her in close to my pasty body and gave her a giant kiss. She was my first love. I adored everything about her. I loved her calm, relaxed demeanor that seemed to embody the California lifestyle. I loved how smart she was and how she'd excitedly try to explain quantum physics to my dumb ass. I loved that she'd make a clicking sound with her jaw when she slept. I loved that she was always happy, like a golden retriever shooing away the darkness. I loved that she'd snuggle up to me as close as she could get any chance she got. I loved that she'd laugh hysterically at all my dumb jokes. She made me feel safe and comfortable just being me. I didn't want to lose her. I couldn't lose her.

I told her that we'd make it work, that she could visit as often as she liked and I'd visit her as frequently as I could. We were already doing the long-distance thing, so she'd just be coming to Salt Lake instead of Los Angeles.

But she was scared. She had never so much as lost a grandparent. She wasn't used to handling anything this intense. She, like the rest of us, wished that my dad had never gotten this fucking disease. Our life together had been an endless vacation, and that vacation was coming to an end. I hoped that this whole thing would bring us closer together, that we'd realize if we could get through this we could get through anything. It would certainly test our relationship in ways that it hadn't been tested before. It's easy to be together when things are good, but when they're bad? That's a whole different story.

I kissed the tears off her soft lips and forced a smile. I pledged that I'd eventually make it back to the good life in California to be with her full-time as soon as I could.

After a bittersweet weekend, I dropped Abby off at the Burbank Airport and kissed her good-bye.

"I love you, babe," I said.

"I love you, too. Don't drink too much," she said.

"Just my usual amount," I said.

"That's too much," she said.

I watched her walk away into the airport shuffle.

* * *

My friends Aria and Henry flew in from Salt Lake to help me with the move. Most of my friends had stayed back in Utah while I went away for college. Utah is a strange place socially because all non-Mormons—no matter your background—bond together. If you aren't Mormon, you are in this secret little club of "bad kids" who drink, swear, and have premarital sex—a blatant reaction to the oppressive religious vibe. Drinking is a huge part of showcasing that you aren't Mormon, so most of my friends from home are heavy drinkers. Anytime I'd come back, it was always a boozy shitshow. My friend Dominic—who we called the Mayor of Salt Lake because of his strong affinity for the city—always made sure I was good and drunk while visiting.

But for help with the move, I decided to ask Aria and Henry. They were my closest, most dependable friends, and shared my dark sense of humor. I'd known Henry since the fifth grade and Aria since the seventh. They were the first two friends who called me when word got out about my dad having Lou Gehrig's disease, so I knew I could turn to them.

I picked Aria and Henry up from the airport, and we rented an eighteen-foot U-Haul with a giant triceratops decal running along the side.

"Wow, this is a complete piece of shit," I said, looking at the monster.

"Yeah, it is. Let's call it 'Big Sexy,'" Henry suggested.

"Perfect. She is big and she sure is sexy," said Aria as he seductively jacked off one of the triceratops's horns.

"God, I wish my parents weren't dying," I said with a deep breath as I kicked one of Big Sexy's big sexy tires, trying out some of my morbid humor on my pals.

"You need to stop saying shit like that," said Henry. "It makes everyone feel awkward and uncomfortable."

"I know. I will . . . But it's true. My parents are dying," I said once more time for good measure.

"We know. You've mentioned it like fifty times in the last hour," said Henry. "We get it."

"I don't think you do, Henry, because your parents aren't dying," I said with a slick smile.

"You're an asshole," Henry said.

We set about filling Big Sexy with my life: clothes, DVDs, some shitty Ikea furniture I had poorly assembled myself. The U-Haul was way too big for what I owned, so everything was bound to slide around, but fuck it. Who cares? Part of me thought I should just run all this junk to the dump and start over completely when I got home.

As we packed, it hit me. When you're first leaving a town, it's sort of exciting, like the opening of a new book, but this book was going to be a tough read—*Infinite Jest* times a million. I was moving from palm trees to pine trees. From beaches to mountains. From assholes to Mormons. From the living world to the dying world. From the selfish world to the selfless world. In L.A., I was on track to achieve society's idea of happiness—independence, a career. I even had a girlfriend I wanted to marry sooner or later. My life was great. What was about to happen to it?

But my sadness was coupled with something else, something bigger. During those last days in California, I felt more pride than regret, because I knew I was doing the right thing. They were, after all, my parents. They had given me the opportunity to live this happy life in L.A. I couldn't continue to ignore that. They had taken great care of me. It was my turn to return the favor.

Henry, Aria, and I loaded up the last few boxes into Big Sexy and slammed down the heavy back door. I hugged my roommate Gabe, who said good-bye with sad eyes.

"Fucking dads," he said, shaking his head, probably remembering his father's battle with cancer.

"Fucking dads," I repeated back. We gave each other a final hug.

I rubbed my hand across Big Sexy's front hood. I'd drive that beast while Aria and Henry followed behind in my out-of-place-given-that-everyone-in-Los-Angeles-drives-a-fucking-sweet-car Subaru.

"Try to keep up with Big Sexy, motherfuckers," I said, jumping into the truck.

I took one last look at my apartment building, at the palm trees waving in the blue California sky. I put Big Sexy in drive and started toward my new life, as ready as I would ever be for the long, shitty road ahead.

MY NEW JOB

Coming home had always been a joyous event. Our house was a relaxing refuge away from the scary real world. It was full of lots of entertainment options, from our tennis court right down to our pinball machines. It was a hub for all our social activities—the place where everyone always wanted to hang out. My high school friends had nicknamed it "The Marshall House of Fun." Usually my arrival was greeted with an ecstatic "Danny's home!" followed by smiles and hugs. Fuck, sometimes there would even be a sign hanging above the garage that read, WELCOME HOME DAN THE MAN. I'd toss my bags at my smiling dad, who would gladly carry them to my room with his fully functional arms, while I fucked around with the dogs and made sure the pantry was stocked with enough pretzels and beer to get me through my stay. After putting my bags in my room, my dad would usually pop a fresh bottle of wine saved for a special occasion and we'd sit in our gazebo, gazing at the Wasatch Mountains and catching up. My mom would bring us more wine and we'd grill up a steak dinner. We'd all eat together and let the food, wine, and company overwhelm us into bliss while thinking, Being rich and drunk sure is nice.

Part of me was hoping coming home this time would be the same as always.

But when I rolled Big Sexy into our cracked driveway, I was shocked to see our house. It was now fully buried in construction work. They had started building the elevator shaft and redoing a few of the bathrooms while widening some hallways. My mom figured that since we were already doing work on the house, she'd also have the kitchen and a couple of other bathrooms updated. The whole place had that ugly midproject look to it: tarps, tools, planks of wood scattered about. Construction workers streamed in and out as if they lived there. There was no WELCOME HOME DAN THE MAN sign. There was no wine. The dogs didn't even run out to greet me. Instead, a cat I'd never seen before and my now bald-from-chemo mother—who wore an old-lady nightgown that made her look like the Ghost of Cancer Past—stood waiting for me at the front door. I hugged my mom's fragile, diseased body as the stranger cat rubbed up against me, getting its germs and hair all over my spoiled white leg.

"Whose fucking cat is this?" I asked, kicking it away.

"His name is Pierre . . . or maybe this one is Pongo . . . I can't remember. It's Tiffany's. Her boyfriend is allergic. Her cats stay here now."

"Where's Dad?" I asked. "I was thinking we'd have a glass of wine."

"He's hooked to his BiPAP machine. He doesn't drink anymore. He gets his food and water from his feeding tube. Remember?" she said.

"Well, fuck me. The house looks like shit," I said.

"Yeah, well, everything is going to hell. Welcome home." She glided away to go lie down.

Henry and Aria pulled up in my Subaru. I had somehow beaten them back despite Big Sexy's size. Henry got out, took one look at the scene in front of him, and said, "Whoa, what happened to the Marshall House of Fun?"

So there I was. Back in Utah. Back in my once happy childhood home, now haunted by a pair of terminally ill parents, construction workers, and strange cats. All my siblings, except Tiffany, were back living in the house, but it wasn't the safe, relaxing nest it once was. It was now a hectic place where it was impossible to get a moment alone. Every morning at six thirty, Jessica and Chelsea would get up for school. Jessica drove herself, but Chelsea was part of a morning car pool the Mormon neighbors had organized. Then my dad and mom would get up. My mom was off to chemo, but my dad needed to be showered, dressed, fed, and looked after for the whole day. He could still walk and would leave the house every day to go to his office or run errands. But when he was home, he was mainly hooked up to his BiPAP machine.

It seemed as though someone was always coming or going. In addition to all the construction workers, visitors would pop by at all hours to check on my mom and dad. Every night, a Mormon neighbor would bring over a meal—usually lasagna. It was strange to suddenly be basking in the glow of neighborly love. Before this our neighbors had wanted nothing to do with us. In fact, when we first moved in, none of the children our age were allowed to play with us; they thought we were bad kids simply because we didn't have the same religious beliefs. But now they were feeding us and driving Chelsea to school? Why? Did they actually feel sorry for us? Or were they using us to win points with Jesus?

I felt as if my life path had somehow jumped off course and was heading into a dark, depressing, alcohol-filled ditch. I was actually doing this. I was really home. My parents were really sick. The playpen that had been my life was closed.

Stana—who seemed to always be hanging around even when it wasn't her day to work—put it best: "Danny, this is you new home. No like old home."

But I tried to remain positive and decided that I was going to work as hard as I could to make things better. I didn't come home to relax and play tennis this time. I came home to help my parents. This was, after all, my new job. I started in.

Like anyone at any new job, I was horrible at it my first few days. I didn't know how to do anything, and even the simplest tasks seemed impossibly hard. I needed a trainer. At first, I thought it'd be my mom. But soon it became clear that she really couldn't care for my dad anymore. The chemo was ruining her as it battled the cancer. Through all the years of watching her go through treatment, I had never seen her this bad. She had already dropped tons of weight. She could barely keep any food down. She could hardly do anything but sleep. She was just a giant lump on her bed hidden beneath her comforter. She needed someone to care for her, too.

Tiffany had started her M.B.A. at Westminster College in Salt Lake. She'd decided to go the business route instead of becoming a lawyer. BCB had opted to stick with the lawyer junk, so he'd packed his bags and was off to the University of Maine in Portland. They'd be doing the long-distance thing. Tiff had a full schedule between her M.B.A., work, and visiting BCB in Maine, so she wasn't around much. Plus, we were still at each other's throats. Ever since the cruise, every encounter between us would spark a fight.

"Finally made it back, huh?" she said as she stopped by to check in one afternoon between work and class.

"Heard your new boyfriend loves you so much he disappeared to Maine," I said, already going into attack mode.

"So when are you going back to California?"

"So who do you think BCB's fucking behind your back in Maine?" I fired back.

Pretty soon after I arrived, Tiffany stopped coming around as frequently. Our contemptuous relationship kept her away. She had too much going on for me to make her feel like shit every time she came home.

Jessica and Chelsea were at school most of the day. When they were around, they didn't help with my parents. They were too young, too confused to really do anything anyway.

"So you don't do anything around here, do you?" I asked Chelsea one night.

"Nope. That's not my job," she proclaimed.

"What is your job?" I asked.

"School, dance, and farting," she joked as she danced off to do her homework.

With my mom, Tiffany, and the little girls mostly out of the picture, I turned to Greg. Once my mom had started fading into her chemo daze, Greg had taken over the caregiving and house-management duties. He had been home for a few months and was doing a great job, but he was already a little burned out—which was understandable. He was only twenty-two. He should've been back in Chicago nailing dudes he met at gay bars. But instead, he was home wiping our dad's ass.

Greg and I had always been close—brothers but also best friends. We were only two years apart, and grew up with our rooms right across the hall from each other. As a kid, I had an iguana named Oozy, who escaped his cage, bit my finger, and took over my room. I was terrified of him. So for a long stretch while we figured out what to do about Oozy, I slept in Greg's *Wizard of Oz*–decorated room. We'd stay up late talking about life, tennis, the Jazz, movies, our fucked-up family, etc. Even when we finally caught Oozy and gave him away to a pet store, we still had our brother sleepovers. We did everything together. We wore the same clothes. Fuck, we even had matching Speedos, which we once mistakenly wore to a popular Utah water park called Seven Peaks. "Hey look, it's the Speedo brothers," one bully yelled at us. We retired the Speedos shortly thereafter. No matter what was going on with our family—with the world—Greg and I still had each other.

But Greg was angry with me for taking so long to come home while he trudged through this bullshit alone. He had thought it was going to be more of a team effort. We'd usually talk endlessly, but he was sort of ignoring me, acting a little bitchy and standoffish. After a few days of tension, we finally had a heart-to-heart. I was unpacking a few books and clothes. I decided to set my bed up in the front dining room of our house because it was the only available room that wasn't torn apart by the construction.

"Settling in?" Greg asked, sticking his head in the doorway.

"Yep, there's construction shit all over the room in the basement, and Jess has my old room, so I figured I'd set up shop here."

"Yeah, Jesus, this house used to be so fun. It's a shitshow now," he said.

"Remember the epic Nerf wars?" I asked.

"Oh, man, those were the best," he said. "And *American Gladiators*." In the summer of '93, Greg and I had gotten obsessed with the TV show *American Gladiators*. Greg even called me when I was away at John Stockton's basketball camp to tell me who had won. We were so in love with it that we set up our basement to replicate the *Gladiator* events and would invite our friends over to compete against us.

"I loved *American Gladiators*. You were better than Nitro," I said.

"Though not as gay," he said. "God, all those men in spandex banging into each other, no wonder I loved it." We smiled at each other. It was nice to remember when it was good, when our house had been in its prime.

"Oh, how's your pubic lice, by the way?" I asked.

"Completely gone. I beat it. Only took two months!" he said.

"Atta boy, Gregor." I gave him a big high five and pulled him in for a congratulatory hug. We laughed. I looked at my old pal.

"Sorry it took so long to get home," I said, getting more serious.

"Well, we didn't know it would go this fast with Dad."

"Yeah, really hit the poor guy hard. Fucking Christ. Who knew?" I said.

"It's only going to get worse. God, I sort of hope he doesn't go on the respirator," he said.

"You know Mom's going to hook the fucking thing to his throat herself if she has to," I said.

"Yeah, that's true. Fuck, it's going to suck." Greg shook his head. "Well, glad you're back to help."

"Yeah, me, too," I said.

And just like that, we were best pals again—a couple of American Gladiators ready to face this thing together.

My mom was pretty self-sufficient. She had had cancer for long enough to know how to manage it. She had shaved her head, partially for effect and to shout out to the world, "Look at me. I have cancer," but mainly so she didn't have to go through the process of watching her hair fall out, piece by piece. Several of her friends had agreed to drive her up to chemo and sit with her at the Huntsman Cancer Institute. She'd get ready in the morning, they'd pick her up, and then they'd drop her back at home in the afternoon. She would march up to her bedroom and settle into a long, deep cancer sleep. She had, at some point, become absolutely addicted to yogurt. It was all she was eating, all she could really keep down. All we had to do for her was make sure we always had yogurt in the fridge. But that was it.

Taking care of my mom was easy, but she did suffer from something we called "chemo brain." Chemo brain resulted from her still being a little out of it from the cocktail of lymphoma-fighting drugs they'd given her. Basically she was just really scatterbrained and would say crazy shit. For example, she was really pushing for me to ask for Abby's hand in marriage, even though this was probably the worst time for that. One night while I was watching HBO, she stumbled down to grab a yogurt and started chatting with me.

"So you know how you love Pez?" she said. When I was a teenager, I started a Pez collection to ensure that I would never get laid.

"Yeah, I mean, that was like ten years ago," I said.

"I was thinking you could put an engagement ring in a Pez dispenser and ask Abby that way," she suggested.

"Wow. That'd be an awesome way to scare her away for good," I replied.

"No. She'd love it. You'd just ask her if she wants a Pez, she'd say yes, then the ring would pop out. She'd be so surprised," she said.

"And what if she doesn't want a Pez?" I asked.

"What kind of monster turns down a Pez."

"Okay, great suggestion. I'll go pick out a ring and Pez dispenser tomorrow," I said sarcastically.

"Great!" My mom then floated away with her yogurt.

We were always on the lookout for chemo brain and would warn each other when she had it. "Watch out, Mom has chemo brain," we'd say. We'd know to ignore anything she said at that point.

The main focus was on my dad. His arms were gone. Well, not really gone—they were still attached to his body; he just couldn't use them. His diaphragm was getting weaker and weaker by the day, making breathing very difficult. He needed to nap while hooked to his BiPAP machine at least a few times a day. He couldn't dress himself. His speech was slow and labored, his voice so soft you could barely hear him. He required three feedings a day. He was done with regular food. Just water and cans of Promote, all injected into his stomach through his G-tube. Once his breathing got bad enough, he'd go on the respirator, at which point he would be permanently hooked to a machine and bound to a wheelchair or bed.

There was very little talk of hiring an aide to help with some of my dad's more intimate care. My mom insisted that we just do it. I brought it up only once.

"Shouldn't we hire some asshole to at least get Dad ready in the morning and handle some of the bathroom bullshit?" I asked my mom just before she left for chemo one morning.

"No, it's not that bad. God forbid you lazy kids actually do something around here. A little hard work won't kill you," she said.

"But a little hard work also wouldn't kill a hired aide," I said.

"Shut up. Your dad doesn't want some ugly aide touching his penis and watching him shit. You kids can do it. He's your father," she said, slamming the door and ending the discussion.

It was official. We would provide all the care. And my mom was right. A little hard work wouldn't kill us. We were unemployed. We could handle it. It was time to roll up our sleeves and just fucking deal with this. So Greg and I became our dad's little helper monkeys—Greg taking the lead as head helper monkey.

Greg started training me to be the assistant helper monkey by teaching me what to do when our dad needed to go to the bathroom. Though he could still walk, getting him up and down was a hassle, so we started using a bedside urinal, which was this disgusting plastic container that looked like a Nalgene water bottle gone horribly wrong.

"Now, you place his penis in the urinal so he can pee," he said, while placing my dad's penis in the urinal.

"And he's okay with a gay person touching his penis?" I joked.

"Your gay jokes aren't funny anymore, and he doesn't care who touches it at this point," Greg said.

"So long as it's not an ugly girl," my dad said. I had already helped him take a shower, so I felt strangely okay helping him pee in bed. My cherry had been popped. I mean, it was still weird as shit, because it was my dad's penis, but it was just something that had to be done. There was no getting around it.

The feedings were next.

"You just take this syringe and stick it into his G-tube. Then you pour in a glass of water, three cans of Promote, then another glass of water," Greg explained.

"And you just have to watch it go in, all slow like that?" I asked as I watched the yellow goop slowly drain into my dad.

"Yes, you can't fill Daddy up too fast, or he'll pop," explained Greg. Greg called my dad "Daddy" sarcastically, when he was in goof-around mode.

The hardest part of the new job was the BiPAP machine.

"You have to put the mask on first. Place it over his nose and mouth, and tighten the straps around his head. Then you turn on the machine. Once it's humming, you can swing him into bed," Greg explained, swinging my dad into bed like a pro. "Then be sure to give Daddy a big kiss on the forehead, and tell him how much you love him," Greg said, with a little sarcasm. "LOVE YOU SO MUCH, DADDY."

"Do I have to do the kissing part?" I asked.

"Yes. It's the most important part," Greg said, planting another kiss on him.

"God, you're so gay," I said.

"Not funny," Greg said.

"Dad would laugh, but he's hooked to this fucking machine," I said.

Greg eventually trained me to do a pretty good job caring for my dad, and we worked together to look after him full-time. But, even though

Greg and I had some things under control, we were still sloppy in our handling of this mess. There isn't a manual for this sort of shit. So, we made a lot of mistakes.

One day, we accidentally left him on the BiPAP for three hours while he needed to take a shit. He had no way of letting us know that he needed help, and he couldn't get up on his own, so he shit his pants.

"We've got to figure out how to make sure this doesn't happen again," I told Greg as I dug shit out of my dad's pants, missing my life in L.A.—the palm trees, the lifestyle; fuck, even the traffic didn't seem so bad. "We've got to get control of this."

Our stupid solution was to place a cowbell next to his bed, forgetting that he couldn't reach over, grab it, and jingle it like a child on Christmas morning. That obviously didn't work. After the bell, we decided that the best way for him to alert us was to have him kick at the bed when he needed to get up, since he could still move his legs. But his kicks weren't loud enough and wasted a lot of his energy. We're fucking idiots.

Thankfully, our bald across-the-street neighbor, Ralph, stepped in. When we were growing up, Ralph had been one of our mortal enemies, despite the fact that he was the only other non-Mormon in the neighborhood. I was terrified of him. My neighborhood friends Mike and Bob would skateboard in the street right in front of Ralph's house. Ralph hated hearing them out there, so he threw his dog's shit in the road to fuck with them. Mike retaliated by throwing Slurpee cups over his fence into Ralph's backyard. Ralph responded by saving up those Slurpee cups for months and then setting all fifty-something of them at Mike's door as a warm "fuck you."

Things got really bad with Ralph after one of Mike's friends mooned him as he drove by in his self-made car. (Ralph was an engineer who built things he wanted, like cars.) Ralph swerved into Mike's driveway, got out of the car, and charged toward the ass-flasher, saying, "I'm going to tear your fucking head off and shove it up your ass." He then asked a simple question to the group while rolling up his sleeves. "You ladies ever get your asses kicked?" We were about fifteen years old at the time, so Ralph had the foresight to back off, maybe picturing the headline BALD 60-YEAR-OLD ENGINEER SHOVES 15-YEAR-OLD'S HEAD UP OWN ASS FOLLOWING MOONING.

But the incident still scared us. We were so scared, in fact, that we would hide in my backyard and launch water balloons at his house. We even got to the point where we filled the launcher with some of the shit he had tossed on the street and tried shooting it back his way.

But when my dad was diagnosed with ALS, Ralph underwent a transformation. I guess there's good and bad in everyone and tragedy can amplify either. While some will shy away from the challenges tragedy presents (as I did initially), others give a William Wallace–esque scream and charge toward it with whatever weapon they can round up. Ralph was in the latter category. He said, "I don't like many people, but I like your dad." I mentioned that it's virtually impossible to hate my dad, and he responded by saying, "I know. I tried. I couldn't. He's a good man. Couldn't be a better guy to get this horrible, horrible disease."

Thankfully, Ralph was a handyman, and though he didn't have any hair, he had a lot of tools. In fact, he had a whole back room in his house full of them. Having only ever used a hammer for killing ants on the sidewalk, I was pretty amazed by both the number of his tools and his ability to use them.

Ralph would help out however he could—all while sporting an angry, judgmental scowl. I complained to Ralph about how my dad couldn't alert us when he needed something, and told him about the bed shitting.

Ralph shook his disappointed head and said, "You guys really don't know what you're doing over there, do you?"

"Not really. There's not a manual for this sort of shit, so we mess up a lot," I said.

"Yeah, yeah, yeah. I've heard the whole 'manual' speech from all of you. I think it's just important to use your head, be logical. This stuff isn't that hard," he said. "He can't be shitting the bed."

So Ralph built a doorbell for Dad to ring whenever he needed anything, sort of a "Please come help me" button. Genius. It wasn't that fancy, just a doorbell button screwed to a piece of wood that emitted a single, pleasant DING when pressed, but I could spend the rest of my life trying and never make something like that. I can hardly make a fucking sandwich.

We set the doorbell next to my dad's hand, and it worked great. He had enough strength to hit it. It seemed to bring a lot of order to the house. My dad would ring it whenever he needed to get up, then we'd go help him. All Greg and I had to do was sit back and listen for the bell.

Part of the job required that Greg and I watch my dad during the night. The bell made that easier. We'd take listening shifts. We called it "Daddy Duty," which is also what we called the massive shits he'd take. While on Daddy Duty, listening for the bell was all encompassing. Since my parents' bedroom was on the top floor, hanging out and playing pinball, drinking alone, or watching TV in the basement was not an option. I'd started smoking cigarettes, because that seemed like the right thing to do in this situation and because I'm an absolute moron, but those were out now, too, since we couldn't hear the bell outside.

Once the bell rang, Greg or I would sprint to my dad's bedside. We'd sit him up—which was getting easier and easier since he was losing so much weight—then take the BiPAP mask off. He'd take a second to collect himself, swallowing a couple of times and taking a few deep breaths, before making his request. He'd keep it pretty simple with one-word utterances.

"Pee" meant he had to urinate. We'd grab the bedside urinal, get his cock out, and he'd have a little piss right there and then. We also kept some Kleenex bedside for the wipe up. The urine would be dumped on my sleeping mother. Just kidding. It would go in the toilet with any used Kleenex. We'd flush and wash our hands.

"Bathroom" meant he had to shit. This involved standing him up and helping him walk to the nearby bathroom. We'd usually stay toilet-side and watch him, making small talk about the Utah Jazz or all the cats that were now running around our house. He hated the lack of privacy, but, hey, we hated having to watch our dad shit, so it all balanced out. When he was done he'd say something like, "I'm done," and we'd wipe him up, pull his boxers back up, smack his ass, and put him back to bed.

"Nose" meant he needed to have his nose wiped. For whatever reason, the BiPAP would always give him a runny nose. Since he was a marathon runner, I'd make jokes like "Your little nose is running a marathon there." He wouldn't laugh at my shitty joke. We'd grab a Kleenex and he'd blow his nose load into it.

"Up" meant he wanted to get up. This usually was the request issued at the start of the day or if he'd been napping. We would help him get up and go to another part of the house to sit and struggle to breathe.

"Kill me" meant he wanted to die because the pain of slowly losing the ability to move, breathe, and talk was becoming too much. We'd grab the bedside gun and fire a round into his head. Even this loud noise wouldn't wake my mom from her cancer sleep. We'd use the Kleenex to wipe up the blood and remove the fingerprints from the gun.

I got good enough at caring for my dad that I didn't need Greg's help. So, we started divvying up the Daddy Duty so that one of us could have a life on nights off. We were both too tired to activate our social lives, so we'd mainly just hang around the house, lounging and eating leftover lasagna. Whoever wasn't on duty would rub it in.

"What are you up to?" Greg would ask.

"What? I can't hear you because I'm too busy not listening for Dad's stupid doorbell," I'd say as I reclined on the couch reading the sports section for Utah Jazz news while listening to music, a half-eaten plate of lasagna at my side.

"I just asked you what you're doing," Greg would say.

"Just relaxing. Reading. Listening to music. Eating lasagna. Not wiping Dad's ass. You?" I'd say.

"I just had to wipe Dad's ass," Greg would say.

"Bummer. Sucks to be on Daddy Duty tonight," I'd say while folding up the paper. "If you need me, I'll be in the basement drinking alone and playing pinball. Fuck, I might even sneak outside for a cancer stick," I'd add.

The nights I was on Daddy Duty were pretty lonely. I wouldn't sleep because I didn't want to fuck up and have him die on me, or worse, have him shit the bed again. I'd find ways to pass the time. And no, that doesn't mean I was masturbating to porn. I actually would have been, but because my desktop computer was in the front dining room, I feared that a neighbor would walk by and wonder if Bob was getting the proper care he needed, only to peer through the front window to see me blasting away at myself.

Instead, I'd usually talk to Abby on the phone. She was still upset with me for not spending time with her out in Berkeley before coming home. Our conversations weren't flowing with the usual ease. It was getting harder and harder to relate to her problems because mine seemed so much more significant. She also didn't seem as sympathetic about the situation as I expected her to be. In fact, it didn't seem like she wanted to talk about it at all. I wasn't sure why. We were struggling.

"I got to the gym and there were no treadmills available. I had to ride the bike," Abby said.

"Well, my dad's arms don't work, and I had to clean shit off his balls," I said.

"My neighbors are throwing a party. I might stop by," Abby said.

"I can't leave the house because I'm on Daddy Duty tonight," I said.

"I hate bugs," Abby said.

"I hate terminal illnesses," I said.

Shit like that. It was really unpleasant for both of us. But we'd always say "I love you" before hanging up, and that's all that really mattered. I figured she'd eventually come around to accepting the situation.

After Abby was off the phone and I was in bed, I'd usually read. Sometimes I'd write. I had written for a comedy magazine in college, so I'd try working on something for them, or I'd write about some of the crazy events happening at home. Sometimes I'd watch a DVD on my computer with one of the earbuds out, so I could still hear that goddamn doorbell. Sometimes I'd listen to the White Stripes—*"I'm thinking about my doorbell. When you gonna ring it? When you gonna ring it?"*—also with one of the earbuds out.

One night, I decided to have a glass of wine and pretend everything was normal. I poured it to the brim and drank it while sitting on a ratty old armchair in my mom and dad's room, watching them sleep as their diseases worked on their bodies, my dad's BiPAP purring along with all the cats. I shook my head. How did things get so fucked up? Why did I have to watch my parents battle terminal illnesses? How is that fair? Is it because my life had been so good up until now? Is it creepy that I'm sitting in their room watching them sleep while sipping on a glass of wine?

I took a giant, delicious sip and closed my eyes. I pictured everything being okay again. The house wasn't under construction. My parents were completely healthy. We didn't have cats pissing and shitting around our house. There was a giant sign that read, WELCOME HOME

DAN THE MAN. We were a big, happy, healthy family. I was on vacation again. I imagined my dad getting out of his bed of his own accord, unhooking himself from the BiPAP, and looking over to me. He'd shake away all the Lou Gehrig's and return to his old, plump, mobile self.

"What are you doing up, DJ?" he'd ask me.

"Oh, just enjoying a glass of wine. You want one?" I'd say.

"Absolutely. I love wine, and it'd be nice to catch up," he'd say as I poured him a matching glass to the brim that he'd grab with his fully functional hands and begin gulping down without spilling a drop.

We'd go out to the gazebo in our backyard. He'd talk about all the running he was doing, and about how he found the hobby to be a relaxing and rewarding escape. I'd tell him about my job in L.A. and ask him about strategies for how to start saving for my own home. He'd give me suggestions. He'd tell me about all the traveling he'd do once he decided to retire. I'd tell him about how much I loved Abby and how well our relationship was going. Marriage was a strong possibility. We'd pour another glass.

"Life is pretty darn good, isn't it?" he'd say.

"Yeah, it's great," I'd say.

We'd listen to the crickets' synchronized chirps and stare at the Wasatch Mountains glowing in the moonlight, letting the wine settle in and overtake us with warmth and happiness. The future would feel safe and certain. We were invincible. Nothing was going to stop us from living long, healthy lives.

DING. DING. DING.

I was pulled back to reality by my dad's doorbell. He needed help. I set down my glass of wine and walked to the bed. I lifted him up and unhooked his BiPAP machine.

"For the love of God, please don't say 'Bathroom,'" I said.

"Pee," he said, struggling to catch his breath.

"One piss coming right up," I replied with forced cheer. I grabbed the urinal next to his bed, helped him get his cock out, and placed it in the plastic tube, which started to fill.

"I'm sorry about all this," he said, looking down at his peeing penis.

"Oh, no worries. Your father only dies once, so I couldn't miss it."

He looked up at me with a tired smile. "Well, thanks for being home, DJ. We couldn't go through this without you. Love you."

"Love you, too. Sorry you have to go through this. And sorry we're not great at this new job yet, but we'll get better. We're gonna try to make your life as good as possible." We both managed smiles. It wasn't the same as sipping wine under the Utah sky, but it was nice to be back with the old man.

I put him on his BiPAP again and laid him down for some rest, remembering, of course, to give him a kiss on the forehead. I grabbed my glass of wine and took a big sip. "Welcome home, Dan the Man," I whispered to myself.

THE LITTLE GIRLS

Of the five of us kids, the biggest victims in this whole mess were my little sisters, Jessica and Chelsea.

Greg, Tiffany, and I had the benefit of having been raised by our loving, normal, caring parents while they were relatively healthy. We had graduated college. We were supposed to be adults now. We had made it through the most vulnerable and impressionable period of our lives with nearly perfect childhoods. I mean, we had season tickets to the Utah Jazz games, took vacations to warm places during the winter, went skiing, rode around on boats. Fuck, we even had one of those Brookstone back massager/vibrator things, which Greg and I eventually discovered we could use for masturbation. Yeah, our mom was battling cancer on and off, so we had to deal with the occasional hardship, but we were mostly spoiled dickheads living in our family's golden age—the byproduct of the American Dream working out for our parents.

Sure Tiff, Greg, and I had our own personal ups and downs in our teenage years. Like the time Tiff accidentally took a hit of acid in junior high school. A couple of "friends" told her it was just a piece of gum, but it wasn't. It had LSD on it. An hour later, some innocent Mormon student found Tiff rolled up into a ball in the bathroom, muttering nonsense and hallucinating some evil shit. A few teachers were able to get her under control, and they called my parents to come grab her. They got her home, then my mom overreacted and took her to the hospital.

The doctor ruled that she just needed to ride out her trip, drink water, get to a safe environment. She was in no real danger and was brought home. My parents contained her in her room, but she got out, found me shooting hoops in the driveway, and accused me of being the devil with lightning bolts shooting out of my head.

She missed the next couple days of school.

When she made her way back, word had traveled within the *Lord of the Flies*–like atmosphere that is junior high school that Tiff was a bad kid, a burnout, a loser, and she was branded with the scarlet letter "D," for "Druggy."

She had also ratted out the girls who gave her the acid. They didn't take well to that and were now threatening to give her a good beating. They shunned her from their social circle, so she was now friendless. She had lost not only a few brain cells, but her whole social identity. She started dressing the part, wearing a black top with black, baggy jeans covered in holes. I'm not sure exactly what that style is called. It was like a bizarre druggy/dropout/grunge/goth combo. She would subsequently attend four different high schools and never truly recover socially.

I was admittedly a giant dickhead to her growing up—a true bully with a mouth like a shotgun. And after the LSD thing, I had more ammunition than ever. I was a nonstop thorn in her side, reminding her of her mistakes and shortcomings and making her life a living hell. She did kick me in the balls in Vegas once, however, so I figure we were even. So yeah, teenage life at school and at home was hard for Tiff and left her with little confidence.

My teenage years were pretty innocent. I was mostly a good kid. I was pretty scared of drugs and alcohol after Tiff's little devil experience, so I focused on school, basketball, making comedy videos in our basement, and masturbation. I did fall in with a group of bored pranksters influenced by MTV's *Jackass*, so we'd occasionally get into trouble. We were all horrible and awkward around girls, so most of our nights were spent trying to mimic the wildness of our *Jackass* heroes. Our best gag was this prank called "Poo Phone," where we'd rub shit onto a public phone receiver, call it from an antiquated cell phone, and watch as some poor bastard answered, only to discover that he had just placed shit in his ear. "You've been poo-phoned," we'd yell into his shit-covered ear.

But I was mainly just a good old boy, living in a simpler time, before things like mass school shootings and Facebook tainted our world.

Greg had his ups and downs in his teenage years. He suffered from a leg ailment, hemiparesis, as a result of his cerebral palsy. It left him with a limp in his right leg that made it tricky to play most sports, though he still managed to move around the tennis court. He had a couple of surgeries to attempt to fix it. For a few years, it seemed like his leg was always covered in a cast. But, instead of sulking, he focused on building his mind. He was an avid reader, was always working his way through a vocabulary-builder workshop, and participated in activities like debate and theater. He loved writing and knew he wanted to be a writer from an early age. He was an innocent kid with a head full of dreams and big words.

He also secretly spent his teens dealing with his own sexuality. He knew pretty early on that he was gay, but he was trying to find the right time to come out. He didn't want to do it while still in Utah. The state just wasn't that gay friendly back then. Greg figured he'd be dragged behind some hick's truck or socially ridiculed. So he waited for the right moment. He decided that moment was when our whole family was vacationing in Palm Desert halfway through his freshman year at Northwestern. Most college kids spend spring break pouring alcohol on their brains and slamming genitals together, but Greg decided he'd liberate himself another way. Greg and I had just seen *Eternal Sunshine of the Spotless Mind*. We were waiting for the rest of the family to get out of some other bullshit movie. So we went into a Borders bookstore, and he told me the news as we strolled through the aisles.

"So, Danny. I have an announcement. I'm gay," he nervously said as quickly as he could, like he was ripping off a Band-Aid. He had told me last because he knew of my bully ways. He figured I'd tease him for being gay the way I'd teased Tiffany for accidentally doing LSD. Little did he know that he was my favorite person on earth, and I'd love him no matter what. I pulled his trembling body in for a giant, brotherly hug.

"Greg. That's awesome. Very cool. When did you know you were officially gay?" I asked him.

"I knew in the fifth grade when I jacked off to Chris O'Donnell in *Mad Love*."

"Jesus, we watched that movie together," I said, a little shocked.

"Yeah, well, I also watched it alone. And jacked off to it," he said.

"Well, I love you and support you no matter who you're attracted to, even if it's Chris O'Donnell," I said, proving what a great and tolerant person I was. It was a load off his mind. I think he was expecting me to call him a faggot and love him less.

His announcement wasn't that shocking. I had suspected he was gay for most of our lives. I mean, he had a cardboard cutout of the Scarecrow from *The Wizard of Oz* in his bedroom standing there like a salute to homosexuality. Only once had he talked about girls with me. It was around his junior year in high school when he asked my advice on finger banging one of his friends. The phrase "finger banging" sounded so clunky and forced coming out of his mouth that I knew it was simply a last-ditch effort to try to appear straight. I was the wrong person to ask. I had had no luck with very many girls before somehow landing Abby.

"Fuck if I know," I had told Greg. "I think it gets wet and you just rub around there, or something. Watch porn," I advised him. "Porn teaches all."

The blind leading the gay.

Greg's other friends from home had also assumed he was gay, so when he came out, he received nothing but love. It was a relatively smooth transition out of the closet. So, though I'm sure he had some inner confusion and torment, he had a pretty great run through his teenage years.

Jessica and Chelsea caught a few years of the Marshalls' golden age, but they were in their mid-teens when our stupid, rich, perfect bubble popped. Having two terminally ill parents is worse than being stuck in the closet with a limp or having a bad acid trip. Well, maybe it's not worse than the bad acid trip. I've never done acid, so I have no idea.

Chelsea turned sixteen a few months after my dad was diagnosed with Lou Gehrig's disease, but she acted like she was nine. She was born extremely prematurely—three and a half months, to be exact—and at birth she weighed in at two pounds, fifteen ounces. One of her kidneys hadn't developed properly, she was deaf in one ear, and she required several surgeries just to keep her alive. She almost didn't make it. But she pulled through and turned into one of the funniest, weirdest people I know. Chelsea and I had always liked each other. I felt sorry for her because she had fought so hard to survive. I took her under my wing, looked after her, ran around being crazy with her, and taught her that farting is just a part of being human. I even gave her a nickname: Moe Ham. "Moe ham" were my first words—my fat-ass attempt to say "More ham." I'm not completely sure why I started calling her that. It just seemed fitting. She just looked like a Moe Ham. I'd later call her Fart Princess, because of her farting. I'm not great with nicknames.

I loved how crazy Chelsea was. I found her unpredictability hilarious. Once, for example, when she was about three years old, she chased my friend Mike around the house with a piece of her shit in her hand. Mike thought it was funny at first but almost broke into tears when Chelsea tossed it his way and it nearly smacked him in the face.

Another time, when she was about four years old, I wandered away from my dad and Chelsea at Toys 'R' Us. As I was searching for Nerf toys, I noticed diarrhea running down one of the model playground slides. I finally found my frantic dad and he said, "DJ, we've got to get out of here. Chelsea just shit down one of the slides."

In other words, she's pretty obviously related to me.

My parents didn't worry too much about the public slide shitting and the shit tossing because Chelsea was just a little kid. "Every little kid does that sort of shit. Give her a break," my mom told me once when I brought up how odd it was. "She probably learned it from you."

They figured she was a little immature because she was born premature. My mom never liked labeling her kids' problems or medicating them. Whenever I suggested that Chelsea should be on something for her hyperactivity or see a therapist for her unusual behavior, my mom would remind me that doctors wanted to put me on Ritalin when I was a kid.

"You were a little spaz, Danny Boy. If I listened to doctors, you would've spent your childhood in a fucking straitjacket. So shut up about Chelsea," she'd say.

Chelsea was also the baby of the family, and we treated her like one. We even turned Moe Ham into "Baby Moe," and still call her that today. We also figured that her behavior was a reaction to our mom having cancer. She was attached at the hip to my mom, following her around the house and talking her ear off about dance. We figured maybe she fixated on bizarre things and acted strangely as a way of coping.

"Give her a break. Her mom has cancer," my mom would tell us anytime we gave Chelsea shit for acting weird.

"But you're our mom, too, and we're not weird," we'd say back.

"Yes, you are. You're all weird," she'd tell us. "In fact, Chelsea's the most normal of the bunch."

But as Chelsea grew older, it was apparent that she wasn't like other kids her age. Once she became a teenager, we officially knew something was up. She was always kicking major ass in school—getting straight A's—but my mom still had to help her get ready every day. She refused to use a fork. She would eat her hair. She couldn't order for herself at restaurants. She'd lick all the salt off pretzels and then put them back in the bag. And she refused to sleep in her own room, electing to sleep at the base of my parents' bed, or sometimes right between them.

Chelsea couldn't keep a friend because she only talked about dance. Plus, she would rip ass and laugh hysterically during a hangout session. Most teenage boys would've found that funny, but girls thought it was gross. She was also incredibly nervous and awkward around strangers. When someone asked her a question, she wouldn't answer them, but would instead look up to us to answer for her. We just thought she was shy, but most of our friends thought that she was mentally challenged.

"So Chelsea's, like, retarded, right?" I remember one of my friends asking.

"Nah, she's just weird," I'd explain. "She likes fart jokes, though, so that's pretty cool."

By the time Chelsea reached junior high school, we couldn't blame her eccentric behavior and social issues on being premature or my mom's cancer anymore. My parents started to do some research and sent Chelsea to a psychiatrist, who suggested that Chelsea might have Asperger's. They started to read more about it and realized that Chelsea was nearly a textbook case. My mom and dad were working on getting her some help, but, just as they started looking into counselors for her, the Lou Gehrig's storm hit. They had bigger things to worry about than teaching Chelsea how to use a fork. She was on her own now.

Jessica was a different kind of mess. My parents had adopted her when she was three days old. Since Greg and I were so close, my parents wanted a sister for Tiffany to play with. Plus, my mom was adopted and wanted to pay it forward. We all loved Jessica unconditionally, but as the one adopted child, she always felt like an outsider in our family. She thought she was the one fuck-up who could never do right. I knew this because while on a family vacation, I was hassling her about doing better in school. She finally snapped, pinched my fat face hard, and said, "I'm not perfect like the rest of you."

She labeled herself as imperfect and struggled through school. By the time I came home to help out, she was in her junior year of high school. My mom and dad had been the ones to help her slide by— meeting with teachers and assisting with homework every night—but now they couldn't provide the supervision she needed to make that final push to graduation.

Socially, she had fallen in with the drinking kids. High schoolers typically don't drink responsibly. Drinking usually means slugging down whatever hard alcohol they can manage to steal from their parents' liquor cabinets. Since she was from a non-Mormon family who enjoyed their alcoholic beverages, Jessica was one of the primary suppliers to her friends. One night, I tried to make a big fat drink and noticed the vodka was mostly water. Jess was attempting to get away with her drinking by using that age-old trick, but hadn't counted on her brother also loving the drink.

She had wrecked her car twice: once when she hit a moose driving down Parley's Canyon from Park City to Salt Lake, and once when some kid took her for a joyride and rolled it into a ravine. She was also caught drinking at Utah's shitty amusement park, Lagoon, over the summer and given a drinking ticket. Her court date was fast approaching.

In addition to the poor performance at school and the drinking, she was also hiding a long-standing relationship with that lacrosse coach she'd been hanging out with—the one we nicknamed Creepy Todd, a thirty-five-year-old Mormon. Creepy Todd's presence in Jessica's life started when she played on one of his teams when she was twelve. He was thirty then. At first it was just lacrosse, but then they started developing a friendship outside of lacrosse. We found out that he was picking her up from school in his truck and would drive her and her friends around to the mall, to the movies, to get Slurpees, etc. He would come to birthday parties. He would call Jessica late at night. They'd chat online, and not about lacrosse. We had no proof that it wasn't all totally innocent, but at the time it still seemed way inappropriate.

One summer night when I was home visiting from Berkeley, Jessica left an MSN Messenger conversation up on the household computer screen. She had fallen asleep on the couch next to the computer. I, being a nosy prick, decided to read it. In the conversation, they said "I love you" to each other, she mentioned that she needed to get her sweater out of his truck, and she asked if she could get a back massage from him. She was fifteen at the time. I didn't want to be a snitch, but I also didn't want my little sister to involve herself in a sketchy situation, so I printed the conversation out and gave it to my parents, figuring it was their job to handle things.

My dad did, sort of. I thought he should have called the cops— even without direct proof of any wrongdoing—pulled Jessica from the lacrosse team, and punched the dude in the nuts, but my dad was too peaceful for nut punches. Instead, he just sat down with Creepy Todd and told him that he wasn't to contact or hang out with Jessica outside of lacrosse. He also had Jessica promise to not see Creepy Todd. I loved my dad and respected the hell out of him, but in this situation I thought he should've done more. It was a rare but giant parenting mistake on his part. But, to our knowledge, they were only seeing each other at lacrosse practice, so I guess it worked. I was still on the lookout for him.

This is all to say that Jessica and Chelsea were already a bit of a mess, even before the whole dying-parents party. And now, my mom was knocked out by chemo, wandering the house eating yogurt and muttering nonsense, and my dad was being rocked by Lou Gehrig's disease. So, in addition to all the Daddy Duties, Greg and I had to manage the little girls and sort of step in as their dysfunctional, fake parents. This meant helping them get out the door to school, picking Chelsea up from school (the Mormons only drove her to school, but not back home), helping with homework, driving Chelsea to dance class, feeding them and keeping Jessica's relationship with Creepy Todd under control. Tiffany refused to help with the little girls, noting that she had been doing this shit for years. It was our turn. Fair enough.

Chelsea, in particular, was a handful. She was used to having my mom and dad run her life. She could still barely get herself ready for school in the morning without my mom's help, and, though she was sixteen, she refused to drive. She was terrified of the roads and wasn't ready to deal with the stress and pressure of operating a car. Greg and I didn't see it like that. We thought if she'd just drive, our lives would be a lot easier; we wouldn't have to run her ass around town.

"You need to stop being such a fucking baby and learn how to drive," I told her, sounding like a deadbeat dad instead of the kind, loving, supportive, nurturing father that she had come to expect in her real dad.

"I don't want to drive," she replied.

"Being a baby isn't cute anymore, Baby Moe. You need to grow up."

"You need to grow up," she retorted with a smile.

"It's just that everything would be so much easier if you just took care of yourself," I said.

"Everything would be so much easier if you just took care of yourself," she mimicked back at me.

"Oh, repeating everything I say. Real mature, Fart Princess," I said.

"You're the Fart Princess," she said.

"I really want to fart on your face," I said.

"I really want to fart on your face," she said. We both started laughing. A fart joke is stronger than any anger I could build up as her fake parent. I drove her to dance.

Occasionally, I would push Chelsea to be more independent. One afternoon, I was feeling particularly worn down. I had been looking after my dad all day, helping him at his office, feeding him, basically just being the best son in the entire world—a true American hero with a heart the size of Texas. I laid my dad down for a nap on his BiPAP, picked up Chelsea from school, and drove her home. Just as I was about to finally relax a bit, she instantly needed another ride to dance.

"Fucking Christ, you need to learn how to drive. You're sixteen years old, and our home is burning to the ground with tragedy," I said.

"Sorry . . . I promise not to fart in the car," said Chelsea, knowing I'd warm up to a solid fart joke.

"I can't stay mad at you," I said as I smiled and grabbed the keys.

As we walked out to the car, I decided it was a good idea for Chelsea to practice her driving. She had a learner's permit, so it was legal. She opposed the idea. I said, "Okay, well, then, I don't know how you're getting to dance class, because I'm not driving." She wanted to go to dance class badly enough to drive, so she reluctantly grabbed the keys and took a deep breath into her tiny, premature lungs.

In the car, I rolled down the window and kicked my feet up. "Shit, it sure is nice to be sitting in the passenger seat."

"Fuck you, Danny," she said as she nervously tried to jam the keys into the ignition, missing a couple of times before finally landing.

It was the first time I had actually been a passenger in one of her wild rides. My mom had warned me that she wasn't a good driver, but no warning could've prepared me. The car made that catlike hissing sound when she turned the key after it was already started. She then tried to reverse the car out of the driveway, but it shot forward instead of backward.

"Wrong way, idiot," I said. "Check your mirrors and put it in reverse." She clumsily put it in neutral before finally managing to get it into reverse. She darted out of the driveway, almost hitting the mailbox and side fence.

"Oh my God, Fart Princess. No wonder you're scared of driving. You're Mr. Magoo," I said as she ran through a stop sign.

"Who's Mr. Magoo?" she asked as she put on her left blinker and turned right.

It was when Chelsea almost slammed into another car during a two-lane merger that I realized that she shouldn't be on the road.

"Jesus, you're going to kill us, and I don't think Mom and Dad should have to sit through their children's funerals, especially in their current state," I said, helping guide the car to the side of the road.

She got out, looking like she was about to pop from stress. I slid over into the driver's seat as cars angrily stormed by. No one honks in Utah, because it's not L.A., but this would've been a prime time to honk.

"So, I guess we're just stuck driving you around. Guess that's just part of the whole dying-parents package. You're the worst driver in the history of driving, by the way."

Chelsea laughed so hard she accidentally farted, which made us both laugh hysterically. I drove her smelly ass to dance.

Though Chelsea was a handful, she was at least fun to be around. Jessica, on the other hand, was a real pain in the ass. It wasn't like she required much of our attention. Actually, she didn't want any of us to notice her. She'd sneak around the house trying her best to go unnoticed. But getting her up and out of bed for school in the morning was nearly impossible. It was a fight every morning. I'd wake her up at six thirty so she had time to get ready, but she'd just go right back to sleep. She didn't give a fuck about school. School was hell on earth. She felt out of place among all the rich white Mormons.

Sometimes we'd get her there, but most days we'd throw up our arms and say, "Fuck it. It's her life."

"Yeah, what are we going to do? Make her go to school at gunpoint?" Greg said.

"That's not a bad idea, but I'm scared of guns. Fuck it. Let's let her sleep. At least someone in this house will be well rested."

More than once, we found her passed out on the kitchen floor or in the basement.

"Damn it, she's taking all the booze," I'd say.

"Come on, let's get her to bed," Greg'd say back.

"There's still a little vodka in here," I'd say as I finished off the bottle she'd been drinking from. Greg and I would pick her up and plop her into bed, so she could rest up for her big day of not going to school. I'd thought drinking too much was going to be my job. Jessica was sort of stealing my thunder.

I knew Jessica was acting like this because she was scared about what was happening with our dad. She loved him more than anything. She was in pain. Some of the drinking was simply an escape. I felt endlessly sorry for her, but I didn't know how I could help. I had talked to Jessica about her drinking before, and school counselors were meeting with her on a weekly basis, but it obviously wasn't working. It was useless bringing it up while she was still drunk, so I tried to get her one morning while she was hungover. She had already decided to not go to school that day and had come downstairs to dig some food out of the fridge.

"You know how your head hurts and you feel like you might die? Well, that's from the alcohol," I said as she opened the fridge.

"I didn't drink," she said, having forgotten about the night before.

"Greg and I found you passed out," I reminded her.

"So?" she said, still giving me attitude.

"So, you know how you can stop feeling like shit every morning? You could stop drinking and start focusing on getting through the eleventh grade," I said.

"K," she said as she slammed the fridge.

I instantly felt bad for trying to parent her, so I tried to wrangle her in for a hug, figuring maybe she just needed a little love.

"Come here and give your loser brother a hug. I love you," I said. But she gave me a dirty look instead and stormed upstairs with a plate of leftover lasagna.

Acting like her dad felt incredibly strange to me. I didn't like it. I wanted to go back to being her cool brother. I didn't want to be barking criticisms at her. But I didn't know what else to do. I was concerned Jessica was going to permanently fuck up her life. I wanted to shake her and demand that she stop screwing up, but I also wanted to console her and tell her that everything was going to get better. The problem was that she wasn't responding to either approach.

The good news was that my coming home appeared to have scared Creepy Todd away. He knew that I wasn't cool with Jessica hanging out with him. It was probably because anytime I'd see the guy, I'd stare him down and raise my middle finger. "Stay away from my family, you creep," I'd mumble. I was like Robert De Niro in *Meet the Parents*, and he was like Ben Stiller, only I wasn't Jessica's real dad, and he was a creepy lacrosse coach. I had also told Jessica that my tough friends and I would kick his ass if we caught him hanging around. Realistically, I would've done nothing because I'm a pussy. But they didn't know that.

So, all in all, Greg and I were doing the best we could, but it felt like the dam was about to break open and fuck up the whole town, and we were just a piece of gum preventing disaster for but a few brief moments. The girls needed their real parents. They were confused, lost teenagers trying to figure out how to manage this big, scary world and their road maps were fading. It wasn't supposed to go like this. They were supposed to graduate high school with two healthy parents smiling in the audience. Their dad was supposed to take them on college tours and help guide them into the next phase of their lives. Instead, Greg and I were at the helm of the ship, steering them right for the iceberg.

My poor dad had to watch as Greg and I fumbled around and tried our best, all while the Lou Gehrig's disease continued its relentless conquest of his life. It must have tormented him; the disease made it so he could no longer parent his children the way he wanted to. He could no longer drive them to school. He could no longer patiently help them with their homework. He could no longer proudly stand on the sidelines of a lacrosse match or in the audience of a dance recital. He could no longer wait up worrying at the window as they went off to prom. He could no longer scare off boyfriends. He was now fighting his own battle. He could no longer fight the battles for the people he loved.

But he was still our dad. He wasn't dead yet. He was still capable of flashes of greatness, flashes of his old self.

It was a pleasant October day. Fall in Utah is glorious—the calm before the messy, gross, endless storm that is a Utah winter. The temperature had dropped, but not enough to make it uncomfortable. The mountains were colored by the changing leaves. Jessica was due at the courthouse for her Lagoon drinking ticket. My mom was at chemo, so she couldn't go. Greg was exhausted from being on Daddy Duty the night before. So I figured that I'd go with her, stand in as her fake father.

We were about to leave when my dad said, "Wait, I'm coming with you."

"Really? Why don't you rest up so you can try to not die later today?"

"I want to go. Jessica needs me," he said.

"Are you sure? You're in bad shape there, Papa Bear," I said.

"Just get my jacket. I'm going," he insisted.

So I put a jacket on his bony shoulders and got him loaded into the car. He was still walking, but he looked like he was about to keel over at any moment, so I grabbed the manual wheelchair that someone had donated to us and jammed it into the trunk. We got to the courthouse, and I unloaded the wheelchair. Jessica looked terrified—like a scared kid closer to childhood than adulthood. My dad looked over to her.

"Look, we know you messed up, but I'm here for you, and I love you," my dad managed to say. "We all make mistakes. It'll be okay."

"Thanks," Jessica managed to reply.

I got our dad out of the car and into the wheelchair. "Probably good we brought the wheelchair. They'll feel extra sorry for you," I told Jessica.

"Yeah," nervous Jessica said.

Once we were in the courtroom, we made sure to sit right in front of the judge so he was sure to see our dying father. He wouldn't punish a girl whose father was on the brink of death, right? Surely he would take mercy on her and understand the need to escape into numbness that brought about her drinking. Maybe Jessica and I would be seen as heroes (of sorts) fighting the good fight, and we'd actually leave the courtroom with a Golden Medal of Courage or something.

"You two are so strong. Stay strong and keep him strong," I imagined the judge saying.

"Thank you, Your Honor. Our lives are complete shit right now, but we'll do our best to find a way through this mess. No more drinking for Jessica. I'll see to it," I imagined myself saying. "Though I might have a drink or two myself," I might joke, sending the judge and possibly the whole courtroom into fits of laughter.

"You're a good man, and a funny son of a bitch," the judge would say.

"Hey, my mom's no bitch," I'd reply, causing more laughter.

"You rascals get on out of here. And don't forget your Golden Medals of Courage," he'd say as he placed the pure gold medallions around our tired necks.

That's not what happened.

Instead, the tired and matter-of-fact judge ran through the list of petty thieves and recreational drug users that decorated the Utah courtroom. He finally got to Jessica.

"Jessica Marshall, looks like you had a little too much fun at Lagoon," he said. Jessica nodded back. "Looks like you're a minor. Do you have anyone here with you?" he asked. "Anyone here for support?"

The courtroom was silent for a second. The judge stared at Jessica, Jessica at her feet. I was about to say something like "I'm here. I'm Jessica's fat, budding alcoholic older brother." Then, with all the strength in his weak body, my dad rose out of the creaky wheelchair.

"I'm Jessica's dad," he managed to say. All heads turned to him, shocked by his resurrection out of the chair. He stood there like a proud parent, his weak legs barely able to hold him up, watching after his little girl, making sure she knew he still had her back. "I'm here to support her."

The judge looked my dad over. "Okay, and are you okay, sir?" he asked.

"I have Lou Gehrig's disease, but we're trying to manage," my dad said. The judge solemnly nodded back at him and made a few notes.

Jessica got out of the ticket. She just had to do forty hours of service, which the judge said she could do by helping out at home. We weren't awarded any Golden Medals of Courage, but Jessica left knowing that her dad was still looking after her. Even if he could barely do it, he stood up for her.

"The wheelchair really did the trick," my dad said as he smiled at us. "We really fooled them." I smiled at my dying dad. He had flashed back to who he was before Lou Gehrig's disease, if only for a brief moment.

"Come on, let's get the fuck out of here," I said as Jessica and I wheeled our dad out of the courthouse and into the crisp fall air.

STANA'S CAT HOLOCAUST

Before the Lou Gehrig's disease, my dad did a great job of maintaining our house—keeping it looking fresh and modern, making us appear to be a family in its prime. The TVs worked and functional batteries weighed down the remotes. There was always an abundance of beer in the fridge. The yard looked like the cover of a magazine that specialized in beautiful yards that were never littered in dog shit. Lightbulbs were replaced the instant they burned out. There were multiple shampoo and conditioner choices in the showers. Rolls of toilet paper were at least an inch thick. The grill had a never-empty propane tank connected to it and chicken shish kabobs sizzling on top. The garage was swept and didn't smell like a combination of dog urine and cat urine, with a splash of drunk-Dan urine. There was chalk next to the pool table. No leaves floated in the pool. The tennis court had a net. The cars were washed and had gas in them. There were no spiders in our basement.

Then the ALS shitstorm hit.

Suddenly, our house was transformed into a war zone. There were weeds on our dirty tennis court. Dog shit and dandelions marred our yard. HBO worked on only a couple of our TVs. The hot tub smelled like balls and teenager piss. Cobwebs haunted our windowsills and spiders ran our basement like a 1920s speakeasy. Rooms were unevenly lit or just darkened by dead bulbs. Keys on the computer keyboard were missing. The grill functioned as a recycling bin for unfinished 3 a.m. beers instead of the place where meat was made delicious. Two of our three pinball machines no longer worked. The mini-fridge in the basement had more types of mold than beer and wasn't even plugged in anymore. Door handles jiggled. Locks didn't lock. Our cars were filled with Del Taco wrappers, Red Bull cans, sunflower seeds, hardened pita bread, banana peels, and glasses lined with week-old orange juice residue. No new pictures went up on the wall. Cat piss yellowed our carpet. Cigarettes and weed were smoked in the backyard. Raccoons danced in our trees and shit on our trampoline.

We had lost the man of the house, and his absence amplified how much he had formerly done for us. Greg and I were left to try to fill in and keep the house up and running. But we were so used to having our dad do everything that we didn't know how to do anything. For example, once it took me forty-five minutes to change a lightbulb. I thought an old one had broken off in the socket. I had read somewhere that a potato could grip the bulb and spin it out. I started there. The potato didn't work. Before I knew it I had an apple up there, then a banana, then a cantaloupe, then a Fruit Roll-Up, and then I went back to the potato. It turned out that all I had to do from the get-go was screw in a fresh bulb. In the end, the whole fixture was destroyed and smelled like the produce section of a grocery store.

To add to the deterioration of our house, there were way more animals running around than we could handle. It was a zoo. In addition to the two golden retrievers, we now had four cats: Brighton, Bailey, Pierre, and Pongo. Brighton had been around our house for years. She must have been fifteen years old. Cats are a reflection of their surroundings, and growing up in our house was chaotic and intense, so Brighton was rather skittish. Plus, she didn't get along with any of the other cats. Anytime another cat would approach, she'd make that terrifying hissing noise and even take a swipe at them. Bailey was our second-oldest cat. My mom had apparently rescued him from traffic on State Street. Bailey also kept to himself, and didn't really interact with us or any of the other animals. Tiffany had dumped Pierre and Pongo on us after BCB turned out to be allergic. They were brothers, so they sort of ran the show, ganging up on Brighton and Bailey and taking over the best nap spots. All the cats were territorial, and they were engaged in a rather epic piss battle, leaving stains everywhere and making the majority of our house absolutely reek of cat urine.

The combination of the loss of the man of the house, Greg's and my inability to fill his shoes, and the cats' piss war amounted to our home slipping into total dysfunction and decay. And with the construction in full force, half the house was covered in tarps, dust, and construction gear. It was mayhem.

* * *

No one noticed the deterioration of our home more than Stana. Stana had worked for our family for as long as I could remember. She was in her seventies, but tried really hard to look like she was in her fifties. She had a wrinkly face, was about five feet tall, wore glasses, and had dyed blond hair. Her backstory was caked with tragedy. She was born a Jew in Poland just as things were heating up with that asshole Hitler. When the Nazis stormed her family's house and pulled her parents out, they somehow missed Stana, leaving her alone in their ransacked home. She was two at the time. Neighbors discovered her and raised her.

My mom, being a cancer survivor, naturally took a liking to Stana. "She's a survivor like us, and survivors are always good to have around," my mom once explained. Plus, Stana was short and feisty, like my mom, and hated Mormons more than anything on earth. Well, maybe except for the Nazis.

Because my mom had a soft spot for Stana (survivor sisters for life!), she didn't seem to mind that she wasn't a great cleaning lady. Instead of actually cleaning, Stana seemed more interested in the house gossip. I guess she was looking for a replacement family. So we took her in, and she became a sort of grandma figure in our lives. Fuck, she even attended birthday parties and some holidays. She was a friend first and a cleaning lady second.

I always liked her because she was funny. Funny goes a long way in my book. She swore up a storm ("son of a bitch" was her go-to) and would call people out if they were fucking up. I admired her honesty and bluntness, even when it came at my expense. When I visited home after my first semester at Berkeley, Stana took one look at me and said, "Oh, Danny, you is havin' fat face now." It hurt my feelings, but it was true. I was havin' fat face after a semester of eating shit, drinking beer, and never exercising, as college students tend to do.

Stana had her flaws, though. She, like our real grandma, was a not-so-closet racist. I always thought it was strange to hear a woman who survived the Holocaust discriminate against anyone who wasn't a Nazi, but she did. For example, though it was only October 2007, preparations for the 2008 Democratic primary elections were kicking into high gear. Hillary Clinton and Barack Obama were neck and neck. When I asked her whom she liked for president, she said, "Danny, I is no likin' Obama. No be president."

"Why not? Obama's super cool and he likes basketball."

"Danny, it is because he is black. No black president. This is, how you say, ridiculous," she explained in her adorable broken English.

I didn't know what to make of that, so I said, "Well, I like him. He's really smart and is a welcome change from that dipshit George W. Bush."

"There is no way this man is president. Black people no get good jobs," she retorted as she swept our hardwood floors, not recognizing that maybe she didn't have the best job.

Stana, though she thought she was really smart, couldn't read or write in English. One year, she gave my mom a birthday card that had on the front the words "I give you my deepest sympathies in this your time of mourning." So she was an illiterate, unrepentantly racist Holocaust survivor, but we still loved her like one of our own.

Though Stana wasn't great at it, she tried her best to make our home look orderly and warm. While the dying-parents mess was happening, Stana was trying to figure out how she could put a stop to the decline of our house. She noticed the obscene amounts of cat piss popping up all over the place and started blaming the cats for everything.

Construction in the basement had finished, so I moved from the dining room down into the basement. One Monday morning, Stana darted into my basement room—one of the cat-piss hot spots.

"Danny, you is up?" Stana yelled through my door as I lay in bed, still in my boxers, rubbing the sleep out of my eyes, trying to figure out what to do with my morning wood.

"Yeah, I am now."

"You is come with me. I is showin' you what son of a bitch kitties doing," she said, pulling me out of bed.

"Did they piss again?" I said.

"I showin' you," Stana said.

"I bet they pissed again," I said, now awake.

Stana guided me to a corner of the living room where a fresh batch of cat piss had been pissed. "See, Danny. Son of a bitch kitties goin' pee all over here," she said.

I shook my head in disbelief and asked if I could go check on my dying father. Stana continued to stare at the piss, shaking her head and muttering "son of a bitch" under her breath.

Her loathing of the cats grew so fervent that she eventually started describing ways in which she would brutally murder them.

"Danny, I is takin' kitty in backyard and hittin' with hammer on head."

"Danny, I is takin' kitty and leavin' in middle of traffic."

"Danny, I is takin' kitty and runnin' over with my car."

"Danny, I is buyin' gun and shootin' kitty."

"Danny, I is throwin' towel over kitty head and squeeze until no more kitty."

She would have acted on any of these ideas had it not been for my mom's love of animals and unwillingness to take on any more death and tragedy. Mom had a particular love for Brighton. Brighton mainly hung out on my mom's bed, nestling up to her after brutal rounds of chemo. "She's my chemo kitty, and she's not going anywhere," Mom said. When she had the energy to do so, she would plead with Stana to stop complaining.

"Stana, please. We're dealing with so much right now. We can't worry about getting rid of the cats," my mom said.

"But Debi, kitty is ruinin' home. This is no home for kitty. Daddy is no healthy and kitty is makin' pee-pee all over bedroom," Stana said.

"I know, Stana, but I can't stand losing anything else right now. Not even the cats," said my mom.

"Stana take care of. I is takin' kitty in backyard and hittin' with hammer on head," said Stana as she made a little hammering motion with her hands.

"Not today, Stana, please. I really need to lie down. I just had three hours of chemotherapy," said my tired mom as she headed off to bed to get some postchemo rest.

Stana subtly announced her dedication to ridding our home of piss-easy cats when she showed up one morning with a large animal cage. She set it in the garage and woke me up.

"Danny, I is bringin' cage for kitty. You is catchin' and puttin' in cage and Stana is takin' kitty far, far away," she said excitedly.

"It's six in the morning, Stana. Can I go back to bed?" I said, not able to match her enthusiasm.

"Okay, but when you is wakin', I is showin' you kitty pee in Mommy's room and we is catchin' son of a bitch kitty," she said.

Though initially I had no problem with the cats, Stana slowly convinced me to hate them as much as she did. I found myself flipping them off anytime I saw one. I would occasionally catch one and shit-talk it for five to ten minutes. "You better watch yourself, you fucking cat. We're on to your pissing. Next time I catch you in the act I'm going to take you in the backyard and hit you over the head with a hammer, and then there is no more kitty." The cat would usually mistake the aggression for affection and begin rubbing its head against my face with a solid purr.

When people brought dinner over, I found myself escorting them around the house, showing them all the places the son of a bitch cats had urinated. "And look at this corner. The cats pissed all over it. Those fucking sons of bitches," I would exclaim.

"So, you're putting in an elevator?" they'd ask, trying to change the subject.

"Yeah. It's so my dad can get around the house. Don't know why he'd want to, though, since most of it is covered in cat piss," I'd say as I was escorting them to another corner of the house. "Look at this area behind the couch. Those sons of bitches."

"Um, okay. So where do you want me to put this lasagna?" they'd ask.

To me, the cats started to symbolize more than just a yellow marking on the carpet. They started to represent selfishness. Here my siblings and I were moving my dad's arms, wiping his ass, speaking for him, reading to him, showering him, and these lazy cats were running amuck in our house—pissing, sleeping, killing birds, playing with the curtain strings: everything we wanted to be doing ourselves, instead of the aforementioned Daddy Duties. Fuck those cats. Fuck those cats hard.

My siblings agreed with Stana and me. The cats were a big, disgusting problem. Chelsea was fixated on the fact that the cats were here because of BCB's allergy.

"It's just bullshit that Big Cock Brian can't be around cats, so we have to deal with them, ya know," said Chelsea as she licked the salt off a pretzel.

Greg didn't like all the fur everywhere. "Living with this many animals is just sort of gross. We've got to get rid of them," he said.

We asked Tiffany to take them back since Brian had moved to Maine, but she still refused. "Guys, Brian can't be around cats when he's in town. He's fucking allergic. Just fucking deal with it."

Greg and I decided we needed my dad on our side if we were ever going to get rid of these cats, especially since my mom was no help. We convinced him that the cats were way worse than Lou Gehrig's disease. It got to the point where we would say, "What should we do with the cats?" and he would say, "Kill 'em."

Stana had Greg and me so riled up one morning that we pledged that today would be the last day our house would be subject to cat piss. We were to wait for my Humane Society–loving, yogurt-eating, hippie-bitch mom to leave for chemo, and then we were going to catch those cats come hell or high water. Stana was going to lead the charge.

It was as though we were going to war. The only problem was that Greg and I were scared that the cats would catch on to our scheme and collectively decide to claw out our eyeballs. To curb our fears, I rounded up some old racquetball goggles for us. We teamed those with construction gloves I found among all the tools and gear, plus three layers of sweaters. We felt good and protected against the cats' piss-stained claws.

Stana didn't wear anything special. Just her regular cleaning uniform. She decided that all she needed was a large sheet to throw over the cats and then, "We is takin' son of a bitch kitty and puttin' in cage."

My mom left for chemo and we started our hunt. We were able to chase Brighton into my parent's bedroom. Once she was cornered, Greg and I thought it best to focus on this son of a bitch kitty while Stana patrolled the halls for additional cats. Greg and I were terrified and having trouble seeing out of the foggy racquetball glasses, but we were determined to get this cat. Brighton had cleverly placed herself beneath my mom and dad's king-size bed, where she sat poised to claw the lord out of our eyeballs. Greg was on one side. I was on the other. Stana entered.

"Me is no findin' other kitty. We is focus on this son of a bitch," she said as if she had been on the evil side of World War II instead of the tragic side.

Stana suggested that Greg and I lift the bed while she waited with her sheet. We lifted the entire bed. We couldn't see the action unfold and only heard Stana yell, "Son of a bitch, shithead kitty!" followed by the sound of a swooshing sheet and a struggling cat. We dropped the bed and looked over. She had Brighton wrapped up in the sheet. Poor Brighton struggled and made a meowing noise that sounded like "help."

This is the part where we fucked it all up. Stana walked the cat over to me and said, "You is put son of a bitch kitty in cage." As she tried to hand her over to me, Brighton squirmed loose and darted off. We didn't see her for another week, but eventually found her in our backyard storage shed. She was still shaking and clearly hadn't eaten. If cats could write, I'm sure she would have written a poetic, Anne Frank–like journal entry about hiding from her oppressors.

Before we could plan another attack that day, my mom came home. The game was over. "Why am I wearing these construction gloves and racquetball goggles? Well, Mom, because of all the construction dust, of course. I suggest you do the same, especially since you have cancer."

Stana, Greg, and I were all disheartened. Stana said it best. "Son of a bitch kitty. Danny, we is be so close."

The next week, Stana seemed to have lost her motivation. She didn't show me any cat piss. She focused on mopping the floors, washing the dishes, doing the laundry. I was tempted to grab her by the arm and guide her around to all the cat piss spots staining our carpet as she had done with me, but she seemed uninterested.

Wednesday rolled around and I realized that I hadn't seen two of the cats—Pongo and Pierre—for a few days. I asked other family members if they had seen them. "Not that I give a fuck, but have you seen Pongo or Pierre?" I inquired nonchalantly.

They realized that they hadn't seen them either. I figured that maybe they had had a powwow with Brighton and decided to take off to another house that wasn't ruled by terrifying dictators hell-bent on eliminating them.

Thursday came. No Pongo. No Pierre. I walked through the house inspecting the piss stains: none of them were fresh.

It was surprisingly depressing. If nothing else, the cats were a nice distraction from the dying parents. With no new piss sprouting up, I felt like I had to return my focus back to my dad. No more fun and games. No more trying to kill cats with Stana.

Later that night, Tiffany came bursting through the front door holding the two cats. "So some lady brought Pongo and Pierre over. She found them in the middle of the Salt Lake Valley, by State Street," Tiff explained.

Apparently pets are now required to have electronic ID chips implanted just below their fur so that, if lost, a vet or other local animal authority can identify them and return them to their rightful owners. Pongo and Pierre were both registered to my sister's address.

"What the fuck were they doing in the middle of Salt Lake?" asked my sister as she filled the cats' dishes full of water and food.

I knew. I knew it was Stana. I knew that she had decided to take the law into her own Holocaust-surviving, illiterate hands. I knew that she had gone behind our backs, rounded up the two cats in that cage she had brought over and left them to fend for themselves in the middle of Mormontown.

But I played it cool. "I have no idea. That's so strange. They must have run away or gotten lost."

Tiff looked puzzled.

"Well, it sure is nice to have them back," I concluded, petting one of them really hard.

We were all surprised to see the cats again, but no one was more surprised than Stana. On Monday morning, when my mom was too far away to hear, she approached me. "Danny, how is the kitty here?" she whispered.

"What do you mean?" I asked.

"Danny, I is catchin' kitty and takin' soooo far away," Stana explained.

"They have these ID chips in their necks. Someone brought them back," I said.

Stana shook her head and said, "Son of a bitch kitty. I is no believin'," as if the cats had thought up the whole ID chip idea themselves.

Later, my mom caught wind that Stana had taken the cats. She loved Stana but wasn't happy about this. My mom knew that I had been supportive of Stana's anti-cat ways, so she bitched me out to the point where I decided to love cats again, and then she decided to write Stana a long-winded note about how it is "my house" and that Stana "had no right to take those cats, even if they were peeing on our carpet."

After my mom had delivered the letter directly to Stana's mailbox, I broke the bad news. "Mom, Stana can't read."

MEET MIKE, MY DAD'S NEW VOICE

The loss of my dad's voice was the next step in the Lou Gehrig's grind. He could still talk, but his breathing was so weak it was really difficult to understand him. He was also about to go on a respirator, so there was a chance he would never talk again. We thus decided to buy him a fancy communication device, the ECO-14. The ECO would become his voice if it got to that.

My dad wasn't very excited about the thought of communicating through a computer. He was trying to hang on to the things he could do for as long as he could. He wasn't ready to give up his voice yet, so he saw the ECO as a tool to be used down the road, and only if completely necessary.

But I was pretty excited about it. Not because I wanted my dad to lose his voice, but because I viewed the ECO as a new toy. The second I heard that my dad was getting a computer that could talk for him, my face lit up. My palms got sweaty. I smiled for the first time in weeks. I couldn't wait to program phrases into the computer and hear it say them back in a Stephen Hawking–esque voice. I had always wanted to hear Stephen Hawking say, "Fuck my anus, you heavy-cocked whore," and with the ECO, I finally could.

The ECO was a large, bulky device with a touch screen—though the touch screen proved to be almost useless since my dad could barely move his arms. He would eventually have to navigate the ECO using an infrared sensor and a silver dot placed on his forehead. The ECO Web site advertises this feature with the following cheerful description:

PRC's new ECO-14 ushers in a new generation of Augmentative and Alternative Communication (AAC) devices by combining advanced

communicating and robust computing in a single device! This sleek, large-screened and versatile device is an AAC aid and Windows® XP-based computer rolled into one, allowing for powerful, independent AAC communication plus convenient, state-of-the-art computing on-the-go.

I liked the "computing on-the-go" part. As if my dad would be bouncing along on the subway, double espresso in his hand, needing to shoot an e-mail back to corporate before his racquetball match with his mistress.

My parents had purchased the ECO before I came home, but they hadn't figured out how to get it up and running. It was a bit esoteric. So my dad, Greg, and I took the device down to this geek named Bart at the place where they bought it. Bart knew everything there was to know about the ECO, just like I knew everything there was to know about wiping my dad's ass. He was a prototypical nerd: bacon breath, glasses, an autodidact, referred to computers as "her," full of McAfee antivirus jokes, way happier than I'll ever be. But the geek knew his communication devices, so meeting with him was the only way we were going to learn how to get Stephen Hawking to call my mother a racial epithet.

At the time we went to see Bart, my dad looked like a walking skeleton. He was getting lots of Jesus-Christ-that-guy-looks-like-he's-about-to-die looks from strangers. Utah is an especially tragic backdrop for physical decay because it's filled with a bunch of smiling Mormons pretending life is perfect. Their cheery demeanor only seemed to amplify the bleakness of my dad's situation. The tricky part about taking my dad anywhere was that we couldn't stay long. He needed to get back to the BiPAP machine, where we all felt he had a reduced chance of dying. Plus, Greg or my dumb ass would always forget to bring things like extra Kleenex or a change of pants in case God sent us an angel in the form of a diarrhea shit. The Promote made him constipated, so my dad had started taking a laxative with his morning feedings, which turned him into a real shit monster.

We rang the bell and asked for Bart. He was in the back room training for the Doritos-eating contest my imagination had entered him in. They took us to a large room in the back of the building that was filled with computers. Bart didn't move from his chair. I guess laziness can be as crippling as Lou Gehrig's disease.

"Hey, Bob," said Bart as he reached to shake my dad's hand, but then remembered that he couldn't move his arms and settled for a shoulder pat. "You got the ECO-14, right?" My dad nodded his head as much as he could. Conversations were pretty awkward now, very one-sided. "Great device. Let's take a look at her."

Bart poked around the screen for a bit, cracking a couple antivirus jokes, before realizing that we had put the computer in the wrong mode. What dumb-asses. He tickled the screen back into submission and set it up so that an alphabet appeared.

"That was easy," Bart said like a hotshot, a booger hanging from his left nostril.

We began playing with it. I started to type in "Greg is gay," but stopped after the "ga" to write "gallant" instead. Greg responded by starting to type "Dan is fat," but stopped after the "fa" to write "fantastic at basketball." We decided to get my dad involved in the joke, so I started to type "My dad is dying," but dropped after the "d" and wrote "dandy." He managed a slight smile.

In other words, we were quickly learning how to fuck around with the thing.

But I wanted to get into funnier options—things like changing the speaker's voice to a woman's, or to a very deep-voiced black man's. I pictured my dad speaking with Karl Malone's Louisianan twang and laughed.

"I wanted to be traded yesterday, but don't today. I've done a complete three-sixty," I imagined my dad saying through the computer as Karl Malone.

We couldn't screw around too much, though. We were here to learn, and, as I mentioned, we never knew when diarrhea would slide into the picture.

"How do we change the voice?" I asked.

This machine was replacing our dad's voice, so we tried to find one that sounded sort of like his, but it was difficult. They were all very computery—a chorus of bad first dates, each with a name and gender. There was "Will," who sounded like he had a bad cold. There was "Rod," who was a little too chipper. We didn't want my dad to sound too excited about having ALS. There was "Micah," who sounded like a tired donkey. There was "Saul," who seemed to have been pulled out of a meth den. We finally settled on "Mike," whose voice was a little softer than the others, the most normal from the list.

"Fuck my anus, you heavy-cocked whore," Mike's voice said in my head.

We also wanted to know how to preprogram buttons to say certain things, so my dad didn't have to go through the arduous task of spelling everything out one letter at a time.

"Oh, you mean Quick Hits?" asked Bart. "Go into the toolbar here and push Modify Page, then select the button on the page you wish to modify. And then you just type in whatever you want said. You can also change the icon using this picture option here and type in whatever you want it to say. Let's try one. How about we do one that says, 'Hello, my name is Bob Marshall'?"

"Stupid," I wanted to say.

"Sure, Bart, let's try that one," I actually said.

"Hello, my name is Bob Marshall," Mike boasted.

Right as we were programming the second Quick Hit, my dad leaned in and notified us that he needed to leave, that he was about to shit his pants, that maybe we could come back later. So we raced home. Greg handled the shitting and put my dad down for a nap. I went straight to the device to work on some more amazing Quick Hits.

"Fuck my anus, you heavy-cocked whore," Mike said, finally letting me get that out of my system. Relief washed over me, as if I were a heroin addict finally getting his fix. With that out of the way, I started to think of practical things my dad would actually need to say. So I started programming.

"I need to go to the bathroom."

"Can you move my arm?"

"I need a nap. Can you help me with that?"

"I need to go to bed."

"Leave me alone."

"Could you scratch my back?"

"I'm hungry. Can you feed me?"

"I need some water."

At this point, I was bored out of my mind with this bottom-of-Maslow's-hierarchy-of-needs bullshit. So, I started to ease into funnier, more risqué quips.

"The dogs are barking. Can you get them to shut up?"

"Please don't smoke around me. My lung capacity is at eighteen percent, you inconsiderate asshole."

"Don't look at me. I am not a monster."

"How am I doing? I have Lou Gehrig's disease. How do you think I'm doing? Unbelievable."

"If you loved me, you would put three shots of gin into my feeding tube."

"Please give me five dollars. I have Lou Gehrig's disease and you can still do all the things you love."

"There's a knife downstairs. Please kill me."

I also thought my dad would probably want to thank me, so I programmed a few ways he could express his appreciation.

"Thanks for all your help, Danny. You are the single best thing that's happened to this family."

I then did one that was a slight alteration to Lou Gehrig's famous speech at Yankee Stadium back in 1939.

"For the past two weeks you have been reading about the bad break I got. Yet today I consider myself the luckiest man on the face of this earth, especially since Danny is my son."

But saying "thank you" isn't funny compared to something sexual. Because sex is funny, right? I continued to program.

"Wow, that was a great round of sex. Let me rest for five minutes and we'll go for round two."

"Boy, I could use a blow job."

I placed a picture of a limp penis as the icon for the "blow job" button and a picture of a vagina for the "sex" button.

After a couple hours of programming my nuts off like a little Bart wannabe, my dad finished his nap. I brought him down to sit in the kitchen—the heart of our house. He had always sat at the head of the table. He was still the man of the house, the head of the pride. I wanted to show him all the quick hits I had programmed.

"And this is if you need to go to the bathroom," I said, hitting the bathroom button to cue Mike's voice.

It didn't take long before my dad noticed the limp penis dangling halfway down the screen. He pointed with his nose at the penis icon, and cleared his throat enough to speak. "What's that one? The penis?"

"Oh, this little guy?" I smiled, anticipating the payoff for my programming labors.

CLICK. "Boy, I could use a blow job."

You can't laugh when you have Lou Gehrig's—it's one of the rules—but you *can* call over your wife and tell her to listen to or watch something, signifying that something is funny. So my dad called for my mom, who ghosted to the table in a nightgown, a yogurt in her hand, her permanent frown intact. I clicked again.

CLICK. "Boy, I could use a blow job."

Her permanent frown flatlined, her version of a smile. When you've had cancer for fifteen years, you can't laugh—it's one of the rules. But you can call over your daughter. Chelsea came over.

CLICK. "Boy, I could use a blow job."

Chelsea erupted with laughter and asked what a blow job was. She was too obsessed with dance and school to know anything about sex. Jessica entered from the TV room and asked what was so funny.

CLICK. "Boy, I could use a blow job."

She smiled. Being a popular seventeen-year-old, Jessica knew what a blow job was. Greg walked downstairs next, having just woken from his daily nap. He was wearing a robe and heading straight for the fridge. I told him to listen up.

CLICK. "Boy, I could use a blow job."

Greg was well versed in both giving and receiving blow jobs, so this really hit home with him. He chuckled as he made himself a giant plate of lasagna.

Tiffany entered through the front door, making a rare appearance, and set her keys, coat, and cell phone down on the kitchen counter.

"Hey, guys. What are you up to?" asked Tiff.

"We're just fucking around with Dad's new communication device. Check it out," I said.

CLICK. "Boy, I could use a blow job."

Even Tiffany managed a smile.

I noticed that the whole family was here. The past few years had pulled us in different directions, so it was hard to find a moment where we were all together, even under these our-parents-are-dying circumstances. And when we were together, we were always at each other's throats. This was one of those rare moments that we weren't. Everything seemed right again. Sure, the situation was different. We weren't all together on a family vacation sitting by the pool in Palm Desert applying sunscreen and reading Dan Brown novels. But Dad was back at the head of the table—in the heart of the house, his little bald wife by his side, his children resting their hands on his shoulder. We all took in the moment. I knew my dad wanted to stand up and give a Lou Gehrig–esque speech.

"We have been through a lot over the years. We have recently encountered an unprecedented amount of bad luck that all decided to hit at once. Shit has piled up pretty deep. But we are all still here *now* and I want you to always be there for each other, to be part of one another's lives, because when it comes down to it, family is all that you have, and all that's truly important in life. I love you all very much and am so proud that you are my family," I imagined him saying.

But there was no way he could rouse such a benediction from his weak body. Mike spoke for him now. I turned the device over to him.

"Go ahead, Dad. Say whatever you want," I said.

With all his remaining strength, he lifted one of his long, pointy fingers and hit a button.

"Boy, I could use a blow job."

CANCER COMEDIAN

My dad was a morning person. Before the Lou Gehrig's disease, he'd get up around six and go for a long run. Then he'd come home, sit outside in our gazebo looking up at the Wasatch Mountains with a cup of coffee and listen to the world wake up. He'd thumb through the *Salt Lake Tribune*, reading more than just the sports and entertainment sections, unlike the rest of us dumb-shit philistines. He'd think about what he'd done yesterday and what he had to do today. It was his alone time before his wife and kids flooded his life with activity and useless drama.

But now, my dad always had someone with him. No more alone time for Bobby Boy. His whole focus was survival. He'd wake up with a breathing mask velcroed to his narrow face. He'd ring his doorbell so whichever one of his loser sons was on Daddy Duty could sit him up and take off his mask. Then, once he caught his breath, we'd help him piss, shit, shower, and dress. It was a far cry from running through our neighborhood streets and sipping coffee alone with his thoughts and the mountain view.

On this morning, I was the loser son on Daddy Duty. Greg was still asleep, probably dreaming of feeding a naked Chris O'Donnell some lasagna. I had actually managed to get Jessica up and out the door to school, so she and Chelsea were gone. My dad was dressed and showered, his thinning hair slicked to the side in my attempt to make him appear as if everything was in order. We were going to go down to his office to get some work done, but he needed breakfast first. He sat at the end of our big kitchen table in front of a cup of coffee. Though he couldn't drink coffee anymore, he still liked the smell, so I'd pour him a cup. It meant morning to him.

"Ready to load more shit and piss into your dying body?" I asked as I approached with three cans of Promote and some Miralax to be injected into his murky feeding tube. This was his new coffee. He managed a slight smile.

I sloppily loaded the Promote into him. I'd always try to feed him as quickly as possible, because I'm an impatient person. Some of the Promote dripped on the floor. Our oblivious dogs lapped it up with their big, ass-licking golden retriever tongues. We always made small talk during these feedings, usually about the Jazz or the stock market. But he and my mom had paid a visit to their shrink, Robin, yesterday, so I figured that I'd ask him about that. I was a psychology major, so I was always really intrigued by therapy.

"How'd it go with old Robin yesterday? What'd you talk about?" I asked.

My dad cleared his throat to speak. "I just talked about how frustrated I am that I can't do all the things I enjoy doing anymore. I miss running and walking the dogs up Millcreek. I miss drinking coffee. I miss gardening. Now all I can do is sit here."

"I know. It's hard. Seems like you're losing your life piece by piece."

"And she had a couple of good suggestions. She suggested I try to spend more time with Jessica and Chelsea so they're not so freaked out," he labored.

"Yeah, probably a good idea," I said.

"So it was a good meeting," he said, trying his best to stay optimistic. Poor guy. He was frustrated, but still so calm and collected about everything.

Just then, my mom floated down the stairs. She was already in her coat. Sitting atop her bald cancer head was a cartoony moose hat with antlers. I had purchased the moose hat several years prior at a costume shop in Berkeley, and had dressed as a moose for every Halloween since. Apparently, my mom had spotted it and decided to wear it as some sort of joke.

"What are you two assholes up to?" she asked.

"I'm just feeding this asshole," I said.

"Sounds fun," she said.

It was rare to see her up and at 'em. She wasn't a morning person, and she had been rather elusive lately—sleeping all day, only getting up to take a chemo shit or to wander to the fridge for more yogurt. But today she looked perkier than I'd seen her since I'd been back home. She seemed in good spirits, almost happy and full of life. She didn't seem to have chemo brain.

She plucked a couple of yogurts out of the fridge and took a seat across from us.

"Why the fuck are you up so early?" I asked her, not acknowledging the moose hat. I like to deny people attention when they're clearly seeking it.

"I have fucking chemo again today," she said.

"Great. Well, Dad and I are going to the office," I said.

"I need you to take me," she said, spooning an especially big yogurt-load into her mouth.

"But isn't a friend driving you?"

"They canceled."

"But what about Dad?"

"Fuck your dad for a day. I have cancer. It's not all about him," she reminded me. She always got jealous when I brought up caring for my dad. She wanted us to care about her and her cancer, too.

"But . . . Dad, what do you think? Shouldn't I stay with you today?" I pleaded.

He collected himself, took a deep breath, and said, "Take your mom to chemo. I'll be okay." He was always the decisive vote in any argument, the kind voice of logic and reason in this chaotic house of shitheads.

"Get your ass ready. I've got to be there by nine thirty," my mom interjected with a sly victory smile.

I had taken my mom to chemo a few times over the years and generally wasn't a big fan of the experience. Sure, the infusion room at the Huntsman Cancer Institute had a snack cart with bags of mini Rold Gold pretzels, Sun Chips, and Cheez-Its. They also had an unlimited supply of tea and coffee. It was a dream place from a free snack and beverage perspective. The major drawback was that you were surrounded by cancer patients—a collection of the misfortunate and unlucky, all getting pumped full of chemotherapy, all battling it out and hoping for the best as their concerned loved ones held their veiny hands.

Although I was sort of used to it, I didn't really like to see my mom have chemicals blasted into her frail body. It didn't seem right. My mom was supposed to be there to love me unconditionally, to support me, to spoil me, to help me feel safe and confident enough to pursue my dreams and make the most of my life. She wasn't supposed to be saying crazy shit and running to the bathroom every few minutes.

It's never good to see your parents vulnerable, and she always looked so vulnerable at chemo.

Greg wandered in and stuffed some turkey in some pita bread. Breakfast of champions. My mom came back downstairs. She still wore the moose antlers.

"Come on, let's get the fuck out of this depressing house, Danny Boy." She grabbed a few more yogurts from the fridge and packed them into her giant purse.

"Don't die while we're gone, Dad," I joked as I poured his full cup of coffee into the sink and followed my moose mom out.

"I'll try my best," he managed to joke back.

We got in my mom's Lexus RX 350. She had purchased it upon hearing that my dad had Lou Gehrig's disease. It was like she had realized that life is a long, painful journey until death, so why not drive around in something with soft leather seats and a sunroof? "I got myself a nice car before Dad dies," she explained when she first told me about it. "It has heated seats," she bragged. It was nicer than any car we had ever had. The best part was that my mom was able to get a handicap-parking pass because of my dad's disease. Who said there aren't perks to terminal illnesses!

"You want your seat heated? This car comes with that," Mom proudly reminded me.

"Fuck yeah," I said, loving all the luxuries of my life.

She pushed a button and twisted a knob, then did the same for her seat. I could instantly feel the heat on my spoiled ass.

"So, did you notice anything new about me today?" my mom asked while adjusting the moose antlers.

I looked her over. "Let's see. What could it be? It's not that you don't have cancer anymore, because you look like you're about to die and I'm driving you to chemo. Oh, are you trying a new brand of yogurt?"

"No, same brand. Do you notice anything else?" she said, now pointing up to the hat with her beloved yogurt spoon.

"Did you do something different with your hair?"

"I don't have any hair. It's the moose hat, you smart-ass. I'm wearing your moose hat."

"I thought that thing was just a side effect from the chemo," I said.

"I found it in one of your boxes." I hadn't completely finished unpacking. Part of me thought that if I didn't entirely settle in at home

I'd get back to the good life in L.A. faster. I clearly hadn't fully accepted this situation yet.

"You sure you really want to embarrass yourself with that hat up at chemo?"

She got a little defensive. "For your information, the nurses get a real kick out of me," she said. "You might not think so, but your old mom is actually pretty funny."

We pulled up to Huntsman—a new state-of-the-art cancer treatment facility complete with gorgeous views and valet parking. "I've got to shit before my chemo," she said. "I'll meet you inside." My mom scurried out of the car to run to a bathroom.

I handed the keys over to the valet guy. He was around my age. I wondered what other people my age thought of me. I mean, here I was pulling up in a rich-bitch car on a workday, so I figure they thought I was a piece-of-shit loser still sucking off my parents' collective tit. But, on the other hand, I was accompanying my dying mom to chemotherapy, so maybe they saw me as a hero (of sorts). Or maybe they were just as confused by the whole thing as I was. "My dad also has Lou Gehrig's disease. I gave up a real job to do this, so stop judging me," I wanted to yell at the valet unprovoked.

I entered Huntsman's lobby carrying only the notepad I had brought along so I could scribble down some poignant observations about life and dick jokes while my mom got bombed by chemo. I was directed to the infusion room up on the second floor. I took the elevator. Fuck stairs. The elevator was full of nurses, doctors, and even a couple of cancer patients. "So cancer, what a piece of shit disease, am I right, you guys?" I wanted to say, but instead I just stood there looking sad like everyone else.

The doors dinged open. I walked through the waiting room—where a few tired caregivers distracted themselves by putting together puzzles—and toward the infusion room. I thought I'd see my old mom already curled up in a chair asleep, dreaming about being young and healthy again and having a husband who wasn't on the brink of death. But instead, there was a group of nurses and doctors all circled around her, laughing their asses off.

"I'm so fat I probably look like a real moose," she joked. They all roared with laughter. She had lost a lot of weight, partially because of the chemo and partially because she was only eating yogurt, but she still called herself "fat" for some reason. She wasn't actually fat. "I told

Bob that if he stays living, I'll give him a blow job in the moose hat to cheer him up," she added, sending the crowd into even bigger fits of laughter. I was disgusted, picturing my mom sucking my dad's dying dick, the antlers bobbing over his crotch like a moose trotting through a forest.

"Oh, Debi, you are just too much," giggled one of the nurses. "What a sense of humor."

I sheepishly approached. I'm always a little shy around strangers. I especially didn't like being around my mom and strangers because she loved to embarrass me. I'm a big blusher, and she got a kick out of watching my face turn red.

She spotted me and smiled.

"This is my son, Danny. He went to Berkeley but moved home to help since Bob and I are now dying, bless his little heart," she proudly said. I waved and managed a shy hello. I was thankful she had introduced me with the good items on my résumé instead of the bad. She didn't embarrass me. My face remained its normal color.

"This is the son who ate his own shit out of his diaper when he was two."

My face turned traffic-light red as everyone burst out laughing.

"Jesus, Mom, stop," I said.

But she was just getting started. "We were playing hide-and-seek, and I couldn't find him, but then I found him under his crib with his diaper opened, eating his own shit with a GIIIIIANT smile on his face. Hadn't ever seen anyone that happy." Everyone laughed harder and harder as I wished I could disappear into nothingness. The crowd was getting bigger, all centered around my mom. It was as if we were suddenly in a comedy club. I half expected a microphone to shoot up out of the floor and for waitresses to start shelling out overpriced drinks.

"Another funny shit story. Danny had some trouble with potty training, so my dad told him that he'd give him a dollar every time he shit in his little potty-training toilet. My dad even made him a little box where he could keep his money. He called it his 'kaka box,' because my parents are Basque and 'kaka' means 'shit' in Basque. And Danny, bless his little heart, would wait for a large crowd, then he would pull out his little potty-trainer, then he'd take a shit in front of everyone." The nurses were in stitches as my mom continued. "Then he'd go around with his kaka box and collect a dollar from everyone. He was making twelve dollars a shit."

My face was so red it was about to explode. "All right, let's get some chemo in you," I said, reminding her why we were there.

"Maybe one of the nurses can find you a potty-trainer and you can make some money, Danny Boy. Should've brought your kaka box," she said. All the nurses laughed.

"Sooo funny. And I just love your hat. Oh my goodness," said one of the nurses.

We finally got situated in one of the chemo chairs. The infusion room window looked out on a hill, maybe to metaphorically remind patients that their fight with cancer was an uphill battle. Parts of the building were still under construction. The windows were tinted, so occasionally a construction worker would come piss against the building, not knowing that there were dying cancer patients on the other side.

"I wonder if we'll see a pissing construction worker today," joked my mom. "I like to think it's good luck. Like seeing a leprechaun or something."

The nurses giggled as they got her comfortable. They started hooking IV things into her port. She had had a port implanted in her chest because her veins were so shot to shit from all the chemo. She was in her fifteenth year of treatment, after all. They gave her some pain pills, and she curled up in the blanket, her moose antlers still intact.

Just as it looked like she was finally cozy, I said, "You are such an asshole."

"What do you mean?" she asked, digging some yogurt out of her purse, her eyes now half closed. It looked like the chemo and pills were already fucking her up.

"All the shit stories. It's embarrassing," I said.

"Oh, please. It's not half as bad as all the horrible shit you say about me," she said. She had a point. I was always really hard on my mom. That's the thing with parents: you can act like the worst piece of shit on earth and they still have to love you. It's their punishment for bringing you into this world. I had always taken advantage of this rule with my mom. We were always extremely close and loved each other very much, so we knew we could get away with bashing each other.

"Still, Mom, I didn't come home from California so you could tell strangers that I ate a diaperful of shit," I said.

"Whatever, Danny Boy, you did it. You should embrace it," she said. "It was really impressive, actually. A little boy eating that much shit."

I shook my head. "I'm going to track down the snack cart," I said. "Does your cancer-ass want anything?"

"If they have yogurt, grab as many as you can carry," she said as she deep-throated a bite of her own yogurt.

"Do you eat anything besides yogurt anymore?"

"Well, I was hoping we could stop at Shivers on the way home. I usually get a Diet Coke from there. It's my chemo treat." Shivers is a little shit-in-a-box local fast-food restaurant that my mom loved for some reason.

"Maybe. I don't know if we'll have time. Should probably get back to Dad, since I love him more," I said.

"Fuck you and fuck your dad. We're stopping."

"Probably not," I said as I got up.

I found the snack cart with ease. If nothing else, I'm great at hunting down snacks. I grabbed three bags of pretzels and a bag of Sun Chips, because why the fuck not? I also made myself a tea. As I did, I noticed a few of the nurses eyeing me and giggling. "Sorry we're not serving diapers full of baby shit," I expected them to say.

They didn't have any yogurt.

I went outside to call Abby, hoping her sweet, angelic voice would soothe me. She was due to visit in a week or so, so I figured we could start planning her stay. I wanted to get out of the house for a little bit, as I was spending virtually all my time there. Right before my dad was diagnosed, he had purchased a condo in the resort town of Park City. So I figured we could go up there, drink wine, sit by the fire, and lounge around like a couple of in-love assholes. It would be a nice break. Abby answered after a couple of rings.

"Hey babe, what's up?" I said.

"Not much. Heading up to the lab." Part of her Ph.D. required that she work up at the Lawrence Berkeley Lab on some laser, or particle accelerator, or some crazy shit I'll never understand.

"Great, I'm up at chemo with my mom. She's acting like an asshole, so I figured I'd talk to you about your visit, because that'll make me happy," I explained.

She was quiet on her end, then finally said, "Listen, I decided I'm not going to be coming next weekend. I have Jody's birthday party to go to." Jody was one of her new classmates.

"What? Fuck Jody," I said.

"Well, it's important that I'm there for her."

"It's important you're here for me. I'm going insane out here. My life is turning into shit. I need you. I miss you," I pleaded.

"Listen, I'm almost at work. I'll call you later." She abruptly hung up. I was shocked. I didn't see that coming. Abby seemed to be acting more and more distant about all of this. I guess she had her own life up and running, but still, I just wanted to see her. To crack jokes with her. To kiss her. To listen to her patented jaw clicks as she slept. To wake up next to her instead of a pissing cat.

After attempting to put a couple of puzzle pieces together while I burned through a bag of pretzels in the waiting room, I finally came back and sat next to my mom. I pulled out the notepad to jot down some thoughts. Some of this shit was just too weird to not write down. I wrote, "Boy, Mom can sure be a loudmouthed bitch," and under-lined it twice. I was still pretty angry and embarrassed about the shit stuff. It was one thing for her to wear the antlers, but to turn me into a prop?

I looked up at the loudmouthed bitch. She was asleep, already snor-ing lightly, her now brittle body working with the chemo chemicals to fight off the cancer. She looked so fragile, so vulnerable, as if it could all end at any second—which would leave me without a mom to tease me about eating shit.

Sometimes I forgot that she went through all of this—all the chemo, all the surgeries, all the ass-pounding diarrhea—just so her kids could still have a mom. That was always her goal. "Cancer isn't going to win. You kids need a mom," she'd always say. "Plus, I don't want your dad out there fucking some other woman who you guys like more than me," she'd add.

I think it was so important to her to be there for us because her own biological mother had left her at an orphanage in Blackfoot, Idaho, to be put up for adoption. Apparently, my mom's mom already had five children and just couldn't handle any more. I guess life can get overwhelming anywhere, even in Blackfoot. The nuns at the or-phanage started calling her Debi and raised her for the first few months of her confusing, parentless life.

Eventually, some angels came along in the form of my grandpar-ents, Rosie and Joe Mendiola (pronounced Men-dee-ol-a)—a couple of bighearted Basques from Twin Falls. Grandpa Joe ran a gas station, a Texaco, on the edge of town, and Grandma Rosie worked a variety of different jobs to help with the bills. They were simple blue-collar Catholic people who loved drinking beers and smoking cigarettes with their extensive Basque family, who all lived in Twin Falls or in neighboring towns. My grandma Rosie's ovaries were broken, so they couldn't have kids. They'd spent a few years crying about it before deciding that they should just adopt. After an expansive search, they finally came across the orphanage in Blackfoot. They and my mom were a perfect match: they wanted a child and she needed parents. They wanted to name her Francesca and call her "Frankie" for short, but since the nuns were already calling her Debi, they decided to stick with that name.

My grandparents later tried to adopt another kid, but couldn't. It was always just them and Little Debi, Little Debi Mendiola.

My mom didn't love being an only child, but she fought off the loneliness by making her best friend, Julie, and her next-door neighbor, Brook, her surrogate siblings. When she wasn't hanging with them, she'd read books and write. Being an only child at least helps build your imagination.

Because she was abandoned by her biological mother and an only child, she always felt like an underdog. Consequently, my mom developed a real me-versus-the-world attitude. "Little Debi versus the world," I'd always say to her when she was in a fight with someone. She thought everyone and everything was out to get her. She turned into a very feisty and opinionated person who never fully trusted anyone. When she was diagnosed with cancer in 1992, she used that "Little Debi versus the world" attitude to fight it, pledging that cancer would never beat her or prevent her from being our loving and supportive mother.

When she was first diagnosed, I was such a sympathetic son. Anytime she got home from chemo, I'd go into our yard and pluck a rose off a thorny bush, not knowing how to show that I loved and supported her, that I had her back during this new fight.

I'm a very superstitious person. During all Jazz games I would rub an old rabbit's foot and wear a pair of purple Jazz wristbands. I wouldn't let anyone else so much as touch them. One year when my mom was starting chemo back up, I gave her the rabbit's foot and wristbands to hold as good luck charms.

"You need these more than I do," I told her.

She started to cry, knowing that I was giving her some of my most treasured possessions.

"It's brought the Jazz lots of luck," I said.

She pulled me in for a hug and pressed her wet-from-crying face against mine. "This means so much to me. I'll bring it to every chemo, Danny Boy."

"Just, please keep on fighting, Mama Bear," I said, also crying now.

"I will. I promise," she said, her body shaking from the sobs.

I'd sit by her bedside, always telling her to keep on fighting, to push through so I could keep having a mom.

And she did.

Being a mom is hard work. Being a mom with cancer is even harder work—the hardest work. All of her limited energy went into being our mom, and she was wonderful. My dad did a lot of stuff, but she'd still cook dinner for us every night and make sure we had a nice, big steak at least once a week. She'd spoil us on birthdays and Christmases, turning what should've been minor happenings into grand events. "This might be my last Christmas, so we've got to have a big one," she'd say as she unloaded presents under the tree. "We love you, Mom. Don't die," we'd say. She was there for every special moment of our lives, right by our sides, encouraging us no matter what. Fuck, I remember her coming to all my basketball games throughout the years, even when she was going through treatment. She'd sit at the top of the bleachers with a turban atop her head and a surgical mask on her face, away from all the other parents because her white blood count was so low. "Way to go, Danny Boy," she'd yell through her mask as loud as her little cancer lungs could manage.

As the years clicked by, she was still standing. But my siblings and I became desensitized to how amazing it was that she continued to fight. She had been telling us that it could be her last Christmas/her last birthday/her last Mother's Day for several years now. It started to feel like a boy-who-cried-wolf situation. It seemed that she was never going to die. Our mom had cancer. So the fuck what?

"I have cancer, you know," she'd sometimes remind me.

"Yeah, yeah, yeah. I'm sick of the cancer spiel, Little Debi," I'd say back.

But the point remained. She did still have cancer. She was still our mom. She had managed to stay alive. And now the poor thing was losing her husband to Lou Gehrig's disease, facing a future where she'd have to continue to battle the disease/the world alone, as if she were an orphan again. She was in panic mode, not only about what

life was like now, but also about what life was going to look like for
her in a year or so. If she survived the cancer, she was going to potentially be faced with a whole new set of challenges. It was really going
to be Little Debi versus the world. She was going to have to learn how to
operate in a world without my dad at her side. My siblings and I couldn't
stay around here forever. She would have to learn how to run the house.
Pay the bills. File the taxes. Take care of the dogs. She had gone
through hell, was going through hell, and had even more hell to go
through.

And here I was, calling her an asshole, not giving her the support
or love she needed, that she had earned and deserved. I needed to be
more grateful.

I looked at the poor thing nestled into all the blankets. She looked
worn down by life, her face like the fingertip of a kid who'd been in
the swimming pool too long, her eyebrows like they'd been rubbed
away by a giant eraser, her head all marked up like a damaged pump-
kin from having various skin cancer spots removed.

I looked back down at my "loudmouthed bitch" comment.

Jesus, Dan, have a little sympathy, I thought.

I crossed out the comment, then ripped the page out, tore it to
pieces, and tossed it in the garbage atop latex gloves, bandages, and
syringes. My mom wasn't a loudmouthed bitch. She was a chemo war-
rior, a hero. If I ever got cancer I'd probably be like, Welp, guess I'm
going to die, then ungracefully die in the most shameful and embarrassing bout with cancer ever recorded.

But not her. She cared about being our mom way too much to give
up. So what if she made fun of me to the nurses. So what if she brought
up that I used to shit in front of people for money. She had few joys
left in her life. I couldn't take this one away from her. She had paid
her dues. She liked to make people laugh. So what if it was at my
expense.

My mom adjusted in her chair, causing the moose antlers to fall to
the floor. I picked them back up, dusted them off, and placed them
back on her cue ball head.

As I did, she woke up and half opened her eyes. "Hey, Danny Boy,
you're still here, sweetheart?" she managed to say, her voice now
groggy, as if she'd been asleep for a decade, as if her body were too
weak to focus on anything but the fight with cancer.

"Sorry I woke you. Just putting your antlers back on," I said.

She managed a smile. "Guess what I still have?"

She held up my old rabbit's foot I had given her years ago. "I bring it to every chemo. You were such a little sweetheart for giving it to me. And it's working, because the old bag is still kicking."

I smiled back at her, a little teary eyed. "I know chemo sucks ass, but you'll fight through this round," I said.

"Yeah, I can't leave you kids without a mom," she said.

A nurse just starting her shift came over to check on all the tubing and machines and add a new pouch of chemo drugs. "I just love your moose hat," she said.

My mom smiled as big as she could manage. "Thanks. Oh, this is my son, Danny."

"Nice to meet you," I said, now a little friendlier than before.

"He went to Berkeley . . . but he's not as smart as he looks. One time I caught him eating his own shit out of his diaper," the Cancer Comedian said.

The nurse and I laughed as I nodded to confirm the story, my face red again. "You are too funny. My goodness, Debi. What would we do up here without you?"

"And he used to shit for money," my mom said as she smiled and closed her eyes to go back into her chemo coma. "He made twelve dollars once."

The nurse looked at me as if I was insane. I just shrugged.

"She's a real fighter. You should be proud of her," the nurse said.

"I am."

I stopped at Shivers on the way home and got her the biggest Diet Coke they sell.

A VISIT TO THE QUEEN B

My dad and I were spending a lot of time around his office finalizing some things before the ALS tsunami completely swept through. He was still in the process of selling his newspaper business. He had a buyer, so they were just working through the last details. Over the years, his newspaper business not only earned him a nice living, but also kept him occupied and gave him an excuse to get out of the house and away from his wife and his little asshole children. His work had also been his dream. His father had been in the newspaper business. He was in the newspaper business. Plus, he was good at it. It was sad to see it go. If only he were as good at not getting Lou Gehrig's disease as he was at his job, we wouldn't have been in this damn mess.

Although we now had the communication device, my dad didn't like using it. It was more for down the road, so he could talk like Stephen Hawking when he started to look like him. Our family could understand him, but strangers couldn't. A lot of "What?"s and silences greeted anything he said. So, at the office I ended up acting as a translator while he talked over the phone to the lawyers and businessmen about selling the papers.

"We received the noncompete forms and will sign them," my dad would say.

"What?" the lawyers and businessmen on the other end of the phone would say.

"We received the noncompete forms and will sign them," I would say.

"Who's that?" the lawyers and businessmen would ask.

"That's my son Dan. He's helping me around the office because I can't speak or move very well," my dad would then labor.

"What?"

"I'm Bob's son Dan. I'm just helping him out around the office because of the Lou Gehrig's disease and whatnot. I'm a hero of sorts," I'd say.

"Oh, hi, Dan," they'd reply. "So did you guys receive the noncompete?"

"Yes, we received your ridiculous noncompete forms, though I'm not too sure you have much to worry about, given that my dad has FUCKING LOU GEHRIG'S DISEASE. If he somehow does live long enough to compete against you, and wins, your business should probably not exist," I wanted to say.

"Yes, we got them! We'll sign them and mail them back!" I actually said.

After a long day of getting a lot of really, really big business deals situated thanks to my amazing, herolike help, we received a call from my aunt Sarah. She informed us that my grandma Barbie wasn't doing so hot, and that the doctors were expecting her to last just a couple more weeks.

"Well, add another piece of shit to this feces burger we're munching on, am I right?" I said to my dad after we hung up with Sarah.

He had few working neck muscles, so his head always hung, but even if he hadn't had Lou Gehrig's disease, I'm pretty sure his head still would have drooped. Death was hitting him on all fronts: the poor guy was losing his mother while he was losing himself.

"I guess we're both losing parents. We finally have something in common besides our love for the Jazz." He looked like he was about to cry. I shouldn't have said that. I'm a fucking idiot. Maybe I should learn how to keep my fat mouth shut. He took a deep breath in, probably wishing he had the ability to raise his hand and smack me upside the head, but instead said, "Let's get home. I've got to shit."

We'd known my grandma's death was coming. She was eighty-four. She had casually smoked and drunk most of her life. She had been in decline for years, unable to walk on her own. In fact, she wanted to die. She, like my grandpa Wendell—who shot himself in the head with a sawed-off shotgun when his health started to deteriorate in 1994—thought that there was a certain quality of life that needed to be maintained. If that quality of life dropped below a certain level, then death was the best option.

It was a trait that most members of my dad's family seemed to share: the desire to have life end before it got too horrible. It was the opposite of how my mom thought, the opposite of how my siblings and I were trained to think. I remember when we were at a wedding on Lummi Island—a tranquil spot off the coast of middle-of-nowhere northern Washington—my dad, then healthy, and I had talked about his mother's health. While we stood watching the clear, nearly motionless water slowly roll onto the rocky shore, he mentioned that there were quality of life issues related to Grandma Barbie, and that she had the right to determine when she'd had enough. To him, death shouldn't be a long and painful event. It should be handled with grace and poise. He called it "dying with dignity."

"Yeah, but hopefully she doesn't blow her brains out like Grandpa Wendell, just from a cleanup perspective," I'd wanted to say.

"God, it's really beautiful up here, isn't it?" I really said, changing the subject from death to not death. I didn't like talking about morbid things back then.

My dad looked around and took a breath of fresh air. "Yeah, it truly is." He would be diagnosed with Lou Gehrig's disease two months later and never return to Lummi Island. It was his last look at the place. Too bad he had to spend part of it contemplating the end of his mother's life instead of taking it all in.

Since Lummi, my grandma had been in waiting mode, sitting in her fancy house along Pocatello, Idaho's Juniper Hills Country Club Golf Course, hoping that something would go drastically wrong with her ailing body so she could elect to not treat it. Nothing life threatening was happening, though. Sure, her knees were ruined, and I think she had something wrong with her hip, and I think she also had something wrong with her bladder, or some other body part that I didn't want to think about, her being my grandmother and all. It seemed as though she had been waiting for a couple of years now.

Finally, finally, finally—praise the good lord—her prayers were answered. Her kidneys started shutting down.

"Well, shit, Dad. What awful timing, right?" I said while he pumped out a ten-pound grizzly bear shit back at home. He nodded his head as much as he could.

"What do you want to do? You want to run up there and visit her? I'm sure we could find some sort of AC power adapter to run your

BiPAP, and I drive real fast. Still got some L.A. in me," I said. He nodded his head as much as he could.

"ROAD TRIP!" I yelled as I extended my hand for a high five, forgetting about his disability.

We planned on leaving for Grandma Barbie's house the next day.
I was able to round up a power adaptor for the BiPAP at Radio
Shack. I didn't even know Radio Shacks still existed, but they did,
and man, are they a great place to pick up supplies for a road trip
with the terminally ill. Maybe that should be their new angle. I also
loaded the car with diapers, baby wipes, a spare pair of pants, the
urinal, cans of Promote to keep my dad alive, and pretzels, sunflower
seeds, and beef jerky to keep me alive. I also brought my dad's communication device, not so he could use it, but so I could showcase all
the jokes I had loaded into it to my dad's family.

Greg decided to accompany us on this journey. It would be nice
to have him aboard. My mom had never gotten along with my dad's
family, and it had been even worse since she shunned them at the
Boston Marathon. In particular, she hated my grandma, going as far
as referring to her as "The Queen B," the B standing for Bitch. So
there was no way she was coming. And the little girls had school. Tiffany agreed to keep an eye on the ladies of the Marshall clan while
the men were in Pocatello.

Greg and I helped my dad get his near-limp body into the car, set
him up on the BiPAP, turned on the car, and started the two-and-
a-half-hour drive to Pocatello from Salt Lake. Greg hummed Disney songs. I slammed sunflower seeds and beef jerky into my fat
mouth. We were just a pack of dudes on a road trip, rolling alongside the beautiful Wasatch Mountains up Interstate 15 as if we were
invincible.

Though my mom didn't get along with my dad's family, I enjoyed
hanging with my aunts, uncles, and cousins. Most of them were up there
playing golf, drinking, and hanging with the Queen B while she slowly
died. I always wished my mom and my dad's family could find a way to
get along. Because of the hatred, we unfortunately weren't very close.
I knew the circumstances of this visit were shitty—the death of my
last living grandparent and all—but there is no better way to forgive
and forget the past than through birth or death. It reminds us that
most of our problems are self-made and that the only real problems

are centered around trying to stay alive for as long as possible. So, part of me thought that maybe between my grandma dying and my dad dying, we'd find a way to patch things up and all get along like a big, happy, loving family.

We rolled into Pocatello with ease. It was a simple drive. I think my dad only needed to piss once, which wasn't a big deal since we had the urinal with us. The big thing was that he didn't shit. What a blessing!

Though I was looking forward to seeing my grandma, aunts, and uncles, I could tell my dad was sad. I didn't know if it was because he was upset about seeing his mom for the last time or if he was worried about showing his family exactly how much damage his disease had already done to his body. Though there was nothing he could do about it, he felt guilty for the way the disease made other people feel, especially his family. It was an interruption to their life-is-a-vacation mentality. They wanted nothing to do with it.

We arrived at Grandma Barbie's and sat in the car looking at the house. It was a single-level residence to make getting around simpler. Apparently, stairs suck for old people. When we're born, life is really simple. It's all about keeping the stress to a minimum. As we grow into adulthood, we just complicate our lives with junk: kids, mortgages, marriages, cars, insurance, jobs, drugs, stairs. As we start heading for death, it's all about making things simple again. No more stairs. Big, safe, easy-to-drive cars. We only engage in a few simple, mindless activities that relax the brain. No jobs. No sex. No problems.

"You ready for this?" I asked my dad.

My dad took the deepest breath he could muster and said, "Yeah. Let's do it."

Greg and I got out first. Greg was in charge of carrying things like the BiPAP machine and the urinal. I was in charge of moving the communication device and the old sack of dying bones that was our father.

"Why'd you bring that stupid thing?" Greg asked about the communication device.

"I don't know. Jokes. Plus, I think they'd like to know that Dad will still be able to communicate with them even after shit gets really bad," I said.

I got him out of the car and we started the long walk into the house.

Every walk is long when you have Lou Gehrig's disease, but this one seemed especially lengthy. I rang the doorbell.

"Just open the door," my dad said.

"Oh yeah, I forgot you could do that with family," I said. We opened the door and went in.

All my aunts and uncles carry that drinker's weight and have faces that seem to be permanently stained red. Sure, we were walking into my grandma's living room, but we could've very well been walking into a frat party where everyone was thirty years older than they should be. Right in the middle of it all was Grandma Barbie, the Queen B.

She looked pretty good. She had a few nurses caring for her, so she was dressed and put together. She even wore makeup, which almost made me cry. Here she was about to die, but she couldn't let go of that pressure to always look her best. And she did look her best. In fact, she looked beautiful. My grandma had a lot of good and love in her—even if my mom couldn't see it. She had, for example, paid for all of her grandkids' educations, which were not cheap.

"Hello, everyone," we said, forcing smiles.

They all lifted their drinks to say hi. I set my dad up right next to my grandma so they could talk and hold each other's hands. My dad had always been my grandma's favorite, so they shared that warmth and togetherness that only a favorite son and a mother could.

"You look really good, Mom," my dad said.

"So do you," my grandma lied. My dad looked way worse than her. We weren't taking as good of care of him as my grandma's nurses were taking of her. She rubbed her old hand over the top of my dad's bony hand. His fingers were starting to sort of coil up. She managed to uncoil her boy's fingers and run her motherly hands up and down them, probably something she used to do when my dad was a child.

"You're very brave and a very strong woman," my dad said.

"No, you're the brave one, Bobby," she said. She always called him Bobby. That was his childhood name.

"This all sucks, doesn't it?" my dad said.

"Yes, yes it does, but let's have a drink," my grandma said, fighting back the tears. My grandma's boyfriend, Walter, made my grandma a strong gin and tonic. Her favorite. She grabbed it with her liver-spotted hands and took down a gulp big enough to kill her. She probably shouldn't have been drinking, what with the kidney, but oh well. Fuck it. My dad didn't have a drink. He couldn't.

Everyone else refilled their glasses. I let my dad and grandma chat it up and share their last moments together while I talked to some of my aunts and uncles. They said they were grateful that Greg and I had taken some time off from our lives to help with my dad. In some ways, it meant that they didn't have to. My aunts Sarah and Ellen, in particular, were very sweet about it, thanking us repeatedly and telling us what good sons we were. That's always nice to hear.

My dad needed to go on the BiPAP for a little bit, so I laid him down for a nap. Then Greg and I went and sat down next to our grandmother.

"Well, Grandma, sorry you're dying and all. It's hard to see," I said.

"Me, too," she said, with a little hint of bullshit in her voice. She wanted to die, after all. All these extra good-byes were just extra pain for her.

"Thanks for paying for my college. It led to a pretty good job out of school. Though I had to leave it because of Bobby Boy's Lou Gehrig's shenanigans . . ." I said.

"I'm glad you got a good education," she said. She took a big sip of her gin and tonic and looked me over. "We never really got to know each other, did we?"

"Yeah, if only my mom and you weren't in a bitch fight my whole life," I wanted to say.

"No, we didn't, really," I really said. "It's too bad. I think we could've been pals."

"Well, maybe there's still some time," she said. But we both knew there wasn't. We'd never have a relationship. "Let's have another drink," she said, draining everything in her glass but the ice. She motioned to Walter to get her another round. Everyone else refilled, too. I guess dying with dignity involves a lot of drinking.

I didn't really know what to do once the conversations ran out. I couldn't get drunk because I had to drive home. Driving drunk in the dark would most certainly elevate our chances of dying. I wanted us to live. I wanted to see how all of this played out. I was curious. So, instead of drinking, I just wandered around my grandma's house. Greg was chatting with my aunts, so I started to explore. It wasn't their family home, so it didn't quite have the history I was hoping for.

I couldn't go sit in my dad's childhood room and smell his old clothes, or anything creepy like that. But my grandma had a lot of photos up. I looked at a few. Since we were the outcasts of the family, there weren't many of us; just a few of me in my old basketball uniform, or Greg dressed as the Scarecrow from *The Wizard of Oz*, or Chelsea in her dance leotards, or Jessica with her lacrosse stick, or Tiffany holding her snowboard.

Then I wandered into my grandma's room. On the wall closest to her bed—presumably the one she looked at the most—were her most prized pictures. There was one with her mom and sisters. One of my grandpa Wendell and her in Sun City, where they had a second home. The rest were of my dad and his siblings. I was drawn to the pictures of my dad. I looked at one of him as a high schooler. He had gigantic ears, a chipped front tooth, and was going through a shaggy-hair phase. He looked like the type of guy you'd want to be your friend: not a jock, but not a complete nerd. Just a good guy. Strange to think that this good guy was destined to get Lou Gehrig's disease later in life. I sort of wanted to take out a stamp and stamp TERMINALLY ILL across my dad's boyish face. I wondered if they sold stamps like that.

There was another photo of my grandma and my dad hanging out at my grandma's house on Camano Island in northern Washington. It was the house where my grandma had grown up, but it had turned into a vacation home later in life. My dad must have been in his teens then, and my grandma in her forties. Every summer, my grandma would take her kids up there. They'd read, they'd swim, they'd lie out in the sun, they'd pick blackberries. My dad and his brother Jack would stay up late talking on the front porch, where they also slept. My dad had his first kiss along Camano's rocky shores with one of the neighbor girls he had a crush on. It was a special place for him.

I found a picture of my parents' wedding. It was back when they weren't terminally ill. They looked like a couple ready to take on the world. There's nothing more beautiful than youth—the feeling that anything is possible, that your life is an exciting mystery full of hope. Here these two were, having just teamed up, a look of invincibility in their eyes.

I found another picture of my grandma and dad, now much older, sitting with Chelsea on the back porch of the Camano house. My dad was now a man—a proud father—trying to pass along his love for his favorite childhood place to his daughter. He had always been our compass, directing us through life.

Another picture featured my dad as he crossed the finish line of the Salt Lake Marathon, his arms triumphantly raised—a healthy and capable athlete, but also a man who had mastered his hobby.

All the pictures were like a quick tour of my dad's journey through childhood, into adulthood, into parenthood, and then into midlife. I knew there was never going to be a picture of him in old age. His life was going to be cut short. There would never be a photo of him holding a grandchild, or one of him buying a home in a retirement community. But it helped to know that he had lived a very full life, achieving all these milestones with a smile on his face. It made the Lou Gehrig's disease seem slightly less tragic.

Seeing all the pictures of the good times my dad had had and knowing there would be no pictures of good times ahead made me depressed. Living in the past makes you sad; looking to the future makes you happy. It always seemed to me that depressed people are depressed because they can't move on from the past. Happy people are happy because they're excited about something in the future. I needed to stop this trip down memory lane, live in the now, have some fucking fun. So I walked out of my grandma's bedroom and straight to the communication device. I decided that I'd show everyone the ECO-14 to lighten the mood. After everyone refilled their glasses, I gathered them around and hit a few of the buttons.

"If you loved me, you would put three shots of gin into my feeding tube," the ECO said. Everyone laughed and raised their drinks. Heavy drinkers love jokes about drinking alcohol. Makes them feel like it's okay to drink so much.

"Please give me five dollars. I have Lou Gehrig's disease and you can still do all the things you love," the ECO joked. Everyone laughed again. It was as though the communication device was doing stand-up comedy—and killing. Maybe I should take this thing to some open mics. Even my grandma was chuckling. Maybe the ECO's jokes would help my grandma and me quickly become the best friends in the world, and make up for all the lost moments we had missed out on over the years.

Just then, my uncle Jack noticed the icon with the penis on it. "What's that one do?" asked my uncle.

"Oh, don't worry about that one," I said as I grabbed for the device. But it was too late. My uncle hit it.

"Boy, I could use a blow job," said the ECO.

Everyone was stunned to silence. They all lifted their drinks for a big sip. "Oh, my," my disappointed, dying grandma said. Guess blow job jokes aren't what your rich grandma wants to hear on her death-bed. Guess I wasn't going to turn around our relationship. Oh, well. You can't be close with everyone you meet in this life. Guess you should just appreciate and cherish the people you are close with. I missed my mom and my sisters. At least they thought this was funny. I hit the blow job button again. "Boy, I could use a blow job." Nothing.

My dad woke from his nap and I sat him down next to his mom again. They didn't say much. It was getting late and we still had to get back home, as I'd promised my mom that we'd have our dad back alive by bedtime. I gave my dad that we-better-get-going look. He got teary eyed.

"Well, Mom, I've got to go, but keep on fighting," he said. "Maybe I'll see you again."

"You keep on fighting, too, Bobby. I love you very, very, very much," she said.

"I'm glad you were my mom," he said.

"I'm glad you were my son," she said.

They both cried and held hands for a couple more minutes, taking in their last moments together, wishing they were both young and healthy again, sitting on the porch at their house on Camano Island back when life had seemed endless. Everyone else cried, too. No mother wants to see her son die. Shit, maybe that's why she wanted to die so bad. Maybe she couldn't bear the thought of watching her little Bobby go before her.

After all the tears were dried, they gave their last smiles to each other. I helped my dad up. We walked to the car with the ECO-14 tucked beneath my arm.

"Maybe I'll see her again," he said, looking back at the house and tearing up.

"Yeah, well, maybe. Maybe not. Miracles can happen, even if they've never happened to us," I said.

Greg and I put my dad in the car. I popped some sunflower seeds into my mouth and took one last look at my grandma's house. "You know what would be a true miracle? If you didn't shit your pants on the drive home."

"Let's not ask for too much," he said, smiling at last.

My grandma passed away one week later.

THE AMBULANCE, BRO

It started as a typical Friday in our household. I had been drinking more lately and having no sex, so I woke up hungover with a boner. Everything smelled of cat piss. My dad still had Lou Gehrig's disease. My mom still had cancer and was always sleeping—waking only to down yogurts and ask silly questions like "Do you want dinner?" at eleven in the morning. My sisters were MIA. Greg was planning on either running on the treadmill or riding the stationary bike between shifts of Daddy Duty. The usual shit.

My dad was supposed to have a tracheotomy and go on a respirator a few days earlier, but we canceled the surgery because my grandma's funeral had been the weekend before. My dad just wasn't feeling up to it, so we pushed it back one week. It had been a big fight. My mom insisted that my dad get the surgery as soon as possible and seemed convinced that he was going to die if he didn't. But he didn't want to do it yet. It was a big decision. Being on the respirator meant that he'd be hooked to a breathing machine for the rest of his life. It meant that he'd probably lose his voice. It meant that he would basically be immobile. It also meant that he'd need twenty-four-hour, around-the-clock care. He thought he could hold off a little longer.

We had all just returned from the funeral, where my siblings and I all cried a lot—not necessarily because we'd lost our grandma, but because of the whole shitty situation. We'd take any chance we got to cry these days. Greg cried for an hour straight—one of those really gross cries where you have snot and tears all over your face. It got so bad that an uncle told him to get his shit together. I said, "Wow, Greg, I didn't know you loved Grandma Barbie so much."

"I didn't," he said. "I'm crying for Dad. Look at the poor bastard." I looked at the poor bastard staring at a photo of himself and his mom when he was a teenager, when times were happier, when life was bright. Our dad was too skinny for his suit. It looked like he was a young kid playing dress-up. He was really wearing down. He didn't stand a chance against this fucking disease. Poor guy.

My mom had a slight smirk on her face throughout the funeral, proud of herself for outliving the Queen B. Since she was supposed to die years ago from the cancer, anytime she lasted longer than someone she didn't like, she saw it as a giant victory.

With the canceled surgery, the day was shaping up to be chill and relaxing compared to what it could have been had the trach operation gone down. The weekend was approaching—the time when young adults celebrate their youth by consuming alcohol and fantasizing about connecting genitals with strangers. I wanted to focus primarily on the "consuming of alcohol" part, since I still had a girlfriend I loved, even though she wouldn't visit me out in Salt Lake. I understood why she didn't want to come. Shit was depressing. I didn't want to be here either. Why should I subject anyone else to this?

My social life since moving home had been basically nonexistent. I was spending all my time taking care of my family's bullshit. I figured it was why I was home—that I hadn't come back to Utah to fuck around and party with pals, like all the times before. But I was beginning to realize that I needed the occasional break to protect my sanity.

I'd started watching football and drinking beers with my friends Henry, Aria, Mike, Tigg, and Bob. I'd also been hanging out with my party animal friend Dominic. Dom has a dead dad, so we loved getting drunk and talking about how unfair life could be. I found I could form an instant bond with anyone who had lost a parent. We were suddenly in a weird, fucked-up club. Dom and I called it the Dead Dad Club, though I wasn't officially a member since mine was still hanging on. I actually liked telling old friends why I was home. In high school, I had a reputation for being an asshole—for a stretch my nickname was Dickhead Dan. I wasn't a full-on bully, but I was prone to saying really blunt and offensive things. Now that I was back taking care of my dying parents, people started to treat me like I was a tragic figure with a heart of gold, instead of a dickhead. I loved feeling like a good person for once. Maybe I was losing my dad, but I was gaining a heart.

Everything was running as smoothly as it could, so it was looking like I could sneak away from home for a little bit. I called Dom. Plans were made. We would be going out on the town. Alcohol would be consumed. Fun times would be had.

I laid my dad down for an afternoon nap next to my mom, who had fallen asleep with a yogurt in one hand and a spoon in the other. I showered and found a nice shirt to wear—one that gave my arms the freedom to easily lift drinks to my mouth. I sprayed myself with cologne, trying to hide the smell of dying parents and cat piss. I was all ready for a great night. I'd start with a bit of wine and finish with a flurry of gin and tonics and maybe a few late-night beers out on the gazebo. Perfect.

As I was about to pour myself a glass of wine, my dad rang his bell. I ran upstairs, pulled him up from his nap, and removed his BiPAP mask.

"I can't breathe," gasped my dad.

"Okay, well, I'm going to have a glass of wine. Ring if you need anything else," I joked. Him struggling to breathe wasn't out of the ordinary, so I figured everything was normal.

"DJ, please," he managed. I took a closer look at him. He was for real. He didn't look good at all. He was white as a Mormon. He was struggling. At a recent doctor's appointment, we were told that his lung capacity was down to 18 percent, meaning he needed to take five breaths of air to get a normal breath. At this point, the five-breaths-for-every-one was more like seven. He looked like he was about to die. I stopped dicking around and got serious.

"Shit, do you need to go to the hospital?" I asked.

He didn't answer. He was too focused on breathing. I rushed over to my mom and tried to jostle the yogurt in her hand loose—a process that wakes her up 98 percent of the time. She jumped from the bed with energy I hadn't seen out of her in years.

"Don't touch my fucking yogurt," she said, her spoon held like a pistol. She looked more like John Wayne than a cancer patient.

"Dad isn't breathing well. What should we do?" I asked the cancer patient. She walked over to my dad.

"Bob, are you okay?" she asked. No answer. He could only focus on his breathing, with a look of absolute fear in his eyes.

"Fucking answer me. Just because you have Lou Gehrig's disease doesn't mean you can act like an asshole," she said.

"No, not okay," he managed, the rate of the breathing intensifying.

"Mom, call Dr. Bromberg and figure out what we should do," I said.

I hooked my dad back onto the BiPAP, sure that if we didn't do something immediately, he would die.

My mom spoke. "I fucking told you assholes that we should have done the surgery on Tuesday, but no one takes the cancer patient seriously." She closed her eyes. "I fucking told you."

"Mom, call Bromberg. Dad can't breathe. Jesus Christ," I yelled back.

She opened her eyes, picked up the phone, and slowly dialed the number. I heard her hang up the phone a couple of times, probably because she misdialed or something. She finally held the receiver to her ear.

"Hi, we're trying to get hold of Dr. Bromberg. This is Bob," said my mom. There was a pause as the receptionist said something. My mom closed her eyes. It looked like she was about to fall asleep. It didn't look like she was in the middle of an emergency. "No, this is Debi, his wife. Did I say it was Bob?" my mom laughed. There was another pause as the receptionist said something. "Okay, so he's in Africa? What part?"

This was getting nowhere, so I snatched the phone away from my mom. "Mom, give me the phone. What part of Africa? Are you fucking kidding me? Like that matters."

"Hello this is Robert's son, Daniel. My father is having a lot of trouble breathing and may need to go in for an emergency tracheotomy. What should we do?" I asked.

"Well, just call 911 and they'll take him up to the hospital," she said.

"Okay. That makes sense . . . Is Dr. Bromberg really in Africa or was that my mom's chemo talking?" I asked.

"He's really in Africa," she said.

"Oh, what part?" I asked.

Of course! Why hadn't we just called 911? Instead we were sitting there like a couple of idiots with yogurt spoons up our asses. I called 911. I was amazed how calm the operator was. So smooth. So in control. So nonchalant. Probably fairly sexy. Who knows. I tried to match her calmness, but couldn't. I was a frantic mess. She managed to get my address out of me, and said she'd send over the paramedics right away.

Right after hanging up the phone, I heard the sirens. They were for real. They didn't mess around. I bet they didn't make a joke about drinking wine. They understood the magnitude of the situation.

Greg and Chelsea were the only other people home. Tiffany was still at work and Jessica was out with friends. Greg and Chelsea came upstairs. They weren't as frantic as I was. Chelsea was carrying her math book, a finger holding her place. She had been doing homework like a good nerd, even though it was a Friday.

"Is everything okay?" Greg asked casually.

"Dad can't breathe anymore," I explained. "He might die."

"Oh no," said Greg as he went over and placed a hand on our dad's shoulder.

"Could someone help me with math homework later?" Chelsea asked.

"Your fucking dad is fucking dying, you little fucking idiot," I yelled at Chelsea, reactivating the Dickhead Dan in me. She giggled and left to go attempt her math homework by herself.

"I told you guys we shouldn't wait. You all think I'm crazy, but I'm the smartest one here," said my mom through a mouthful of yogurt.

"Now is not the time to act crazy, Mom," said Greg.

A fire truck, an ambulance, and a strange truck emblazoned with the words UTAH UNIFIED FIRE DEPARTMENT showed up. All of our bored Mormon neighbors started to collect outside our house, trying to figure out what was going on. One small boy, probably eight or nine, kept casually riding by on his Razor scooter like he was just enjoying the sunlight instead of waiting to see a corpse exit the front door. Fucking Mormons. So bored all the time.

Four paramedics came up into my dad and mom's room. They began asking me a series of questions, from simple to complex. Greg and my mom stood off to the side.

"What's his name?" one asked.

"Bob Marshall. Middle name Wendell, after his father, who shot himself in the head with a sawed-off shotgun when I was in the fifth grade. That was also on a Friday and also messed up my weekend plans," I wanted to say.

"Bob Marshall," I really said. "Oh God, I hope he doesn't die."

"How old is he?" one asked.

"Only fifty-four. Can you believe that? He should be out enjoying life, drinking wine in France and compiling a reading list for when he retires. But instead, he's a prisoner in his own body, not able to do the things he loves. Skiing. Running. Visiting friends. Holding conversations without people having to say 'What?' every two seconds. Lou Gehrig's disease can go fuck itself," I wanted to say.

"Fifty-four, I think," I really said.

"Does he have heart problems?" one asked.

"Nope, he's really lucky in that area. He's actually a really healthy man—minus the Lou Gehrig's, which has crippled him and blessed him with the inability to push that crucial element we so casually refer to as 'oxygen' in and out of his body," I wanted to say.

"No," I really said.

They were good, very professional. One of them focused on taking my dad's vitals (oxygen level, blood pressure, pulse, other shit I don't know about). One guy focused on asking me the questions. One guy talked on his walkie-talkie. But one guy roamed around the room looking at photos, not really doing anything, saying things like "Nice house." He was no help. I bet the others hated working with him. He kept asking them questions, but not helping out himself. He also used the word "bro" a lot, as if he were sitting around a bong waiting for an awesome, meat-covered pizza to arrive. He would say things like "Did you take his pulse, bro?" or "Did you activate his oxygen, bro?" or "Should we run him up to the University of Utah, or would St. Mark's be the better choice, bro?" or while looking at a picture of us in Hawaii, "Where was this picture taken, bro? Looks like Hawaii."

My mom sat there with her yogurt, shaking her head. "I told you fuckers he needed it on Tuesday. And now he's going to die."

"Shut the fuck up, Mom," I told her in the politest voice I could manage.

"You're the absolute worst person to have around in an emergency," said Greg.

Because my dad's vitals were so low, they decided that running him up to the hospital was the only thing that could keep him alive, bro. He'd stay up there until they could perform the life-altering trach surgery on him, bro. Assuming, of course, he made it until then and didn't die, bro.

Construction was starting to settle down, but our elevator was still being built. We needed to take the stairs. "Grab the transfer chair, bro. We're going to have to carry him out of here," said the dipshit paramedic.

They got the transfer chair and gathered around my dad.

"One. Two. Three. Bro." He was lifted.

I was in a state of absolute panic, but it was sort of relaxing watching other people care for my dad for a change. It had been a rough couple of months.

The paramedics carried my dad out with ease and kept asking if he needed to be intubated. Intubation is the process of jamming a breathing tube down a patient's throat and into his or her lungs, which would be incredibly painful, unless you were some sort of deep-throat champion, which I assumed my dad wasn't.

"You want to be intubated, bro?" asked the casual medic.

"Fuck off and get me to the hospital, bro," I imagined my dad saying. But he couldn't talk. He could only focus on breathing, not shitting himself, and enjoying the last moments he would spend in his dream home without a respirator breathing for him.

Somehow, in the mayhem of it all, I ended up in the ambulance with my dad. The neighbors swarmed. "Is he okay?" asked one.

"He has fucking Lou fucking Gehrig's fucking disease and he fucking can't fucking breathe so we're fucking taking him to the fucking hospital, you fucking fuck fuck!" I wanted to yell at the top of my lungs.

"He'll be fine. He's gonna live forever," I really said.

We settled into the ambulance. It was actually quite cozy. I mean, I wouldn't throw a sleepover party in there, but I could certainly nap in it. I sat holding my dad's hand, now withered and cold. I told him over and over again that it was going to be okay. I didn't know what else to do. He just stared back at me with a look of terror in his eyes.

"It's going to be okay. It's going to be okay. It's going to be okay," I repeated on loop, more for me than for him.

As we were sitting, I looked over at the medic who had said "bro" a bunch. He was drawing doodles on his latex glove, like a bored fourth grader sitting in science class. I guess the whole "My father is dying" thing didn't pique his interest.

"Bro, the Forty-fifth South Bridge is closed. You got to take Thirty-ninth," he said.

Though the circumstances that find you in an ambulance are always shitty, it's a pretty slick way of getting around town. No wonder it's so expensive. Everyone pulls over for you and lets you zoom by. It's like being royalty. One car, however, decided that they would follow us—apparently seeing the ambulance as a way of beating the thick Salt Lake traffic. The "bro" bro took notice. He hit one of the other paramedics on the arm. "Bro, check out this asshole," he said while shaking his head. "What an asshole that asshole is."

The ride took only about ten minutes. I was thankful the "bro" dude didn't ask to stop at Wendy's so he could raid the dollar menu.

When we arrived at the hospital, two of the medics picked my dad up and carried him toward the hospital's emergency room.

"It's going to be okay. It's going to be okay. It's going to be okay," I said a few more times for good measure. My dad gave me an ever-so-slight smile, as if to say that it would be okay, that he would pull through and keep on fighting this shitty fight. I gave him a smile back and said, "It's going to be okay," one last time before they wheeled him off and he disappeared into the hospital's busy clutter.

His life was now in the hands of professionals. He would go on a respirator. A machine would now breathe for him. He would never be the same again. This horrible disease was slowly taking everything.

I figured it was time to go outside and start making phone calls to family members and canceling plans with friends. No drinking for alcoholic Dan tonight. Going out would be way too messed up, and for sure place me in hell. Tonight would be the first of many spent at a hospital praying to the God that doesn't exist that my father would live another day, bro.

Tiffany had missed Grandma Barbie's funeral because she was out visiting her boyfriend in Portland, Maine. I thought missing the funeral for a vacation was incredibly shitty. I had consequently been extra mean to her this week. So I decided it would be a nice gesture to call her first. Maybe it'd patch things up and we'd be best friends forever.

"Dad's in the hospital," I said.

"No shit," she said.

"Whoa, you don't have to be a fucking bitch," I said.

"I'm not, but I know when my dad's in the hospital. Greg called," she said.

"Sorry."

"Well, I'm coming up. Do you want anything from Starbucks?" she said.

"Coffee drinks give me diarrhea," I said.

"So do you want anything?" she asked.

"I'll have a nonfat vanilla latte."

I hung up and called Abby. No answer.

I put my phone in my pocket and found myself standing next to the "bro" guy. It was awkward standing next to each other and not saying anything, so I figured I should make some sort of effort.

"What's up, bro?" I said.

"Not much, just chilling, bro," he said.

"Well, thanks for helping save my dad's life," I said, even though it seemed like he hadn't done shit, assuming drawing doodles on latex gloves added no medicinal value.

"I was glad to help, bro," he said as he patted me on the shoulder and lit a cigarette. "I've seen a lot of shit in my day, and your dad seems like a tough dude, so I'm sure he'll be chill. Hang in there, bro."

"Thanks, bro," I said, hoping he was right.

This was all such a close call. Had we not called the ambulance, had we fucked around any more, had my dad not elected to go on the respirator, this could've been the day Lou Gehrig's finally got its hands around my dad's throat and strangled him to death. I was glad it wasn't. Though watching him struggle with this horrific disease was the worst thing I had been through, I didn't want it to end. I still wanted to have a dad. I still needed to see that rare smile. I still needed to hold that bony hand. I still needed my road map. I wasn't ready to become an official member of the Dead Dad Club just yet.

I took a deep breath and headed into the hospital, ready to start the next stage of the Lou Gehrig's grind, thankful that my dad was still ticking.

REHABILITATION

M y dad's surgery was scheduled for November 13. The doctor couldn't push it up, so my dad had to wait four days in the intensive care unit until he had the tracheotomy. During that time, he was intubated, so he couldn't talk, and they didn't want him moving around at all—not that he was very mobile anyway. So he just had to lie there with a fuck-my-life expression on his face, staring at the hospital's stained ceiling. He looked terrified, as if he wasn't sure all this pain was worth it. After all, the surgery wasn't going to cure Lou Gehrig's disease. It was simply going to prolong his life another year, maybe two, maybe three. His days of running marathons through the streets of Boston, or alongside the Green River in Moab, were fading further and further into the distance. He had a whole new life now. I felt bad for my dying pal.

I visited him in the hospital every day. The Jazz season was starting up, so I figured we could put the game on the hospital TV, hang out. Fuck, maybe I'd bring us a couple of cold beers and some popcorn. Maybe I could manage to jam that shit into his feeding tube. Before the Lou Gehrig's disease, anytime we were watching a game together and the Jazz scored, we would exchange a high five. We couldn't do that anymore.

"I wish I could high-five you," I said after Deron Williams nailed a three. My dad didn't say anything. But he did raise his foot as much as he could. I looked at it, a little confused. Carlos Boozer slammed down a jam. My dad raised his foot again. I finally put it together. "Oh, you want to do foot high fives?" He nodded his head as much as he could. I pulled my chair up to his bed, and we exchanged foot high fives every time the Jazz scored. It wasn't exactly like watching the game together in the Delta Center, but it was better than nothing.

The surgery finally rolled around. It was a routine tracheotomy.

Nothing special. The doctor was pretty ho-hum about the whole thing. He talked about it as though he were piercing my dad's ears or something. The operation basically involved cutting a hole in my dad's trachea, putting a plastic tube called the trach tube through the hole, and then hooking the respirator to it. The doctor had done hundreds of these surgeries before, so it was just another Tuesday for him. For us, though, it was a life changer.

The surgery was successful! Everything went great! My dad is the luckiest man on earth!

My dad was moved to the postsurgery part of the hospital for a week, and then to the Neurological Rehab Center at the University of Utah. The purpose of his stay in rehab was for their professionals to train us, his shithead family, on how to care for him. Insurance wouldn't cover the cost of a home nurse, and my mom insisted that we continue to care for him, so we had no choice. It was our duty as his children. I didn't mind, but caring for him was now going to completely change. We'd have to learn how to operate and manage the respirator. This involved suctioning the mucus out of his lungs with this gross plastic tube, changing his tubes, and maintaining certain pressure levels. We'd have to learn what all the parts and buttons were, and what all the various alarms meant. Someone would have to be there to monitor him at all times, just in case the tubing came loose or the respirator began to malfunction.

He would also no longer be as mobile as he once was. He would be hooked to a machine via two external respirator tubes: a blue inhalation tube and a white exhalation tube. So we needed to learn how to move him around without messing up the tubes. This proved to be harder than it sounds, because one wrong tug on one of the tubes and it would pull on his trach tube, possibly ripping it out of his throat. "That would be pretty painful," explained the doctor. "No shit," I wanted to say.

Since my dad was mainly restricted to a bed, we'd also have to learn some physical therapy exercises and how to rotate him so he didn't get bedsores. When he wasn't in bed, he'd be in a power wheelchair. He had been fitted for a chair before the respirator, but it was still being built at the magical wheelchair factory. Some generous guy from the Muscular Dystrophy Association (MDA) found us one we could use temporarily. We'd need to know what all the controls and buttons on it did. Additionally, we'd have to learn how to transfer my dad from his bed to the wheelchair, and vice versa, without killing him.

He'd now be in diapers. He wasn't happy about that. They made him feel too helpless and too much like a baby. I guess lying around shitting yourself is sort of the definition of helplessness. So, though he had to wear the diapers (which one nurse made us call "briefs" to try to protect some of his dignity), my dad insisted that we learn how to transfer him from the bed to a bedside commode, so he could take a shit there instead.

Our hope was that we could figure this whole thing out, adjust to my dad's decline, and get him into a Stephen Hawking situation where he lived a long, long time. We figured that having our dad in this state was better than not having him at all.

The good news was that he could talk. We were worried that the surgery would destroy his vocal cords, but it didn't. He had a small balloon in his throat called a cuff, which blocked the respirator air from leaking out of his mouth. It was used to assure that my dad got as much oxygen as possible. To talk, he had to have his cuff deflated so air could pass over his vocal cords. His voice was raspy and had a constant hum, but we learned how to understand him. Small victories.

Our mom was still getting pounded with chemo three times a week. But that just didn't seem like a big deal anymore. Had she not been bald, we probably wouldn't have even noticed her cancer. Dad was the star of the show. He was the closest to death. He got all the attention. This continued to upset our mom, because she was used to playing the lead in *The Marshall Family Tragedy*, given that she had been battling cancer for fifteen years. She started to get a little jealous of all the attention my dad was getting, especially now that he was in the hospital. I knew it pissed her off, so I really played up the attention I gave my dad.

"How are you doing today, Dad?" I asked as I walked into the hospital room, completely ignoring my mom, who was eating yogurt next to the hospital bed.

"You know, I'm sick, too," my mom said.

"Yeah, but you can move your arms, scratch your own nose, wipe your own ass, walk, breathe, talk. You're practically the healthiest person on earth by comparison," I said.

"Yeah, but I have cancer, and my bones hurt, and I'm tired, and I wouldn't mind having someone else wipe my ass," she said.

"Yeah, yeah, yeah. So anyway, how's Dad?" I asked again.

We were all pretty nervous about this next stage of the Lou Gehrig's battle. With the caregiving pressure increasing, we needed to step up to the plate with the game tied and smack the baseball out of the park. Most of it was still on Greg and me. Tiffany was still wrapped up in school and work, and would visit BCB in Maine about every other weekend, it seemed. She was so stressed and overwhelmed that she looked as though she was going to have a nervous breakdown. My mom was still too out of it to actually do any caregiving. If she were in charge of my dad, he would most certainly die. The hope was that we could get her through the last push of chemotherapy (she was almost done) and healthy enough to help us out a little more. Then, maybe things would get better. We could reclaim some of our personal lives. We could get real jobs. I could actually leave the house. And maybe I could eventually move back to California to be with Abby. I'd be happy again, and on my way toward living forever!

Greg and I both had the free time to be up at the hospital. Greg had taken a job at Franklin Covey selling day planners, but was only working a couple of days a week. He wanted to get a job just to get out of the house. Plus, all his friends from college were working, so he was starting to feel like a loser. Nothing gets you down like not having a job. He had the "our parents are dying" excuse but didn't feel even that was an adequate enough reason for not working.

I was heading in the opposite direction. I had just let my boss in Los Angeles know that things were too hard at home for me to return. It was a difficult conversation to have. I had been really hopeful going into this situation that I could eventually come back. I was coming to see how unrealistic that notion was. I felt that my old life was starting to disappear completely. All that work building a career was just consumed by this disease. I was now living an alternative life I never saw coming. I just hoped that after it was all over, I could get back on track.

Initially, Greg and I took the training seriously. We'd drop my mom off at chemo at Huntsman, then go to the rehab facility. Luckily, the two were adjacent. We learned how to change our dad's diapers. He had changed our diapers back in the day, so I guess what goes around comes around. We learned about his wheelchair. We learned what all the tubes on his respirator meant.

But we slowly started to shift into goof-around mode. We were supposed to drop my mom off at chemo, show up at the rehab facility by 9 a.m., and stay until 4 p.m.—a seven-hour day. Instead we would roll out of bed around ten and question whether we should even go in that day, treating the whole ordeal as a vacation. We had been taking care of our dad intensely over the past couple of months with no assistance. Having him at the rehab facility was a nice break. He was hooked to machines with a nursing staff at his beck and call. He wasn't going to die. He was fine. He practically didn't even have Lou Gehrig's disease anymore.

Home without my dad there was much more relaxing. There was no Daddy Duty. There were no doorbells. There was no waking up in the middle of the night to help my dad shit. We could just hang out and be degenerates in our awesome house. "I might just sit in the hot tub and watch *Curb Your Enthusiasm*," I said upon waking up from a twelve-hour sleep one morning, still in my robe, munching on a plate of lasagna for breakfast, because why the fuck not?

"Yeah, I'm probably going to play tennis and look for vests at Thrift Town," Greg said.

"Where's Mom?" I asked.

"She's at chemo."

"Who drove her?" I asked.

"I was supposed to, but I was reading about *There Will Be Blood* online, so she drove herself. I'm so excited for that movie. Daniel Day-Lewis is so hot. I would definitely fuck him," he said.

"Shit, I might even fuck him," I joked.

"He'd be a big upgrade from Abby," Greg replied with a smile.

"Man, we should've probably driven Mom to chemo," I said. "Ah, fuck it. You want to grab a burrito?"

The rehab facility was a sad place full of patients trying to adjust to their new, horrible lives. Most had been in car accidents. Some had had strokes. My dad was the only person up there with Lou Gehrig's disease. The hallways were full of wheelchairs and there were constant beeps from all the medical devices making sure all the patients stayed alive. It was a place where you tried to feel optimistic and have a positive outlook, but it was hard to not feel sorry for everyone there.

I also felt guilty. Why was I able to walk around, eat, fuck, live, while all these poor souls were imprisoned in their own bodies? It just didn't seem fair. I felt the weight of a great imbalance in the universe. Why couldn't we all just be okay? My dad's roommate had it the worst. He was a kid from Elko, Nevada, probably nineteen years old. He had been in a car accident. He had severe brain damage and was paralyzed from the chest down. My dad looked like LeBron James next to him—the model of good health and physical prowess. The only thing he did all day was click the button for more morphine. The nurses had to come tell him to stop pressing the button, that he'd already had his daily allotment of the painkiller. And it was only 11 a.m. Once, his friends drove in from Elko to visit. They brought him a Slurpee. He refused to drink any of it. He was too depressed to even drink a Slurpee. Too depressed for a Slurpee? Now that's depressed.

My dad was under the supervision of Dr. Rosenbluth, who looked a lot like Gene Wilder; a physical therapist, Jenny; an occupational therapist, Catherine; a speech therapist, Kristin; a respiratory therapist—usually a fat guy named Geoff who looked like Philip Seymour Hoffman; and a team of nurses. Dr. Rosenbluth would come in soon after we arrived, speak medical jargon for about ten minutes, then ask if we had any questions. We never did, but I always wanted to ask him if he was Gene Wilder in hiding.

The goal was to get my dad home as soon as possible. He was supposed to be in rehab a week, as that is the amount of time it usually takes caregivers to learn the necessary tasks. However, the relaxed mentality Greg and I had at home started to carry over to the training. We dicked around a lot. I think subconsciously, we didn't necessarily want him to come home. It would mean that the vacation was over and that we'd have to go back to being the exclusive caregivers. We weren't quite ready for that.

The medical staff noticed what idiots we were, so they didn't trust us to care for our dad full-time. They refused to discharge him until we had displayed that he was being released into capable hands. So they kept pushing back the date. We got this comment a lot: "Well, *he's* ready, but we should probably get *you guys* a little more trained."

We spent most of our time joking around. We'd drive my dad's new power chair up and down the hallway using the head controls. We'd grab my dad's limp hands, roll his fingers into a fist, and pump his wrist above his penis to make it look as though he was jacking off.

We'd throw small pieces of paper at our mom as we talked to the nurses about how crazy she was when she had chemo brain. We'd joke about dressing our parents up in skeleton costumes as a sick prank. We'd encourage my dad to stop taking the rehab so seriously and instead catch up on the Bourne trilogy.

My dad even got in on the dicking around. We'd unhook his respirator for a couple of seconds. He would fake die, and then we'd fake save his life. When a nurse would ask him how he was doing, he'd often smile and say, "Good, just got back from a long run." We'd even race him up and down the hallway in wheelchairs. We'd always win because he'd accidentally slam his into a wall, having not mastered his driving skills yet. In other words, we were in complete fuck-around mode. At this rate, my dad wasn't coming home anytime soon.

There was a Starbucks on-site, so Greg and I took turns fetching each other drinks. It was closing in on Christmastime, so they had eggnog and cinnamon lattes. We were consequently spending more time walking to and from the Starbucks and raving about the drinks than we were learning how to take care of our father.

The staff started to become increasingly frustrated with us, as they were trying really hard to teach us everything. You could tell Jenny the physical therapist was getting sick of our antics. She would say things like "Okay, guys, this is important, so pay attention," or "Wow, how many eggnog lattes have you had today?" or "Stop throwing things at your mom and listen for a minute."

One day, she sort of snapped. She was stretching my dad's right leg by flinging it over her right shoulder. "Okay, this stretches his semi-membranosus muscles, as well as his gastrocnemius," she said.

I took the last sip of my nonfat eggnog latte, noticed it was finished, and said, "Shit, Greg. My latte is out. It's your turn to grab."

"I'll be back in ten. Nonfat eggnog latte, right?"

"You nailed it," I said.

Jenny shook her head and released my dad's leg. "I'm not doing this anymore until you guys start taking this seriously," she said.

Greg and I looked at each other. We should have apologized and rededicated ourselves to the rehab, committing to getting my dad out of there as quickly as we could. But instead, I smiled at Greg and said, "Oh, actually, Greg, could you make mine a fat latte? I love fatties." Jenny stormed out of the room. It wasn't one of my finer moments. Dickhead Dan strikes again. We looked at my dad and just shrugged.

* * *

Despite undergoing chemotherapy, my mom still tried to participate in the training sessions, but she looked as though she should be lying in the hospital bed next to my dad instead of learning how to care for him. When she wasn't falling asleep standing up, she was wandering back and forth between my dad's room and the cafeteria. She wasn't part of the Starbucks crew, only because they didn't have strawberry yogurt and the cafeteria did. Plus, she already had the shits from chemo, so the coffee would have given her whatever is the next step past diarrhea. She still had flashes of chemo brain. She was constantly pushing for us to get Cheetos for some reason.

"Do you want any Cheetos?" she asked.

"No, I don't really like Cheetos. They make my fingers orange for the rest of the day. Plus, they don't have them at Starbucks," I said.

"Yeah, but don't you want something to snack on, like Cheetos, or something?" she asked again, sort of implying that she wanted some Cheetos.

"No. Do *you* want Cheetos?" I asked back, confused as to why she was so hung up on us getting Cheetos.

"No, I have some yogurt," she said. "You sure you don't want any Cheetos?"

As our time in rehab progressed, Tiffany started to make more of an effort to be around. She'd come up and try to learn the respirator, or do some of my dad's physical therapy stretches, or just drink some Starbucks with Greg and me. I was trying my best to be nicer to her, figuring that I was part of the reason why she hated being around my dad. We needed her help—we needed everyone's help. But she couldn't make it up as often as she needed to. Between the four of us, there was very little learning happening.

But my dad was making progress. He was actually able to still walk with the assistance of Jenny and Geoff. We just had to wrap a gait belt around him, so we could stabilize him and catch him if he fell. He had hardly been able to breathe before going on the respirator. It sucked energy out of his body and color out of his face. The respirator gave him more life and brought a warm, pink tint to his cheeks. He looked better, and he was happy that things finally seemed to be improving.

He'd excitedly tell us about the strides he was making during the day. "I was able to walk to the end of the hallway and back," he told me as I sipped on my eggnog latte.

"That's great, Dad. I'm very proud of you, but which Bourne movie are you on? You better at least be through *Supremacy* or I'll be pissed," I'd joke back.

It got to the point where my dad couldn't stay any longer. Insurance money was running out fast and the staff was tired of Greg and me cruising the hallways in the power chairs, slapping high fives as we passed each other, making sure to not spill our sacred coffee drinks. We had to step it up.

By the middle of December—a month and a week after he had been admitted—the doctors and therapists all hesitantly approved my dad's release, giving us you'll-be-back-because-you're-a-bunch-of-incompetent-shitheads grins. The grins suggested that they didn't trust us, and I don't blame them. I didn't trust us.

In retrospect it seems pretty clear that taking forever to learn how to care for our dad was a defense mechanism. It wasn't that we weren't smart enough to handle it. We were all just scared to take care of Dad on a respirator at home. It's a lot of responsibility to have a fragile life in your hands, especially when you care so much about that life. It was going to consume all of our energy. It was going to take over. It was going to change our changed lives even more.

The rehab center had a practice room that was supposed to simulate what it was like to be at home. No nurses were to care for him unless it was an absolute emergency. Before he could be released, we had to spend the night in this room and show that we were capable of keeping our father alive. This was our last test.

Greg and I arrived around 9 p.m., and the nurses rolled his hospital bed into the practice room. We were slightly nervous about finally taking something seriously. The nurses got my dad situated. Changed his diaper. Suctioned him. Brushed his teeth. Gave him his medication. Put splints on his arms. Placed the emergency button next to his head so he could ring for help. The head nurse looked at us.

"So, you think you can handle this?" she asked.

"Oh, yeah. No problem," I said. "And if we need help, we'll call you."

"The whole point of this is that you don't call us and do it all on your own."

"Right, but if we need you, we'll still call you, because we're not just going to sit there giggling as he dies," I said.

"With you two, it wouldn't surprise me," she said.

"Touché," I said. I got serious for a moment. I didn't think she realized how much we loved our pops. "Listen, I promise we'll take it very seriously. We love our dad very much, and we're smarter than we seem. Greg went to Northwestern. I went to Berkeley. We're not complete idiots."

"All right, well, we'll see. Any additional questions?" she asked.

"Yeah, is Dr. Rosenbluth actually Gene Wilder in hiding?" I asked. She shook her head and headed off down the hospital hallway.

The medication put my dad right to sleep, and Greg and I were left lying in bed with our eyes wide open, staring at the stained ceiling and listening to the rhythmic respirator pushing air in and out of our dad's body. It was like one of our old sleepovers, except now I was twenty-five. Greg was twenty-three. And we were sleeping with our dying father in a hospital. The weight of the situation started to crush us. Could we actually do all this respirator stuff and not be crippled by depression? Was it all worth it? Maybe we should just unhook my dad from the respirator and shoot my mom with a shotgun? Prison couldn't be much worse than this. We had used humor to get through this so far. Could we continue?

I finally broke the silence, wanting to say something that I thought best summed up the whole situation. "Hey, Greg?" I said.

"Yeah?" he responded.

"I want to tell you something," I said, taking a deep breath.

"Anything. We're brothers, after all," he responded.

I lifted up my leg and farted a top-ten-loudest-farts-of-my-life fart. *Ppffumphhhhhhhhh.*

We laughed so hard we woke our dad up. We passed the test that night. We were ready to take him back home.

WELCOME HOME

After almost forty days, my dad was released from the University of Utah's rehab facility and into our slippery, unprofessional hands.

The house was about ready for him. The construction was finally coming to a close. I was happy to have it done for the obvious reasons, but it would also be nice to no longer have all the construction workers wandering in and out of the house while I tried to relax and watch HBO, like a good little rich kid. Having manly men around has always made me feel like a complete pussy.

The last thing on the contractor's to-do list was the elevator, which was, arguably, the most important, since my dad's room was on the top level of our home. They were meant to finish it the day before my dad got home.

I waited for the technicians and crew to arrive, but they didn't. I called the elevator company, which was cleverly called the Elevator Company. After talking to a few middle-management guys, I finally got our project head on the phone.

"Where are you guys? You were supposed to get this thing up and running today," I said.

"Yeah, sorry, Mr. Marshall. We had some scheduling issues, so we can't make it out there until January," the elevator guy said. That meant at least a couple more weeks.

"January?" I screamed back, about ready to toss the phone through a window and cry myself to death.

"Yeah. January. Scheduling issues," he nonchalantly said back.

"That's not acceptable. My dad's coming home from the hospital tomorrow. He has Lou Gehrig's disease. That's a pretty serious disease. He can't walk long distances. He's on a respirator. He's been in the hospital more than a month. Our bills are piling up. We need this done today. This is an emergency. You're not putting an elevator in some vacation rental. We need this fucking thing in there for medical reasons. Life and death. That sort of shit," I frantically ranted.

"Yeah. Well, sorry. It's a scheduling issue. And I don't appreciate you swearing at me," he snapped back.

"Well, I don't fucking appreciate you making our horrible lives even more horrible, and blaming everything on a fucking calendar," I yelled back, then clicked off the cell phone as emphatically as you can click off a cell phone. Bam. One of the remaining manly construction workers was eavesdropping. He gave me a nod of approval after my little outburst. Maybe I was transforming into a man.

So, we were going to have to do this without the elevator. Oh well. At least it was almost Christmas. Maybe I'd have a chance to watch *Elf*.

We had set Tiffany's old room up as my dad's home hospital room. It was a big bedroom on the top level of our house, right in the center, and one of the few rooms that our piss-easy cats hadn't yet destroyed. The medical supply people had actually done their jobs on time. So my dad's new adjustable/retractable bed was all set up. We even had a little rack where we'd hang his respirator—his new set of lungs. All of the respirator supplies arrived in boxes: lots of tubes, humidifiers, extra trachs, sterilization supplies, gauze, bandages, etc. We organized them on Tiffany's old trophy shelf next to ribbons she had won back when she had been an elite swimmer. Her childhood was now covered with the medical supplies that would keep our dad alive.

With the help of Stana, we got the room looking good. Well, not good. But we got it looking like a home hospital room. We put an additional bed in there so whoever was on Daddy Duty could get some sleep. I stole my dad's credit card out of his wallet—which was pretty easy since he was in the hospital and couldn't move—and bought a flat-screen TV with a built-in DVD player for the room so he could watch movies or sports while he lay there dying. Might as well die in comfort, watching HDTV.

A family friend had drawn a beautiful sketch of my dad running in the St. George Marathon. He had a smile on his face. He was happy. No respirator. No Lou Gehrig's. The old Bob. It always depressed me a little because it reminded me what we had lost, how healthy my dad used to be. But Greg had gotten it framed, and we hung it behind his hospital bed along with all the participant medals he had received from running all his marathons. It was like a tribute to his former life as his new one started.

The house was looking pretty good, and we were feeling ready for him. Or so we thought. Then our neighbor Ralph showed up. He had been increasingly critical of the job we were doing managing my dad and the whole situation.

"I feel like you guys are too stupid to figure out how to take care of your dad, especially now that he's on a respirator," Ralph said.

"Hah, yeah, probably," I said, ignoring him. Though he had been a big help with certain things like the doorbell, he was a bully when it came to getting our act together.

"Fine, just ignore me," Ralph said.

"I know it looks like a mess from across the street, but we've really got it under control, Ralph," I said.

"Doesn't look that way. You idiots don't know what you're doing," Ralph said.

Ralph was right. We didn't know what we were doing. He seemed to represent the logical voice of reason from the outside—a voice that we needed but didn't take seriously. We were sure that everything we were doing was right, mainly because we didn't know if it was wrong. We were learning an unlearnable job on the fly.

Right as we got his hospital room all set up, Ralph asked why we hadn't just made our front dining room the hospital room. That way we wouldn't have to get him up and down in the elevator in case it broke or was never installed. It was a great idea. We could just build a ramp up the front steps and that would be that. But we were too stubborn to listen to Ralph. We insisted that Tiffany's room would work just fine.

"Well, what about a generator? Do you idiots have a generator? We're having the most severe winter in over twenty-five years. The power might go out, and since your dad's on a respirator, that would be bad," he explained to me as if I was a child. Salt Lake's winters are always up and down. Some years, we'll get a light winter in the valley where the snow never really sticks. Other times, it won't stop snowing. So far, as Ralph mentioned, this winter was a severe one. Snow was piled two feet deep around our house. Our driveway was caked in ice. Icicles dangled from the rain gutters like knives about ready to drop through our skulls. This type of winter requires a little extra pre-paredness.

"Oh, relax. I'm sure we won't need a generator. My dad's portable battery lasts, like, four hours. We're golden."

Soon, Ralph handed me a list of things he thought we needed to grab at Home Depot: flashlights, lots of batteries, lots of extension cords (long and short), a generator, a surge protector, a couple of fans, a dry erase board, and a new doorbell to put at the end of my dad's bed so he could alert us when he needed something. I set the list aside and said that I would eventually grab all the supplies.

"All right, well, it's your dad. Do what you want. Idiots," said Ralph.

I didn't go to Home Depot. We had other things to worry about. Like Christmas! I closed the front door on Ralph and headed to my dad's new TV to finally watch *Elf*. I kicked up my feet and sipped on my eggnog with an extra shot of whiskey, because why the fuck not?

We had initially decided that we wouldn't do a big Christmas cele-bration that year. We wouldn't get a tree or any presents. We'd just be thankful for all the gifts we've been blessed with. "I'm so thankful for Lou Gehrig's disease and cancer, because it's taken my father and mother from me, made me quit my job, and is keeping me away from the girl I love. Cheers," I imagined saying at Christmas dinner, the fire crackling behind me.

However, my mom eventually decided the whole not-celebrating-Christmas thing was bullshit, and that it was a sign that the Lou Geh-rig's disease was winning. She had finally finished her chemo and was feeling better. Now she only had to go to the hospital every three weeks for IVIG blood infusions. The infusions helped her immune system and gave her some more energy so she could do things besides eat yogurt and sleep. The best part was that her chemo brain was starting to fade. She was definitely more with it and active. She started Christmas shopping a ton with Jessica. I think she liked the distrac-tion, and it gave her a reason to get out of the house for a little while.

She also decided to mobilize her friends to help her out. She adver-tised it to everyone as "Bob's Last Christmas," and asked if people could find it in their hearts to help make it extra special. Everyone decided they could. A group of friends put up a huge tree and deco-rated it with colorful lights and sparkling ornaments. Neighbors put up lights on our outside trees and fence, and brought over Christmas cookies and gingerbread houses in addition to the lasagnas. Stana made a special batch of Christmas potato salad with extra potatoes. The house looked good. It was all Christmas-ed out. My dad was ready to come home.

An ambulance picked my dad up at the hospital to bring him home. I went along for the ride. I looked for the "bro" dude, but he wasn't there. I imagined him railing lines of coke and hitting on chicks at the mall, it being Christmastime and all.

The ambulance arrived at our house. I told them all about the elevator. "Those fuckers at the Elevator Company—stupid name, by the way—didn't do their stupid job, so we'll have to go in through the front door. What dicks, right?"

"Not a problem," one of the paramedics said, brushing it off. "We've got a transfer board anyway. Plus, we wouldn't all fit in the elevator."

Fuck. I wish I hadn't made that piece of shit at the Elevator Company feel bad for not getting the job done if we weren't going to even use the elevator. Poor guy was just trying to get through life like the rest of us.

The paramedics got my dad onto the transfer board and started carrying him in. There were a million things that could have gone wrong. I pictured one of the medics tripping over a cat and flinging my dad's limp body onto the Christmas tree. A branch would yank the trach out of his throat, sending blood and spit all over the family portraits in the living room. The respirator would fly through the air and nail my mom on the top of her bald head. She'd fall to the floor like a sack of cancerous potatoes. Something at some point would spark a fire—maybe the Christmas lights. Everything would go up in flames. We'd try to get my limp dad and unconscious mom out of there, but it would be too late. We'd get out and save ourselves, but everything would be lost. All our pictures. All our memories. All our Christmas presents. All our parents. We'd look at the smoking house from the outside and say something like, "Looks like this won't be a very merry Christmas for us." Ralph would pop over and watch the house burn with us. "I told you idiots so," he'd say. Then we'd do something depressing, like eat Christmas dinner at Denny's and talk about how our parents were dead now.

However, nobody tripped on anything. I watched my dad's face as he was carried in. He looked around at the tree and all the decorations in awe—like a little boy experiencing Christmas for the first time. It was crazy to me that only a year ago we were all circled around the tree in our silly pajamas planning for the Lou Gehrig's disease. And now my crippled dad was being carried past it, hooked to a fucking breathing machine. The paramedics continued hauling my dad through our house and up to his new room. They carried him past his favorite spot at the kitchen table, where he would always read the paper and drink his coffee. Past a wall of photos of him and his loving family during happier times: on vacation in Hawaii, skiing at Deer Valley, sitting poolside in Palm Desert. Past the master bedroom, where he and his wife had slept side by side over the years. He smiled. He was glad to be home, glad to be anywhere besides that hospital.

We got him settled into his new room. He looked around.

"Let's hope the cats don't start pissing all over this room, too," I said as I put a pillow beneath his head, already getting to work as his new home health nurse.

His cuff was deflated so he could speak. "I like the TV," he said.

"Yeah, I bought that. Well, you bought it. I stole your credit card," I said.

I noticed he was checking out all the medical supplies and gear that made it look like he was still in the hospital room.

"Sorry it looks like a hospital room. I know you just came from one," I said.

"No. It's fine. It's good to be back home," he said and smiled.

"It's good to have you back. Place wasn't the same without you."

And it was nice having him back home. He was the glue that kept this family together, the pulse that kept our collective hearts beating. No matter what differences the rest of us had, we were bonded by our unconditional love for our dad. His room instantly became the hub of all social activity in the house, the new hangout spot. Friends and neighbors stopped by all the time to visit again. His closest pals came over with some beers and drank with him, though my dad, of course, had to stick to the Promote. The dogs ran in and out of the room, wagging their tails so hard that it looked like they were going to fly off, happy that the house was full of life again. Fuck, even the cats would come and nap in his hospital bed with him, syncing their purrs with the respirator.

Stana said it best: "Daddy is now makin' home happy again."

Jessica and Chelsea hadn't spent much time up at the hospital because they had school, but once my dad was home, they finally got to hang with him. Chelsea would bring her homework up to the room and do her math at the base of his bed. She'd even ask my dad the occasional question by holding the book up to his face. He'd try to answer, but she couldn't understand him very well with his new trach voice. Jessica didn't do homework. She was barely hanging on at school. Instead, she would plop down on the bed next to my dad's and watch HDTV with him.

But having him back wasn't all fun and games. Caring for him was a real drag. A respiratory nurse, a physical therapist, and a speech therapist would stop by once a month, but other than that, everything was our responsibility. He constantly had to be rotated in bed. He needed to be fed three times a day and suctioned about twenty. He was always pissing. And he shit twice a day—once in the morning and once just before bed. The worst part was that one of us had to sleep next to him every night in case something went wrong with the respirator. My mom was still recovering, so it was on Greg and me. No more sitting in the hot tub and sleeping in until noon. No more chatting about fucking Daniel Day-Lewis. Daddy Duty was very much back on.

We duct-taped his doorbell to the base of his bed so his strongest foot could ring it. We'd usually get him to sleep around eleven and doze off ourselves around midnight. It was pretty surreal to me that I was sleeping next to my dying father instead of Abby. He would wake an average of five times a night and ring his bell. When he'd ring it, it was usually for a pee or to be rotated in bed. But sometimes the respirator would go off.

"BEEP. BEEP. BEEP. Wake the fuck up so your dad doesn't die," it would say.

"Fuck you, respirator," we'd say back. I instantly hated the respirator, even though it was keeping Dad alive and giving us more time with our pal. It was always going off. It was like that annoying friend who never knows when to shut their fucking mouth. The beeping usually meant that my dad needed to be suctioned. We'd fire up the suction machine and plunge the little plastic tube into his throat to suck up all the mucus. It was a horrible way to wake up. I've never had to care for a crying baby, but I'm sure this experience wasn't much different.

Regardless, it was still nice to have our dad back home.

During the first week, I was feeling pretty great about the job we were doing: My respirator skills were improving, minimizing the number of times it would beep uncontrollably. We were rotating my dad in bed so he didn't get bedsores and die. We were doing all of his physical therapy exercises. To top it off, we even placed the commode next to his bed and learned how to transfer him onto it so he didn't have to shit his diaper. My dad seemed comfortable and happy.

But then we had a massive snowstorm, and, of course, the power went out. It was pitch black in the house.

"BEEP. BEEP. BEEP. Fucking do something or your dad will die," the respirator shouted. It was freaking out because it needed to be connected to a power source.

"Please, just relax, respirator. We're doing our best. We care so much about our dad and don't want him to die either," we said.

"Sometimes I'm not so sure about that. You seem to be fucking up constantly. BEEP. BEEP. BEEP," it said back.

Using the light from my cell phone, I was able to connect a backup battery to the respirator. The respirator relaxed.

"I'm cool for the time being, but don't keep fucking up," it said.

I called the power company, and they said it could be up to eight hours before the power would come back on. Shit! The backup battery only lasted four. We'd be fucked in four hours. Completely fucked. We'd either have to use a manual Ambu breathing bag to pump breaths of air into him until the power came back on, or he'd die. I searched the house for a flashlight, but all I found was Ralph's list of things I should've already picked up at Home Depot, which included a flashlight. I was about to call the fire department to send over some paramedics. My dad would probably be taken back into the hospital. He'd be removed from his home once again. But, just then, there was a firm knock on the door. I answered it. It was Ralph.

"Didn't I tell you to get a generator?" he said as we walked up to my dad's room.

"I know, I know, I know. We fucked up," I said back. "We all suck at this."

Ralph shook his head at me, then at my dad. "Your kids are idiots, Bob," Ralph said. My dad smiled and nodded in agreement.

Ralph was able to round up a neighbor's gas-powered generator. We set it in the front of our house, and Ralph fired it up. He brought over one of his long extension cords, because we didn't have any, and ran it up through our house and into my dad's hospital room on the top level.

"We could have used a shorter cord if you had made the dining room his room," Ralph reminded me.

"I know. We're fuck-ups," I admitted again.

The power company finally got the power back on. We unhooked the generator and plugged his respirator back into the wall. My dad looked relieved.

"I'm sorry, Dad. We'll do better. That was just a little initial slip-up. You're going to live forever, don't worry," I said. He didn't seem too sure about that.

The next day, my dad got Ralph to drive me to Home Depot to grab a generator and all the other items on the list. As we drove there, I promised myself that I would do better. I would stop being such a child and try to become the man of the house. I would listen to Ralph. It was time to stop fucking around. It was time to grow up and take life more seriously. No more watching *Elf* and drinking eggnog. My dad's life was in my soft, underworked hands. I had to add some calluses to them, toughen them up.

I bought the best generator money could buy . . . with daddy's credit card.

BOB'S MONSTER BUS
OF EXCITING MAGIC

My dad's quality of life would never be what it was. But we all pledged to try to make the time he had left as fulfilling and comfortable as we could. We promised him that, though he was now attached to a respirator, we'd still get him out of the house and take him places. It'd be fun. We'd do a field trip every day. Maybe we'd go to the zoo. Maybe we'd go to a Utah Jazz game. Maybe I'd take him down to a strip club so he could get some tits rubbed in his face. The world was ours!

To keep this promise, we realized that our incredibly expensive luxury vehicles were no longer going to cut it. Lexuses might have heated seats and DVD players and handy compartments and lots of leg room, but they don't have convenient places to host a 450-pound wheelchair with a respirator clinging to the back of it and a near-dead man sitting uncomfortably in it, wishing his life hadn't taken this wicked turn down Fucked-Up Lane. So, we started looking for a wheelchair-accessible van.

My mom and I undertook this project. We didn't know the first thing about buying a wheelchair-accessible van.

"How do we get a van for Dad?" she asked.

"I'm not sure. Maybe we should ask someone who would know," I suggested.

"Who would know?" she said.

"I don't know," I said.

"I know you don't know, but who would know?" she said.

"I'm not sure," I said.

"Me neither," she said.

I started to call around to places with depressing names like Mobility Utah, or Para Quad Mobility, or Freedom Motors, or Freewheel

Mobility. I hate when they try to put a happy spin on something that sucks. It only amplifies the shittiness. It's like a doctor who dons a clown nose to tell you that you lost both of your arms in the car crash. That's right, fuck you, Patch Adams.

All vans—new and used—appeared to cost around thirty-five thousand dollars, but I couldn't find any that had heated seats and DVD players. Plus, my dad sat at about fifty-five inches tall in his chair, making it difficult to find one with a large enough opening for him to be wheeled through; we didn't want him to have to endure both Lou Gehrig's disease and a bonk to the noggin at the same time.

I decided to call Dave Ricketts of the Muscular Dystrophy Association (MDA) of Utah. Dave was a great resource, and knew everyone who had had or currently had ALS in the entire state. He's a prize of a human being. I always wanted to tell him that he put the *trophy* in *dystrophy*, but didn't think he'd appreciate that dark joke. He was the one who had found the temporary wheelchair for my dad.

I had contacted Dave when my dad went in for his tracheotomy operation, knowing it would take some time for a van to be tracked down, even by the master, Dave. He said he would make some calls.

We waited for several weeks without word. I eventually received a phone call from a woman named Michelle who had lost her husband to ALS two years earlier. She was in her late twenties. Her husband had gotten ALS when he was twenty-eight years old—an exceptionally young age for a disease that usually targets men in their forties or fifties. He only lasted about a year. She had been pregnant with their second child at the time. He elected to not go on a respirator, unlike my dad, but they did do the whole wheelchair thing, so they had gotten a van. The van sat in front of her house, a constant reminder of what had happened to her husband—her first love and the father of her children. Now, she was about to get remarried, move on with her life, and forget about all that ALS had destroyed, so she was looking to donate the van.

I asked her how much she wanted for it. She reminded me that *donate* meant *free*.

"Oh, yeah, that's right," I said, wanting to call her a smart-ass, but remembering that she too had been struck by tragedy, making us brothers, or sisters, or friends who have gone through similar shit and thus looked after one another.

"Where do you live? I'll come pick up the van this weekend if that's okay," I said.

"That would be great. I really want to get rid of it. I'm getting re-married, moving on," she said.

"I understand, friend. No sense making life hard and sad forever. So what's your address?" I asked.

"2600 South and 2300 East, in Spanish Fork," she said.

"Fuck," I said.

She paused long enough for me to realize she was probably a Mormon and that the word *fuck* had offended her. Dan, you're a fucking idiot, you fucking fat fuck, I thought to myself. Now, when I called myself fat, it wasn't much of a joke. Because I was so consumed with taking care of my dad's body, I was neglecting my own. I was eating loads of lasagna and fast food and drinking too much, all while also not exercising, leaving me at my peak weight, around 195 pounds. I had always been a skinny kid, so I felt fat as shit.

If you're not fresh on your Utah geography, Spanish Fork is about an hour to an hour and fifteen minutes south of Salt Lake—in other words, not that close to our house—thereby necessitating my use of the word *fuck*. We'd agreed that I'd come and take the van off her hands the next Sunday. I told her that I'd be there around two, so she could attend church and I could get all sorts of fucked up with alcohol on Saturday night.

I stuck to that plan. Saturday night, my buddy Dom and I really tied one on. I woke up more hungover than Jesus after discovering that he could turn water into wine. "I wonder if Jesus could turn twigs into cigarettes," I thought to myself as I lay in bed smelling of smoke. I was fully clothed and felt as though I had dumped a fifth of vodka directly on my brain.

I figured Greg and I would do this one together. We'd drive down to Spanish Fork, listen to some music, stop at Del Taco, talk about how fat I'd gotten, and wonder how long we would be forced to live our sad, parents-are-dying existence. Maybe we'd get to Spanish Fork, our bellies full of spicy chicken burritos, and decide we'd just keep driving south, maybe get to Mexico and eat some real Mexican food. We'd get along swimmingly, as usual. I wouldn't even tease him for being gay once.

"I kind of wish Dad didn't do the respirator," I'd say.

"Me, too," he'd say.

"But not really. You know what I mean. It's just hard. It's a lot of work," I'd say.

"Maybe we should just keep going all the way down to Mexico, run away," he'd suggest.

"We do have bellies full of Del Taco. We'll sit by the ocean, find some women, drink tequila, and be young and not tragic," I'd say.

"Perfect plan, except I'm gay and I don't like tequila," he'd say.

It would go something like that.

But, as I slowly woke up—the previous night a blur in my alcohol-soaked brain—my mom entered my basement bedroom. Greg had been on Daddy Duty the night before, so I had been able to sleep in my own bed. My mom looked especially bald and was wearing a long red coat that looked like a Navajo rug. It covered her perpetually cold body from her shoulders to her toes. She had the bright idea that she would drive the van back, even though she had crashed her much-simpler-to-drive Lexus about six times in the last three months while trying to drive under the influence of chemo brain.

One of my mom's biggest flaws is that she tries to do too much, just to prove that she cares. Though she was still beaten up from chemo, she would sit by my dad all day long. It was a testament to how much she loved him, but she looked exhausted. Visiting friends would advise that she go to her room and rest, but she would say, "I'm fine. Bob needs me," and have a spoonful of yogurt.

"Get up. It's ten. We have to pick up that van," she said.

"We don't have to be there until two," I said, rolling back over in bed.

"But we don't know where Spanish Fork is," she said.

"I know where it is. It's about an hour to an hour and fifteen minutes south of Salt Lake," I said.

"Yeah, but we don't know where their house is," she said.

"I thought Greg and I would do this one. Then maybe flee to Mexico," I said.

"What?" she said.

"Nothing," I said.

"Greg's a bad driver," she said.

"Well, he can drop me off and I'll drive the van back," I said.

"I'm driving the van back," she said.

I sat up in bed, taking the whole thing more seriously now. "You're not driving the van. You're a horrible driver."

"Dan, stop. I'm a really good driver," she said.

"You drove your car into the fence two weeks ago," I said.

"It came out of nowhere . . . Get the fuck out of bed. We're leaving. You smell like cigarettes, by the way," she said.

"You smell like cancer," I wanted to say.

My mom persisted, so she and I got in her Lexus and began the hour to hour-and-fifteen-minute drive to Spanish Fork. I tried joking with her to spice up the drive, but she wasn't in the mood.

"They should call Spanish Fork 'Spanish Food Utensil,' " I joked.

"What?" she asked, confused.

"They should call Spanish Fork 'Spanish Food Utensil,' " I said again.

There was a long pause. My mom started to cry. "What are we going to do about Dad? I don't think I can handle this. How are we going to take care of him?" She had been crying a lot lately. Now that her chemo brain was subsiding, she was smacked with the reality of this grim situation.

I didn't know what to say. I knew that the upcoming months were going to suck some major dick. It wasn't going to be easy. But I didn't really want to talk about it with my mom. I was too hungover. So I repeated, "Don't you think it would be funny if they called Spanish Fork 'Spanish Food Utensil'?"

I probably should've said something else. I probably should've reassured my mom that everything was going to be fine and that we'd make it through this as a family. I should've told her that I loved her and knew things were really hard for her right now. It would've been a nice little heart-to-heart. The two of us needed one of those. I had been hard on her lately. But instead, I said my horrible Spanish Fork line like an asshole.

I was scared shitless that we would get there and my mom would insist on driving the van to the point where I would have to tackle her to the ground in front of strangers to keep her away from the wheel. I would be judged by the Mormons and they would murmur, "He's going to outer darkness," their version of hell, as I pried the car keys from her weak cancer hands. But I would really be saving her life, because if she got in that van, she'd drive it straight into an oil truck, sending blackened pieces of her and her Native American coat a mile into the air before landing on my I-told-you-so face.

Even though the van was free, I had high expectations. My friend

Brian had been in a car accident that left him a quadriplegic, so his family had purchased a wheelchair-accessible van to get him around. It had a DVD player, great air-conditioning, and a nice sound system. Lucky Brian!

I wasn't expecting a DVD player, but I was expecting a bit more than the plus-sized jalopy the van turned out to be. It was the definition of an eyesore. It was disgusting. We got there and my first reaction was "Oh fuck, that better not be it," remembering that I had to drive the thing an hour to an hour and fifteen minutes back.

I don't know why "oh fuck" was my initial reaction. I don't know if it was because the van was baby blue. I don't know if it was because it was the size of one of those school buses for the mentally challenged. I don't know if it was because it probably wasn't worth enough to be traded for a DVD player. I don't know if it was because of all the rust around the tire wells. I don't know if it was because it had no front passenger seat, making road head a near impossibility for safety/logistical reasons. Or if it was because the old wheelchair that a former ALS patient had used before dying was still sitting in the van like an unforgettable nightmare, making it seem haunted. But that was my reaction.

My mom's was, "Do you think it's that blue piece of shit?" which was a bit more precise a response than mine had been.

I thought we should turn around, head back to Salt Lake, fork over the thirty-five thousand dollars, and get a van that didn't look like God's middle finger. We could just tell them that we couldn't find the house and we had to get home because there had been an emergency back in Salt Lake, that my dad's trach had exploded and he was on the brink of death, that we would maybe come back for it if my father survived the trach explosion.

"Mom, we don't really want this thing, do we?" I asked.

"Stop it. It's not that bad. We're already here," she protested back.

"It's the ugliest thing I've ever seen, and I bet it doesn't even work. We take it and then we're stuck with it sitting in our driveway, bringing down the value of our home," I said.

My mom paused for a few seconds, so I thought I had convinced her, but instead she said, "Oh, shut up," and hopped out of the Lexus. We had probably made a mistake by driving a luxury vehicle out to pick up something free, but fuck it. My dad was dying.

We knocked on their door and the young, tragic woman walked outside. She was still in her church clothes.

"Hi, I'm Debi, and this is my son Danny. We're here for the van," said my mom.

I hoped for a second that the blue van in front of their house wasn't theirs, that they had the fully loaded real van in the back with *Lord of the Rings* blaring on all five DVD players.

"I'm Michelle. It's so nice to meet you. It's this blue van out front," she said.

Fuck.

She and my mom hugged. I wasn't sure if I was supposed to hug her. I didn't think the van—given how ugly it was—called for me to sacrifice a hug, even though I was wearing a shirt that read HUG THER-APIST, which is often misread as HUG THE RAPIST.

We looked at each other and silently agreed not to hug.

I was worried that this was going to be a tear-jerking experience for my mom—meeting a woman widowed by the same disease that would eventually widow her. I hoped my mom wasn't going to bring up her illness, that this little adventure could be focused on my father's Lou Gehrig's disease rather than the cancer, and that extra tears would not be shed. After all, Michelle was just trying to take the final step in moving on with her life. We didn't need to cry.

My mom started in. "So your husband had Lou Gehrig's?"

"Yeah, he did. He was twenty-eight when he was diagnosed," Michelle said.

"What a shitty disease," my mom said.

Michelle looked a little offended by my mom's language. She was definitely a Mormon. I could even see a picture of Jesus hanging in her house. But she realized my mom wasn't in a great state of mind, so she forgave her, and said, "Yeah, it's pretty bad."

"I don't know of a shittier disease," my mom said. She then burst into tears, really sobbing hard. "I don't want to be alone," she managed to say.

Though she was twenty years my mom's junior, Michelle was experienced in losing a husband. She pulled my mom in for a hug, rubbed her back. "It's bad, but life goes on. I'm getting remarried soon. That's why I'm trying to get rid of the van. You'll be okay."

"I have cancer," my mom said. "I won't be okay."

We talked for a while longer, mainly about the disease and her husband's battle with it. The whole time I could tell she didn't want to relive the experience. She truly was trying to move on. But my mom was curious and asked all these inappropriate questions.

"How long did he last?"

"Was he able to go to the bathroom on his own or did you have to help him?"

"Could he talk?"

"Did he say 'I love you' a lot?"

"Did he go on a respirator?"

"Are you glad he didn't go on the respirator?"

"How old were your children when he died?"

I had been hoping the van exchange wouldn't involve all this conversation. I knew we were going to be going through all this shit; why talk about it with a complete stranger? I just wanted the keys, so I could go to Del Taco, order two spicy chicken burritos, and get home so I could sleep off my hangover and prepare myself for the newest episode of *Curb Your Enthusiasm*.

Then the father and mother of the dead ALS husband came out. Michelle and her husband had moved in with his parents when he was diagnosed, so they'd have some extra help. I guess they all still lived together.

The mother hugged my mom first and then looked at me. She said, "And this must be tough for you, too." She gave me an awkward hug.

"Well, it is. But let's take a look at the van," I said.

The father was a man's man and knew a shitload more about cars than I ever will. His handshake nearly crushed my baby-soft, never-worked-a-day-in-my-life hand. I could hear my mom continuing with the inappropriate questions while he showed me the van. "So, who are you remarrying? Do you feel like it's too soon? Are your children okay with the remarrying thing? You're moving out of your husband's parents' house, right?"

The man's man was honest and very aware of what a piece of shit the van was. He ended most sentences with ". . . but it still runs." He listed off several things it had wrong with it: "It needs power steering fluid. The oil needs to be changed. The battery needs to be replaced. Sometimes it doesn't turn on. It's top-heavy, so it feels like it's going to tip over when you drive faster than forty. The lights don't always work.

The back left tire has a nail in it. It doesn't pass safety inspections . . . but it still runs."

"Fuck me," I said to myself, worrying about my safety. I figured that this was the way I was going to die. The back left tire with the nail in it would fly off and bounce through the windshield of a family's car, killing them all—the nail going through the youngest and most innocent child's forehead. The top-heaviness of the van plus the missing wheel would cause the fucker to career out of control. I would try to slow down and regain control, but it would be too late; the van's weight, teamed with physics, would send it into a wildly chaotic roll and propel it across the median and onto the other side of the freeway. An oncoming truck carrying cannonballs would approach the van with its horn fully honked. The truck, unable to stop, would hit the van and explode, sending thousands of cannonballs into the air, and then through all the neighboring cars' windows. Everyone in every car within ten miles would die. The paramedics would find me burned to death in the driver's seat of this blue piece of shit and yell, "Why?" as the camera pulled to an aerial shot of all the death and destruction that this ugly, ugly van had caused.

Del Taco was no longer an option.

Michelle recognized the shittiness of the van, too. "It's a bit ugly, I know. But we had some fun in it. Just being able to get him out of the house was priceless." She smiled. "My kids called it the Bus or the Monster."

I hadn't thought of a nickname yet because I was busy concluding the vision about how my life was going to end, but I improvised. "My dad's name is Bob, so we're going to call it Bob's Monster Bus of Exciting Magic."

She paused for a minute, not knowing how to respond. "That's a good name, I guess," she finally said, since she needed to say something. "We just called it the Bus or the Monster."

The man's man started the van, slapped the front hood, and said, "Good luck. It takes diesel, but only one of the tanks works. Also, it's not registered, so be careful around cops. Oh, and make sure you don't go above fifty. It stopped running on us once when we did that."

I looked at my mom. She was still teary eyed. "You still want to drive this thing?"

She looked at the bus and then at me. She shook her bald head and began walking toward the comfortable and safe Lexus.

So, we got a van! And not just a van, but Bob's Monster Bus of Exciting Magic!

I drove home at thirty-five miles per hour the whole way, avoiding forty so it didn't feel like I was going to tip over, and definitely avoiding fifty so it didn't stop running. I stayed in the slow lane and kept two hands on the wheel at all times. The radio probably didn't work, but I was too nervous to check. I repeated, "I'm not going to die," over and over and over again, pausing only to yell "Fucking go around me!" to tailgating cars. My eyes scanned every which way for cops, and I would breathe a sigh of relief every time one passed me without pulling me over.

But all was okay. I always think if I worry about everything and picture the worst-case scenario, it won't happen. I eventually pulled the eyesore onto our cracked driveway. I got out of the car and looked at the van.

"Dad's going to hate this disease even more," I said to myself as I lifted my phone to snap a picture of the piece of shit.

I ran upstairs and told my dad that we had gotten the van.

"Is it nice?" he asked.

"It's okay," I said, not wanting to defeat his spirits.

"What does it look like?" he asked.

I pulled out the phone picture of the van and pointed it his way. He looked at it with squinty eyes, shook his head in disappointment, and said, "We should put a decal on the side of it that says 'Fuck ALS.'"

"I'll look into that," I said. "I nicknamed it, though."

"What?" he asked.

"Bob's Monster Bus of Exciting Magic!" I proclaimed. My dad didn't seem amused, just confused. "Never mind. It's a stupid nickname anyway. Let's just call it the Monster."

"Agreed," he said, glancing at the picture once more. "It's so damn ugly."

WE'RE HERE
FOR THE CAKE

M y mom was a big believer in support groups. She had gone to one for her cancer and it helped provide her with the hopeful, never-give-up attitude that got her through so many chemotherapies. She became instant friends with most of the other members. It gave her a community, a group of people who understood what she was going through, a group of people to cry with, hug, and get encouragement from. They were a giant part of her life when she was first diagnosed.

However, over the years she gradually stopped going. Not because she didn't find them useful anymore, but because her cancer friends started to die. It became too depressing. I guess that's the downside of surrounding yourself with terminally ill pals. Of the twenty-five people she initially attended meetings with, she was one of two who were still alive. It was a sad statistic, but it displayed what a fighter my feisty mom was. She truly was a survivor.

When my dad was diagnosed with Lou Gehrig's disease, Dr. Bromberg suggested he start attending support group meetings hosted by the Muscular Dystrophy Association. My mom—having seen the value of her support group despite losing so many friends—encouraged him to go. So he did.

The meetings were held on the first Tuesday of every month up at the University of Utah's Motor Neuron Disease Clinic. He and my mom attended their first in November of 2006—just weeks after getting the sack-of-shit news—and had been to just about every one since. The meetings would last about two hours and brought together a variety of people affected by the disease in one way or another—either they had it, were with someone who had it, or had lost someone who died from it. Snacks were included. Pizza. Cake. Capri Suns.

Those with ALS would view each other either as warning signs for how bad it could get, or as reminders of how much they themselves had lost. When my dad started attending, he was the fresh-faced guy new to the disease, not showing signs yet. Everyone was worse than him. A guy on a respirator named Vince Senior was the worst. But as the disease progressed, my dad began climbing the ranks.

I found the meetings to be depressing as shit, but my dad enjoyed going, because it made him feel less alone in his battle with Lou Gehrig's disease; it was one of the few places where he could go and say, "At least I'm not as bad as that asshole." He'd open up at these meetings in a way he wouldn't at home and really talk about his fears regarding the disease. The people at the meetings were his friends, his allies, his war buddies—and, though most of them struggled to talk, they really understood each other. He wasn't the only one going through this. Since he enjoyed the meetings so much, once I moved home I promised to take him to every single one until he couldn't go anymore.

Those accompanying the person with ALS to the support group meeting usually looked tired and had more to say than the two hours would allow. Bags under their eyes. Shoulders slumped. Hadn't been fucked for months, maybe years. In other words, I fit right in. These were the people who would really go for the free Capri Suns, cake, and pizza provided by the MDA's scrawny budget. They'd throw caution to the wind. Fuck it, I've got to treat myself since I'm working so hard to keep someone alive, I imagined them thinking as they tried to stab the straw into that tiny little hole that the makers of Capri Suns put on top of the juice pouch in an effort to completely fuck with us all.

Those who had already lost someone looked like they'd had the wind knocked out of them, like they were still mad at God, like they were permanently tired. They were often trying to get rid of all the equipment they had accumulated while caring for a loved one: commodes, urinals, cans of Promote, hospital beds, wheelchairs, communication devices, etc. But these people were always in a little bit better spirits. They'd laugh more, smile more, use the phrase "Believe me, I know" more. They'd been through the Lou Gehrig's mess already. They were in the clear. They were rebuilding. Their lives were starting to return to normal.

The topics at these meetings were as depressing as the crowd. One month, owners of a funeral home came to explain how everyone could save a shitload of money if they prepaid for their funeral and picked out a coffin in advance. Honestly. During this meeting, I was tempted to squirt my Capri Sun at the assholes, but I was unwilling to part with the fruity greatness that is Capri Sun. Plus, it had taken me twenty minutes to get that fucking straw in. I kept looking at my dad with a this-is-bullshit expression on my face. "We helped a woman save over three thousand dollars," bragged one of the assholes.

The meetings would start with everyone giving a quick update about how things were going, what the disease had been recently attacking. The people with ALS would rarely give the updates themselves, instead electing a family member do it.

"This is my wife. She's had ALS for two years now. It's going after her legs, so she's in this power chair," one would say.

"My husband had ALS. He died about three years ago after a long battle. This is my eight-year-old daughter, who will grow up without a father," another would say.

"He was just diagnosed last September, so we're new to this whole thing. It's sort of unfortunate, but we're taking a trip to Italy this summer. He wants to see it before, well, you know . . ." another would say.

The more meetings we attended, the less affected I'd feel by the sob stories, but occasionally I'd hear a new horror story that seemed to top the rest. There was one jovial guy named Shawn in his early to mid-forties who started showing up to the meetings. He always had this bizarre smile on his face and an equally bizarre, happy tone in his voice. He told his story in a crazy, happy voice, saying: "My wife has ALS. She was diagnosed in April of 2007. She's at home now. She can't make it to the meetings anymore. Her breathing is not so good, so she's on the BiPAP breathing machine pretty much all day and night now. She goes off it briefly to eat, though eating is really hard for her. We have three kids, who are also home. They are seventeen, fourteen, and eleven. They're dealing with it okay. She has elected to not go on a respirator or get a feeding tube, so we're expecting hospice to be necessary really soon."

The super-fucked-up-times-forty thing about his situation was that his wife wasn't comfortable letting anyone else but Shawn handle any of the care. It had to be him that fed her, bathed her, changed her diapers, etc. He also worked full-time. Because he was so overworked and so alone, he probably needed the support group more than any of us.

"My wife doesn't let anyone touch her . . . you know . . . privates or whatever. She's too embarrassed. So I have to shower her and change her diaper and all that," explained Shawn, with a smile so big it looked like strings attached to his ears were pulling the corners of his mouth toward them. "I have to do everything."

The room was silent for a moment as the weight of Shawn's situation set in, then another man, Karl, chimed in. "At first I would only let my wife help me with bathroom stuff. Then I would let my kids. Then I would let my siblings. Then I would let my in-laws. Finally, I just let anyone with warm hands do it."

Everyone in the room laughed, Shawn the hardest—so hard, in fact, that he outlaughed everyone by a good thirty seconds. After he finally finished laughing, Shawn's eyes opened wide and he responded, "Yeah, well, my wife won't let anyone but me do it, so I have to do it all." Shawn looked as if he was being tickled. His laughter intensified. "I even have to handle that time of the month for her. You know, her period."

If I'd had anything in my mouth, I would've spit it out in shock. "You're fucking kidding me, right?" I wanted to ask, but I elected to glance over at Greg instead to make sure he was hearing all of this. In the process of caring for my dad and his cock, I had totally forgotten about periods. It made sense. ALS doesn't affect the mind. Why should it affect the vagine? (T-shirt idea.) If my dad were a woman who still got periods, I probably would've been wrist-deep in vaginal waste once a month. I was suddenly grateful that he wasn't a woman. "Thank you, God. Maybe you weren't molded from a large piece of horse shit." I leaned over and rubbed my dad's shoulder. He probably thought I was comforting him, but I was really thanking him for not getting a period.

Shawn continued, "It's actually really funny." He paused briefly to chuckle to himself. "I used to be a tampon salesman when I was younger, so I had to know about all the products, so I knew how a tampon worked—how to put it in, which ones absorb the most. All that stuff. So I'm really lucky. Tampons aren't a big deal for me."

In my mind I was clapping so hard my hands stung. In reality, I sat with a slight smirk on my fat face. This guy was awesome. How could he handle something so tragic with such a positive outlook? We all had something to learn from the tampon salesman. I wanted to stand up and applaud. I wanted to shake his hand. I wanted to throw roses at his feet. I wanted to learn how to whistle so I could do that one loud whistle thing people do when they like something. Thank you. Thank you for looking at your situation with such awkward happiness. Thank you for taking that tampon salesman job years ago even though you were undoubtedly slightly embarrassed and hesitant. Thank you for not bringing your dying wife to the meetings so you could talk about your handling of her period. Thank you for being so strong and such a hero. Bravo. Bravo, my lad.

"But anyway. My wife has decided to not go on a respirator, so she'll do the BiPAP machine for a bit more, and then she'll die," Shawn said, giggling.

It was people like Shawn who made the meetings worth it. It made us all feel we didn't have it so bad after all. Shawn was doing it all alone; he was all by himself on the Lou Gehrig's island. At least we had the help of each other. At least we didn't have to change my dad's tampon.

It was the first Tuesday of February, so we had a meeting to get to. My dad hadn't been to one since October because of all the trach bullshit that had gone down. Since returning from the hospital several weeks ago, we hadn't been out much. The Monster proved to be a real piece of shit, as expected. It still sort of ran, but it was becoming apparent that we'd just have to fork over the money and buy something that was more reliable. Ralph was already helping us look for a new one. Plus, the intense snowing had continued. Just our luck. My dad's wheelchair was pretty awesome, but it wasn't awesome enough to go through snow.

Taking my dad anywhere also required that we make his respirator portable. We were still learning the intricacies of that asshole respirator and didn't have much confidence in our own abilities. My mom's behavior was increasingly erratic. One day she'd be in a panic, the next she'd look all fucked up. We began to suspect that she was overmedicating herself with some of her pain medication. It made some sense; we all wanted to go through this thing comfortably numb. But it made dealing with her really difficult, and it made her a horrible student of the respirator. Greg was never good with technology. He could barely work a Web site to watch gay porn. That meant that the responsibility fell on me.

My dad had a home respiratory nurse, Jeff, who would stop by the house once a month for about an hour to check the machine's pressure levels and change my dad's tubes. Jeff was a short, abundantly happy man who loved his job. He was clearly a Mormon because he was overly nice, and you could see his Mormon undergarments (which we always called Jesus jammies) under his clothes. I liked Jeff because he'd dish out a seemingly endless string of compliments. My fat ass needed a compliment every now and then to combat my growing sadness.

"You're doing such a great job of taking care of your dad. You should be proud," Jeff would say.

"Yeah, we're slowly figuring this thing out," I'd say.

"You're a smart guy, a natural. Heck, you could even be a respiratory nurse like me one day," he'd reply.

"Thanks, Jeff. You're pretty great, too," I said, complimenting him back.

Jeff eventually taught me how to make the respirator portable. I learned how to transfer all the tubes, hook up the portable battery, and mount the thing on the back of my dad's wheelchair. We could get out of the house. We could go to these support group meetings, as I had promised my dad. Hurray!

"You're so awesome. I can't believe how smart you are," complimented Jeff.

Greg and Mom both decided to come along to this particular meeting. I called Tiff to see if she wanted to go. Tiff and I were slowly starting to be nicer to each other, mainly because we didn't have the energy to treat each other like shit anymore.

"You want to come to Dad's bullshit support group meeting?" I asked.

"Honestly, Dan, I would, but I always leave those meetings feeling ten times worse about everything, and I already feel like shit," she explained.

"Yeah, I know. They're fucking depressing. I wish Dad didn't want to go so bad," I said.

"Sorry I'm not coming. But, you know, have fun," she said sarcastically.

So it was just the four of us.

I packed up the respirator. Anytime we left the house, I would also bring the following items:

- One spare diaper
- One spare change of pants in case the diaper and the aforementioned spare diaper didn't do their jobs

- One urinal
- One joke about the urinal being some sort of sick cocktail mixer
- One backup respirator battery
- Wipes
- An Ambu bag to be used if something went wrong with his respirator and we wanted him to continue to breathe
- Suction machine
- Something to write with
- Pocketful of pretzels

As we readied my dad for this adventure, Greg and I pledged that this would be the best ALS support group meeting ever. Lately, whenever anything went wrong, we would say, "Fuck Lou Gehrig's disease," but we figured that this field trip was going to be so wonderful and perfect that we wouldn't need to say it. We got my dad up from his bed and into the elevator—which those fuckers at the Elevator Company had finally finished—with no problem, and only said "Fuck Lou Gehrig's disease" two times: once when we almost dropped my dad getting him into his chair, and once when we accidentally drove the chair straight into the wall.

After a short elevator ride down to the garage level, we pulled my dad's chair onto the driveway and next to the Monster. I pressed the switch to deploy the lift. It didn't budge. The van was broken. It was useless. All that effort to get it in Spanish Fork for nothing. I yelled, "Fuck Lou Gehrig's disease!" so loudly that it seemed to echo through our quiet Mormon neighborhood, rattling its foundations.

Getting my dad to the meeting on the respirator was proving to be a bigger hassle than I thought it would be. It didn't seem worth all the trouble, even for the Capri Suns and for the hilarious period stories from Shawn. So my first thought was FUCK YEAH! We can't go to the meeting! My second thought was Oh shit, Dad's mouthing the words "Let's just take the Lexus."

"Let's just bake the dyslexic?" I responded, purposely misreading his lips. When his cuff was inflated, as it was now, we'd have to read his lips. He persisted, "Let's just take the Lexus." We couldn't say no. He wanted to go, and we'd promised him we'd get him there. Plus, we had to learn how to take him on these field trips eventually. Every bit of practice helped.

So Greg and I transferred my dad into a manual wheelchair that could be folded and stowed in the back of the Lexus. Then we transferred him into the Lexus, resting his respirator on the coffee-stained car floor and making sure we didn't slam any of his tubes in the door. We were loaded. My dad sat copilot. My mom sat batshit crazy in the back, eating yogurt next to Greg, who hummed some Disney songs.

I started to drive. It was then that, having already gone through a huge ordeal to get my limp father into the car, I came up with our entrance line. I always liked to have a line to enter the meeting with so everyone would start laughing and thus be distracted from my thieving of two Capri Suns. I thought the one for this meeting was brilliant: "We're here for the cake." Genius, I hoped everyone at the meeting would realize what a struggle we had gone through, seemingly just to get our hands on a free piece of cake. Greg and I began reciting the line. We practiced saying, "We're here for the cake" in different tones and intonations. We joked that we ought to give each other bloody lips and black eyes to emphasize the struggle.

"We're here for the cake. That's all. Just the cake. It's a mere coincidence that our father has Lou Gehrig's disease," we joked as we drove to the meeting.

We arrived at our destination. All the handicap spots out front were taken by the other fucks with Lou Gehrig's disease, so we had to park in the back of the lot. I transferred my dad from the front seat into the manual wheelchair.

I pushed him toward the building as Greg and I continued to think the "We're here for the cake" line was the funniest thing in the world. We started reciting it in celebrity voices. Jack Nicholson. Owen Wilson. Bill Murray. Chris Farley. We approached the narrow doorway.

Now here's the part where we messed up. As we were reciting the line, now in Brad Pitt's voice from *Snatch*, we misjudged the width of the doorway. Consequently, my dad's respirator tubing—the shit keeping him alive—smashed against the doorframe. Two of the tubes cracked. We had brought the backup diaper but no backup tubes. No more oxygen for Daddy. "Fuck Lou Gehrig's disease."

"BEEP. BEEP. BEEP. Boy, you *REALLY* fucked up this time," said the annoying respirator, always reminding us of our screwups.

We began bagging my dad with the Ambu bag—manually pumping air into his lungs. We were ready to turn around and end this catastrophe when Vince Junior, the son of Vince Senior, came out of

the meeting and approached us. Vince Senior was now a five-year veteran of ALS and a three-year veteran of the respirator. Though his
disease was at the most advanced stage of anyone we knew, he had
plateaued and was now living comfortably. We were hoping to get my
dad into a similar state, so Vince Senior and his family were sort of
our idols. They were pros at managing the disease, while we were still
amateurs.

Vince Junior, a tall, strapping man's man, looked us over and said,
"What's the matter?"

"We broke my dad's tubes," I said.

"Do you have any spares?" he said, talking about it as if my dad had
a flat tire.

"No, but I have some pretzels in my pocket," I said, pulling one out
and offering it up to Vince Junior. He didn't take it.

"Well, we brought some spare tubing. We always bring spare tubing," he said, with a slight smugness in his voice.

"Well, aren't you and your disabled father just a bunch of fucking
professionals," I wanted to say.

"Oh, thank God," I really said. "You and your family are amazing at
managing this thing."

Vince Junior replaced the tubes we broke. Good as new. Oxygen
for Daddy. We'd learned a lesson: we always have to bring backup
tubing on these field trips so my dad doesn't accidentally die. We'd
add that to the list, just below pretzels. More important, Greg's and my
chance of uttering the world's funniest line was saved. We wheeled
my dad into the meeting and smiled.

"We're here for the cake," I said triumphantly.

No response. No laughter. I looked at the food and beverage table.
No cake. I scanned the crowd. No Shawn. His wife had died. This
meeting was a total bust. All that work for nothing, and we had almost
killed my dad. We needed to get better at these field trips. We had to.
We weren't going to let the Lou Gehrig's disease win that battle.

Fuck Lou Gehrig's disease, I thought as I worked on getting the
straw into my Capri Sun.

After the meeting, we got my dad home safely, and I got him back
into bed. As I was doing it, I said, "Sorry we didn't do a better job of
getting you to the meeting. We'll get better at getting you around

town. We promised you field trips. You'll get them, and you won't almost die."

"It's okay," my dad said. "It was good to go to the meeting."

"Yeah, it was. Good to know other people are fighting this thing . . . Shawn's wife died, so I guess he won't be around anymore," I said.

"That's too bad. He was an odd guy, but nice," he said.

"Yeah, the meeting wasn't the same without him laughing it up," I said.

We were both silent for a second, taking it all in, both a little bummed that someone we knew had succumbed to the disease, but also feeling lucky that it wasn't my dad. My dad smiled at me. "Well, I liked your cake line. That made it all worth it."

CHILDREN'S DANCE
THEATER

Chelsea's belief in her dream of growing up to become a professional ballerina was the one constant in her life, besides having dying parents. Most children who participate in an extracurricular activity of any kind have illusions that they will somehow be able to turn it into a profession.

For me, it was basketball. Despite my lack of height and athletic ability, I was going to be the next big thing to hit the hardwood. I was going to make John Stockton look like a fucking D-League player. To a short white kid, Stockton was the perfect idol. He made it seem that if you worked hard enough, anything was possible. Until I was about fourteen years old, I was 100 percent certain I was going to be in the NBA. Then I stopped growing up and started filling out. My only hope was to become better at drinking and making fart jokes than John Stockton.

Tiffany, an early bloomer with tits at twelve, was convinced she'd be an Olympic swimmer. She pushed Greg and me really hard and was sure that we were going to be a family full of gold medalists, just like the Phelps family if Michael had siblings who also won gold medals. She played the role of the hard-nosed, bitchy coach who drove us into the pool by threatening to inflict small amounts of pain or discomfort on us. I played the role of insubordinate athlete who thought his hard-nosed, bitchy coach was a total joke. I often refused to go to practice with her, just to see what small distress she was willing to put me through. One day, we almost came to blows.

"We've got to go to practice," she said, entering my room carrying a glass of milk.

"I'm not going," I said, hoping she'd just leave my room and go to swim practice, so I'd have the house to myself and thus could fine-tune my new hobby: masturbation.

"You're going, or I'll pour this glass of milk on you," she said.

"Yeah, right," I said.

"I'm going to do it," she said, moving the glass closer to me and tilting it to the side, a little milk spilling out onto my blue carpet.

"Don't, Tiff. I'm not going. If you do, I'll tattle-tell the shit out of you," I said.

She did. I chased her from my room with milk dripping from my face. Too bad pouring glasses of milk on your brother because he refused to go to swim practice isn't an Olympic sport, or she'd have a couple of gold medals around her neck.

Tiffany was no doubt a gifted swimmer, setting several Cottonwood Country Club records. That's right, back in the prime of the Marshall clan's existence, we had been members of a country club. But once the other girls developed and caught up to Tiffany's level physically, she appeared to slow down as they sped up. She then realized that her dream wasn't going anywhere and picked up snowboarding. A couple years in, after making the U.S. Development Team, she witnessed a girl break her neck in a half-pipe tournament and decided getting an education was a safer, lower-chance-of-breaking-her-neck route.

For Greg, being gay and all, the dream was acting. He partook in several plays and even joined a traveling acting troupe called Up with Kids. Up with Kids, the child version of Up with People, specialized in performing uplifting and downright awful songs at some of our nation's finest amusement parks and tourist destinations. The group essentially consisted of soon-to-be-drama-nerd fatties, young boys who hadn't yet been injected with that hormonal poison that makes getting pussy a top priority, and Greg. Greg was by far the smartest, best-looking, and gayest member of the troupe, so he stole the show. Whether we were in Disneyland, SeaWorld, Universal Studios, or at the Washington Monument, Greg was in the center of the stage, lighting it up, as my grandma Rosie laughed in the background.

"Goddamn it, this shit is hilarious. Greg is so gay," I'd laugh with my grandma during one of his performances.

"Look, he's putting on a wig," she'd say, bursting into an even greater fit of laughter.

Greg's interest in acting started to wane as he became more self-aware. I also think he started getting embarrassed by my grandma and me yakking it up at all his performances. So, he quit acting and picked up writing.

Jessica dabbled in lacrosse and appeared to be extremely interested in it, but it soon became apparent that she wasn't as interested in the sport as she was in her coach. She sort of gave up on lacrosse around the time she started high school.

For Chelsea, the impossible profession was dance, and her dream was very much still alive, so we were forced to play along and act as though she had a legitimate shot at doing it forever.

"So, what do you want to be when you grow up, besides a fart and shit machine?" I would ask her.

"A dancer. Maybe I'll be in the New York City Ballet," she'd say.

"Yeah, that sounds like a very nice dream. Keep working hard, and keep your hands off your genitals. Masturbating wastes a lot of time and sucks up a lot of energy. I mean, look at me. I get nothing done," I'd say.

Greg and I continued to look after her more than usual during this nightmare year. We were her sarcastic, fake parents. Greg was to handle her emotions and play the role of concerned mother, while I handled the fun stuff—like teaching her how to drive while teasing her about boys. I was the verbally abusive father figure who clearly resented having children because they made him feel guilty for drinking so much. Chelsea didn't take either of us seriously, so the three of us became some sort of a strange family mocking all other families who took being a family seriously.

"You got a boyfriend, you little shithead?" I'd say like a drunk dad.

"No boys like me because I fart," she'd giggle back.

"Well, there's the farting, then there's also the fact that you're a total nerd. Plus, you don't dress like a slut," I'd say.

Greg would walk over, looking like a concerned parent. "Chelsea, that is not true. Don't listen to your drunk father. You *aren't* a nerd and you *do* dress like a slut," he'd joke.

Part of our fake parenting responsibilities also involved supporting her dance dreams. We couldn't let her become aware of the fact that all dreams die once pubes come bursting out of our bodies. We encouraged her and even called her "Dance Princess" occasionally, when we weren't calling her Fart Princess or Baby Moe.

"Fuck, I feel like Chelsea still believes in Santa Claus, and we're forced to play along," said Greg one night in the basement when we were chatting about life.

"Yeah, it sucks. But at least she's not into some stupid acting bullshit."

"That stupid acting bullshit got us into Disneyland," Greg said.

"Splash Mountain is better than sex," I said.

"I'm sure it's better than sex with you," Greg said.

Chelsea was part of a dance troupe called the Children's Dance Theater. Ages ranged from four to seventeen, making Chelsea one of the oldest members. They'd have about four major performances a year, but they practiced nearly every night. Chelsea was still too afraid to drive—mainly because my lessons would mostly end in me yelling at her about how bad she was at driving—so we still had to drive her to her rehearsals. Driving her around was an extra chore, so eventually we started to pawn off the responsibility to the throngs of Mormon neighbors who felt bad about the whole dying-parents thing and wanted to prove to themselves and God that they were good people.

"Let us know if we can do anything to help," a Mormon neighbor would say.

"Drive Chelsea to dance," I'd say.

"Really? But . . ."

"Our parents are dying, remember? God's watching," I'd interrupt.

The actual going to the performance part was one thing that we couldn't pawn off because of the guilt our mom smothered us with. She took a variety of different approaches, usually involving our dying father.

"Come on, her father is dying. She needs you guys. You're all she's got."

"You have to go. It means the world to her, and Dad is dying."

"GET THE FUCK IN THE CAR BEFORE I START GETTING SO MAD THAT I MURDER YOU WITH MY LITTLE CANCER HANDS."

But the most effective line she used involved Chelsea's dreams. "Come on, you guys. Chelsea still thinks she's going to be a professional dancer. You have to support her and play along. She can't lose her father and her dreams in the same year," she'd say.

All these tactics worked to weigh down our souls and cement our asses into seats at the theater where we'd watch the Dance Princess perform.

* * *

As we pushed through the snowy winter, my dad continued to get worse and worse. It was hard to get out of the house. I figured that this would serve as a big enough reason to keep us from Chelsea's upcoming performance.

"I can't go to Chelsea's show. I've got to watch this crippled fuck," I would say as I gestured toward my poor dad. He was my alibi. He would get me out of going. Surely we won't be forced to go under these Lou Gehrig's conditions, right?

There are all sorts of medicines one can use to overcome physical difficulties, but there still isn't one to combat a Catholic woman's use of guilt. Even though my dad couldn't shit, breathe, or walk without another's assistance, my mom still was able to guilt him into going to Chelsea's dance performances. She used a variety of different approaches, usually involving his imminent death.

"Come on, this will be the last chance you have to go to one."

"You have to go. I already bought flowers for you to give her after the performance. Don't let this disease make you into a bad father."

"Chelsea needs her father there because you're going to die soon, and she won't have a father, and she'll be the only girl in the group that doesn't have a father because you'll be dead."

"GET THE FUCK IN THE CAR BEFORE I START GETTING SO MAD THAT I MURDER YOU WITH MY LITTLE CANCER HANDS."

In the end, my dad had to go, and Greg and I were the only ones able to get him there. We had gotten much better at getting my dad ready for a day out, but it was still a pain in the ass. People in hospital beds attached to respirators aren't meant to have active, on-the-go lifestyles.

"Can you believe we still have to go to these things, Dad?" I said.

"Yeah, it's time Chelsea gives up this dream, right?" Greg said.

"Let's just go so Mom doesn't kill us. I don't want to die just yet," Dad said.

My dad was right. He might have been dying, but he still had the wherewithal to know not to mess with my mom's demands and Chelsea's dreams. So we went.

My dad, Greg, my mom, my parents' best friends, Sam and Sue Larkin, and I arrived at the Capital Theater in downtown Salt Lake. We found ourselves among swarms of the type of people who attend mediocre dance performances in mediocre towns: parents, friends, dancers, and perverts looking to catch some camel toe.

Instantly, I knew that this was a mistake. It's one thing to take my dad to a park or a support group meeting, and quite another to take him to a crowded event. Steering a man in a 450-pound wheelchair through a crowd of Mormon glad-handers is quite a task. You have to get used to watching the road and saying things like "Excuse us," or "Pardon us," or "We'd like you to move because you have legs and can easily do that, whereas he is in a wheelchair and can't, you selfish fuckers."

My dad rocked an extremely concerned facial expression that suggested he sort of trusted us, but not really. My mom had piled bouquets of flowers on top of him, which he could deliver to Chelsea after the performance to help her feel special and loved. He looked like he was being rolled into his own funeral.

Once we got into the theater, a nice old man directed us to the absolute worst place in the theater for a wheelchair. Though there was room in the back—close to the exits and the van should something go wrong—he insisted that we sit at the far, front-left corner of the theater, a five-minute wheelchair drive.

"I know you're old and old people aren't as smart because of the wear and tear a human brain takes over the course of our unnaturally long lives, but are you completely stupid?" I wanted to say.

"Great. Thanks. Right in front," I actually said.

We settled into our seats. I sat between my dad, so I could take credit for caring for him and look like a hero (of sorts), and Greg, so we could giggle and whisper smart-ass remarks to each other. He was my new grandma Rosie.

"Is this dance called 'Tights: A Salute to Camel Toe?'" I joked.

"I think it's called 'Look, Little Mormon Girls Can Dance, Too,'" he joked back.

I watched my dad more than I did the dance performance, and kept close tabs on how far along in the program they were. The second we sat down I started asking about leaving. "How long is this fucking thing?" and "When does Chelsea come on?" and "We don't have to stay for the whole thing, do we?"

My mom looked at us and said, "Come on, you're all she has, and this is the last time Dad will see her perform."

Chelsea came on about ten minutes in. We all whispered to each other and pointed to the stage. "Do you see her up there? She's in the back." They always placed her in the back for some reason. She was a graceful dancer—she really does have talent—but her arm swings and leg kicks were always a bit faster or slower than those of the rest of the group, which was fine with us because it made her easier to keep track of. We cheered harder and clapped louder for her. Greg yelled, "Yeah, Chelsea!" which was probably a waste of energy since she's slightly deaf.

I pointed her out to my dad. "You see her up there, Dad?" I asked.

He managed to smile and nod his head. He had made it. It had happened. He got to see his little girl dance one more time. Maybe this horrible journey was all worth it.

After her dance, the performance continued. The theme was something about space, or the future, or technology, or science. The music was sort of futuristic—Space Odyssey, Space Mountain–ish. It was intense. Right as the most intense number with the most intense space-exploration music possible started up, my dad's respirator started to BEEP, letting us know that we had to act or death would soon arrive. It was dark. We couldn't see anything. The respirator continued to BEEP as the music boomed through the theater, loud enough for even the old fuck who sat us to hear.

"BEEP, BEEP, BEEP," it screamed. "STOP WHISPERING SMART-ASS CAMEL TOE JOKES TO EACH OTHER AND SAVE THIS MAN."

Greg and I popped up out of our seats. We saw this as a great time to save our dad's life, but also a great time to use him as an excuse to sneak out of the theater so we could maybe grab a tea and just chill in the lobby. I checked the respirator as Greg tried to comfort him—rubbing his shoulders and checking his tubes. The worst thing that can happen to a person on a respirator besides death is a mucus plug. When he was portable and away from the humidifier, his mucus would start to dry up and could plug the airway, blocking oxygen. That's what was happening: a mucus plug in the middle of a dark theater with space music shooting out of the speakers. Unplugging a mucus plug involved manually bagging him and literally pumping air into him with enough force to push through the plug.

"BEEP, BEEP, BEEP," said the respirator. "YOU IDIOTS BETTER HURRY OR HE'S GOING TO DIE."

"I can't really see anything. We've got to get out of the dark," I yell-whispered to Greg, as I continued to manually pump air into my dad's lungs. A look of absolute panic overtook my dad's face. He was fading fast. We had to act. Death was closing in on us.

So, we started the long journey up to the theater's exit. We eight-point-turned him around and started to panic and swear, much to the chagrin of the Mormon audience trying to enjoy the stupid, whole-some performance.

"Why the fuck did they put us this far from the fucking exit," I yelled as we tried to steer my dad through the dark aisles, banging into seats as we went, while the intense space music blasted through the theater. "Man, if he dies at this bullshit . . ."

We finally got to the top of the theater. The old man smiled and opened the doors for us, as if he was doing us the biggest favor imag-inable.

"If he dies, it's your fault, you old fuck," I wanted to say.

"Thanks for grabbing the door," I actually said.

Greg and I got our dad to the theater's lobby area and started bag-ging him. He was turning blue at this point and was probably starting to think that watching his daughter dance to space music would be his last memory. Greg pumped the bag as I suctioned the mucus out of him. After about five minutes, we had worked through the mucus plug, and everything was back to normal.

We sat in the lobby for the rest of the performance. I sipped on tea and Greg rubbed my dad's shoulders. The flowers still sat on my dad's lap. Soon, the legions of people flocked out of the theater. My mom found us.

"What'd you think? Wasn't she great?" she asked as though Greg, my dad, and I hadn't just taken an epic near-death space voyage.

"We're never coming to another one of these," Greg said.

"It's just too dangerous with Dad. He almost died," I added.

"Where the fuck is Chelsea? We need to get this dying man on wheels back to his home hospital bed," Greg said.

Just then, Chelsea arrived—all made up, still in her dance tights. Her toothy smile beamed back at us without showing an ounce of disappointment. My dad's cuff was inflated, so he couldn't talk. Instead, he clicked his mouth twice to grab Chelsea's attention. She ran to him and grabbed his right hand. He clicked twice again and ges-tured with his eyes down to the flowers sitting on his lap. She picked them up and smelled them. He smiled at her, forgetting about how he had almost just died, forgetting that he was about to die, forgetting that everything had been taken from him but his family and his little Dance Princess.

He mouthed, "Good job," to Chelsea.

She smiled and mustered a quiet "Thanks."

Seeing how proud my dad was, and how happy Chelsea was, I knew we had to keep her dance dream alive. My mom was right. She couldn't lose dance and her dad in the same year. Life was hard enough for our Baby Moe Ham. She needed all the encouragement she could get.

"You're going to be in the New York City Ballet one day," I said, flashing a supportive smile.

"You were by far the best one up there," Greg added, playing along.

"Yeah, I know," said Chelsea, smiling, her dream living on.

We stood there for a minute and soaked in the moment. I finally interrupted. "Okay, great. We did it. Now let's get the fuck out of here."

HIDDEN BROWNIES

Abby finally visited. She hadn't seen my dad since summer—before he had gone on the respirator—so she was absolutely shocked to see how bad he had gotten.

"Oh my God," she said. "He looks like a different person."

"Yeah, well, he has fucking Lou Gehrig's disease. What did you fucking expect, moron?" I wanted to say.

"I know. It's crazy. I love you, babe," I really said.

I wanted to get the fuck out of the house, so we spent a couple of nights up at my family's condo in Park City: we watched movies, lounged around in robes drinking wine, sat in the hot tub, and fucked. It felt like old times again. It was like we were back in Palm Desert, back when everything was perfect—just a couple of young in-love assholes feeling like we were going to live forever.

"Your condo is so nice," Abby said while finishing off her glass of wine in the hot tub, our robes hanging off to the side for when we wanted to go back inside to drink wine by the fire.

"I know. I wish I could live here instead of at my house. Maybe I'll run away from my family and move here," I said.

"You totally should."

"Unfortunately, they'd find me," I said.

And they did find me. Without me at the house, there weren't many capable hands to watch my dad. My mom couldn't be trusted around the respirator. She had replaced her chemo brain with pain pills, and occasionally seemed even more out of it than she had when she was being treated for terminal cancer. Greg was so burned out he couldn't handle it anymore. He had to get on with his life. He had gone out and gotten a full-time reporter job working the entertainment beat at the *Park Record*, Park City's local newspaper. He could pitch in at night but was no longer around during the day. My mom was leaning on me extra hard. She called.

"Dan, we need you back down here. I don't know how to work this fucking respirator and I have an appointment with Dr. Buys up at Huntsman," my mom said. I could hear the respirator going apeshit in the background.

"BEEP. BEEP. BEEP. Your dad's going to die because your pill-popping cancer mom doesn't know what she's doing," screamed the respirator.

"But I'm with Abby. We just opened a fresh bottle of wine," I said.

"Get your ass down here. Your dad is dying. You and Abby can get drunk and fuck each other some other time." She hung up.

So Abby and I put the robes away and drove back down Parley's Canyon to go watch my dad. Abby was quiet. I could tell she missed how things used to be, that she wanted to keep hanging out in the robes and drinking our brains away. She wanted me to get out of this situation. I did, too. But I couldn't. I had to be here. This was my life.

We got back to the house. I ran upstairs and began attending to my dad. I got his respirator under control. Abby sat in a bedside chair watching me care for him. I suctioned my dad, rotated him in bed, and changed his sweaty sheets. When I grabbed his dick and placed it in the urinal so he could take a pee, I almost felt like I was showing off to Abby how good I had gotten at taking care of my dad. She had to be impressed, right? I felt that if she saw everything I had to do, maybe she'd have more sympathy for me and think I was a hero (of sorts). Or maybe she'd see how good I was at taking care of someone else, and view me as a long-term-provider type whom she wanted to spend the rest of her life with.

She didn't.

Instead, she was horrified and incredibly uncomfortable. She wasn't used to seeing my dad like this. She was used to drinking eggnog with him at Christmas, or running with him across the Golden Gate Bridge. She wasn't accustomed to seeing him fill a plastic container full of piss while a machine breathed for him. I was so desensitized to the whole thing that I had forgotten how uncomfortable it made other people.

My dad needed to take a shit, so I had Abby help me transfer him onto the commode. The transfers were getting harder and harder because my dad's legs were getting weaker and weaker—it was always easier with two people. My dad was wearing only his diaper, which started to slip off his bony bottom as we lifted him.

After the experience, I found Abby in the basement crying.

"I can't do this, Dan. I have school and my life. I just can't," she said.

"I know," I said.

"You need some help. You can't do all this alone," she said.

"I know," I said.

"I hate seeing you like this. You're depressed, and you're not taking care of yourself." I'm pretty sure she was referring to the weight I'd gained.

"I know," I said. "But what the fuck am I supposed to do? Just let my fucking dad die? I can't do that, Abby. I can't. He's my dad."

"I know, but . . . this is so hard." She hugged me and cried.

I drove her to the airport the next day. We agreed that if I wanted to see her, I would come out to Berkeley. I was fine with that. It was best if she wasn't here, I suppose. She had a life, a career to worry about. Lou Gehrig's disease shouldn't fuck up everyone's world completely. I gave her a curbside kiss.

"I love you, Dan. You need help at home. Go find help," she said.

"I will," I said. I gave her one more kiss. She went back to Berkeley and I went back to my dad.

I took Abby's words to heart. We really did need some help around the house. My mom had refused to hire an aide initially because she thought we could do it all. As this situation pushed on, it was becoming more and more apparent that we couldn't. We were all tired and on edge, and it was starting to affect the care my dad was receiving. He was unshaved; he looked glossy and unwashed—like a homeless person. He wasn't getting outside enough. He was trapped up in Tiffany's old room, a prisoner to his body and to this house. I was pissed at Tiffany and Greg for having lives of their own. I was sick of Chelsea and Jessica's shit, too. They were young, but they still should've been doing something instead of nothing. Fuck that and fuck them.

"Chelsea, you need to help out more, you little asshole," I told her one night.

"I can't. I have school and dance," she giggled while doing a ballerina spin.

"I'm going to take a dirty shit in your pillow," I warned her.

"I'm going to take a dirty shit in your pillow," she repeated. We laughed.

"How about you, Jessica? Can't you do a fucking thing around here? I mean, you're hardly going to school," I said. She just walked by me and slammed the door to her room.

I was physically breaking down. I just couldn't give any more. I felt like an athlete who runs out of gas at the end of the game. I needed to rest, and I wanted my life back. Depression was taking hold of me. I was forgetting that there was a world outside of my dad's home hospital room. Sure, I'd go out drinking with some pals, but I'd have all my problems waiting for me when I got back home. Lou Gehrig's disease wasn't going to go away. We were stuck with it. I was also starting to resent my dad for the first time in my life. I was all about trying to keep him alive for as long as possible, but this was getting ridiculous. Why did he have to get this stupid disease? Why did he have to go on the fucking respirator? Just so he could torture us?

I finally, finally convinced my mom that I was experiencing "caregiver fatigue," that I was too burned out to be the primary caregiver anymore, that I needed more breaks and more help.

"We need to hire someone to help. I need my life back," I yelled.

"Okay, fine. But I really think we can just do it," she said, half falling asleep as the respirator started its beeping.

"We're hiring help, Mom. That's the end of it."

One of the social workers at the University of Utah had given us the number for a home nursing service. I called them up to see if they could send someone over for Tuesdays and Thursdays, allowing me to escape the house and try to have a little bit of a life. They said they'd send someone over right away. Oh, fuck, yeah!

I called Abby. "We're getting some help, finally," I said.

"Oh, that's so great. Yay!" she said.

"I love you."

"I love you, too." Maybe it was all going to work out and we'd be able to be together, drinking wine and sitting in hot tubs forever.

The first person they sent over was this big, strong Tongan woman named Meredith. The Mormons do a lot of missionary work over in third-world countries like Tonga. They then bring a bunch of people back to Utah to start Tongan-specific wards. Consequently, there's an abnormally large Tongan population in Utah. Meredith had come over to the States recently to be with the rest of her family. She needed a job, but she didn't speak much English, so she started working with the handicapped.

Meredith wasn't actually a nurse, just an aide. Aides differ from nurses in that they can't provide any medical assistance. They help with basic things like sitting with the patient, feeding and showering them, helping the patient go to the bathroom, or going for walks with them. We still had to manage the respirator and suctioning stuff. I was equally concerned about finding someone who got our family's sick sense of humor as I was about finding someone who could provide the best care for my dad.

Meredith's main asset was her size. She could pick up my dad as if he were a rag doll and get him into a wheelchair or back into his bed. With Meredith, we didn't need two people to transfer my dad. She could do it herself.

"Wow, you're gigantic," I said when I first met Meredith, just as she was transferring my dad from his bed to his wheelchair.

"So are you," she said back with a smile, while looking at my growing potbelly. I guess her English wasn't that bad, and she could crack a joke. Off to a good start.

I tested her sense of humor a little more. Since my dad's name was Bob, some random friend had sent over a bunch of Bob-themed T-shirts. One said, BOB'S SON; another said, BOB'S BABE; another said, I'M WITH BOB, with a picture of a finger pointing to the left; another said, BOB ALMIGHTY. The one for my dad said, DON'T WANNA. DON'T HAVTA. I'M BOB. I wore the SON one, my mom wore the BABE one, my dad wore the I'M BOB one, Jessica wore the BOB ALMIGHTY one, and we made Meredith wear the I'M WITH BOB one.

"You have to wear this every single time you're over here, okay, Meredith? This is your uniform," I jokingly told her. But she didn't get that joke and thought she actually did have to wear it. So every Tuesday and Thursday, she'd show up in the shirt. I didn't have the heart to tell her she didn't actually have to wear it all the time, so she just did.

She was very helpful, and even offered up a few solutions to ongoing problems. For example, we were always having trouble getting my dad's shirts on and off. We'd have to sit him on the edge of the bed, unhook his tubing for a brief second, and try to carefully slide a T-shirt on over his bloody trach hole. It wasn't efficient, and the lack of oxygen would leave my dad about dead by the time we got the shirt on his skinny back.

Meredith came up with the solution to cut the backs of the shirts open, so we could easily slide them on and off. She knew how to sew, so she even sewed these little string ties on the back to hold the shirt up. It worked like magic. We didn't even have to sit my dad up, and didn't have to remove his tubing.

"Meredith, you're a fucking genius," I told her.

"What is a genius?" she asked in heavily accented English.

Everything was going along swimmingly with Meredith when we got a call from the home nursing service. They informed us that Meredith had quit, that she thought the situation was too hard and sad. She wanted to find something that wasn't as physically and mentally exhausting. We didn't see her again. She left us. And, to add insult to injury, she took the I'M WITH BOB shirt.

The next nurse to arrive was a young, vibrant girl named Marianella. She was from Argentina, but had lived in Miami for several years. She was a Miami Heat fan, which, being a giant Utah Jazz fan, instantly pissed me off. She had much more training than that big, quitting sack of shit Meredith, so she was quite a bit more professional. She didn't like to joke around, and the chances of us getting her into a goofy T-shirt were very small. She was all business, and even called my dad "Mr. Bob" and my mom "Ms. Debi."

She was so professional, in fact, that she called shitting "BMs," short for bowel movements.

"Don't you mean 'shit'?" I asked upon hearing her say "BM" for the first time.

"We call it a 'BM' in the business," explained humorless Marianella.

"Cool, well, in this 'business' we call it shitting, okay?" I said back.

Though she was professional, she wasn't a great fit for our family. We were too crude and crass for her liking. Lou Gehrig's disease was a serious disease that required serious attention, and in her eyes we weren't taking it seriously enough. Plus, Mr. Bob had a massive BM in the shower that she had to clean up. She didn't like that. She, like Meredith, quit through the agency.

We cycled through a few more over the next couple of weeks. One was giving my dad a sponge bath in his bed, and my dad got a boner.

I didn't even know people with Lou Gehrig's disease could get hard. I guess he still had that going for him. I wasn't there for liftoff, but I found out about the boner when my mom said, "Dad got a boner in front of the aide today."

I looked over to my dad and asked, "Did you really?" He confirmed with a nod and a smile, as well as an eyebrow raise; you know, all the things males do to confirm the validity of a boner story.

"I'm proud of you, Dad. That's great news," I said.

But my mom wasn't proud of him. She assumed that the boner wasn't just a strange chance happening, but was rather brought on by the presence of the aide. She got a little jealous, and consequently, this particular aide wasn't asked back.

Since we couldn't find a permanent aide match, we continued to do the majority of the caregiving ourselves, which continued to wear us down even more. Someone still had to sleep next to my dad every night. I was finally able to get my mom to focus for long enough to sort of teach her the respirator, so she started spending just about every night with him, sometimes even sleeping in his hospital bed. But the night shifts left her exhausted, meaning I had to watch him most of the day.

I eventually sat down with my mom to try to convince her that the aides the service kept sending over were never going to work for us, that we needed to hire someone outside of their system. Plus, the aides were only coming twice a week. We needed permanent help, at least five days a week. Between the construction on the house, the medical bills, and the equipment expenses, the Lou Gehrig's fight was costing us a ton of money, so my mom was being a little more careful than she used to be about spending, but I needed to convince her that the added expense of a full-time aide would be worth it.

"Mom, I love you and Dad and want to help as much as possible, but we need some permanent help," I said.

"But I'm sleeping in there now with him," she said.

"I know, and thank you for that. But still, can't we just hire someone to hang with him during the days? Our lives still suck and we're exhausted," I said.

"I'm not that tired," she said, just about falling asleep with the yogurt spoon in her hand.

"You're just about to fall asleep sitting up, dumb-ass," I said.

"It's too expensive," she argued.

"Having our lives back is priceless, and Dad needs better care. Come on, Mom. Please," I begged her, like a sixteen-year-old kid asking for a new car.

"Fine, but find one who doesn't give him boners." Victory!

So I started to look for someone who could handle our sense of humor and the intensity of the situation, while also being unattractive enough to not give my dad random boners, someone who could come in at nine and stay until five, Monday through Friday.

Before long, we found our match. Her name was Regina. Regina was a Brazilian woman in her early thirties who loved popping zits and plucking ingrown hairs. She had followed her husband to Utah after he converted her to Mormonism on his mission in Brazil a few years prior, though they were now divorced. Despite having a broken heart, she laughed more than Ricky Gervais at a tickle party, mainly about popping zits and plucking hairs. She was exactly what we needed.

I was so excited to get some help. I remember singing in the shower, "I'm getting my life back, and it's all going to be okay, and I'm going to be normal again."

Things were looking up with Regina around. My dad was clean-shaven, his hair combed to the side. His clothes and sheets were washed. He no longer looked like a homeless person. He looked healthier and happier—like he might actually have a nice life in his hospital bed. We were all more rested. I felt healthier and happier. My fat ass even went for a couple of jogs. I was so out of shape that I'd almost vomit.

However, after Regina had been on the job for a couple of weeks, my mom revealed that she hated the new aide. One morning when I asked my mom how she was doing, she replied, "I'm so sick of that fat Brazilian woman sitting around, eating my food and bossing me around."

"Isn't she helping you out, giving you more free time and whatnot?" I asked.

"No, Regina's a fucking bitch and she eats all day long," she replied, like a mean popular girl in high school trying to spread rumors about the new girl.

Wow. Cards were on the table.

My siblings and I were at the age where we'd finally built up the balls to reject our mom's opinions, so we rejected this one. We thought Regina was great. She was very loving, had a giant heart, was fun to talk to, laughed at all my fart jokes, and, most important, had taken over most of the toilet responsibilities. For us, it really helped restructure our relationship with our dad. Instead of wiping his ass and placing his cock in urinals, we could actually sit down and have a conversation with him. Thanks to Regina, he was back to being our dad instead of being our patient in some sick underground hospital we were running. I no longer resented him.

Sure, Regina ate some of our food and often asked, "Where did you get that?" and "Why didn't you get me one?" when I'd bring home a hamburger from a fast-food joint to reward myself after a jog, but who fucking cares. She was great.

Well, apparently my mom did care. She was jealous of Regina. She didn't like another woman showing up on the scene and spending more time with my dad than she was. She wanted to be the one taking care of him. Greg, Tiff, and I just marked all this up to our mom being crazy. Though she had improved her respirator-maintenance and caregiving skills, she had recently been prescribed Fentanyl patches for her cancer pain. We weren't sure who had prescribed them, since Dr. Buys was always really careful about not overmedicating our mom. It must have been some other doctor who felt sorry for her or something. Fentanyl is said to be stronger than morphine, comparable to heroin. So it's some strong shit. Though we found it easier to get along with her when she had a patch glued to her biceps or shoulder blade because she was so zoned out, the patches started to make her a useless caregiver again. She was left able only to eat yogurt and ask us inappropriate questions about our personal relationships.

"Are you ever going to get Abby pregnant? I want a grandchild," she asked. She had given up on the Pez dispenser proposal and was jumping straight to children.

"Bringing a kid into this world seems cruel, especially now," I said.

"I'm gonna start poking holes in your condoms," she said.

"Shut up, Mom. You're nuts," I said.

My mom showed her hatred for Regina in subtle ways. She didn't run into my dad's room with a knife and yell, "Die, you Brazilian slut!" or anything. But she did these little, bitchy things. For example, when guests visited my dad and asked how it was working out with

Regina, my mom usually went into passive-aggressive mode, saying things like "Oh, she's a big help . . . when she's not eating," or "She's so fat it's hard for her to do everything the job requires, like I can," or "She's not bad, but she's getting paid a lot and she doesn't have any college degrees. I got my master's from Northwestern and she's telling me what to do?" or, "Well, she just got a divorce, so . . ."

My mom went as far as getting Stana involved in the shit-talking. Stana and my mom were like a couple of cats ganging up on poor Regina. Stana pulled me aside.

"Danny, I is no likin' this big one. All day, she is eatin' and eatin' and no stoppin'. She is, how called, pig." Stana pressed her finger to her nose, making it into a pig snout to emphasize her point.

"Come on, Stana. Regina's pretty great. We love her. Well, not my mom, but the rest of us do," I retorted.

Stana had also picked up on the fact that Regina was Mormon. Though she couldn't read, Stana liked to dabble into the occasional political or religious conversation. She was talking to me about gay rights or something—using "stupid Mormons" as her main argument—when Regina walked by.

"Mormon is so stupid. They be, how called, brainwash," Stana said loud enough for Regina to hear.

"Excuse me, but I am Mormon. And I don't appreciate when you call us stupid," Regina said in her Brazilian accent. She was weirdly proud of being Mormon, even though she was a convert whose Mormon husband had abandoned her.

"Every Mormon is stupid," Stana said, pointing to Regina with a dirty rag in her hand. "You is Mormon. You is stupid."

"I'm really offended. Please don't talk to me again. You're mean to me," said an innocent Regina.

"You is son of a bitch," said Stana as she stormed off.

Regina would try to ignore Stana and my mom, but at times it would catch up to her and I would have to console her while she popped zits on my dad's shoulder as he sat on the commode working out a big shit.

"Listen, Regina, Stana is jealous of you because you are doing more for this family than she is. Don't listen to her. We love you."

On one occasion, I had my dad loaded into the van. We had gotten a new van, finally replacing the Monster. Ralph helped me pick it out, so I knew it was high quality. It was a gray Dodge Sprinter with a brand-new lift built in the back. It was perfect. We were on our way to the movie theater to see *Forgetting Sarah Marshall*. I had forgotten to pack the suction machine, so my lazy, pathetic ass sent Regina into the house to fetch it. She ran in, then came slowly walking back with the suction machine dangling from her shoulder and Kleenex in her hand. I asked her what the problem was and she answered, "Stana called me a 'son of a bitch.'"

"Jesus, she needs to stop doing that and show more respect," I said.

"I don't say bad words because of my religion, but Stana is the son of a bitch, not me," Regina replied, crying.

In addition to setting Stana loose on Regina, my mom also started asking Regina to do demeaning tasks. At one point, she made a list of things Regina could be doing if she wasn't watching my dad. Regina showed me the list. On the top of it was, "Pick up dog shit in the backyard." Regina asked me if she really needed to go pick up dog shit in the backyard, and I reminded her that she was hired to take care of my dad, not to do degrading chores.

"You don't have to clean up dog shit in the backyard. But if my dad takes a shit in the backyard, that's fair game," I replied.

My mom also started hiding food from Regina. Every Wednesday our awesome neighbor Nancy brought us dinner and a plate of sweets, usually brownies. I walked into the office in the back of our house and found my mom hiding in the dark, snacking on a plate of brownies. I flipped on the lights.

"What are you doing back here?" I said, pretty weirded out that she was sitting alone in a dark room, just chilling, eating brownies.

"I'm eating a brownie," she casually replied, as if it was the most normal thing in the world.

"I can see that, but why back here?" I asked.

She leaned in and whispered, "So Regina doesn't eat any."

"Mom, that's crazy. Regina is upstairs taking care of Dad. You don't need to hide," I said.

"Stana told me she saw Regina eat a whole plate of chocolate chip cookies. What if she comes down and sees me eating the brownies? She'll eat them all," my mom said.

"Jesus, Mom. You're insane. Do you need a Fentanyl patch?" I asked.

"I already have one on," my mom said with a smirk as she slid the plate of remaining brownies into her hiding place.

Hiding food from Regina as if she were some sort of Brazilian Cookie Monster, specializing in brownies? Jesus Christ.

The war had to end, but it seemed like it never would. Regina was now a crucial part of the picture, and all of our lives would be worse and more filled with ass wiping without her. We finally got my dad to tell my mom to back off of Regina. But she was a stubborn woman and wouldn't let up.

"Deb, lay off Regina. We need her," my dad managed to say.

"Yeah, Mom, you need to chill out. Be nice," Tiffany said.

"I personally love Regina. She might be the best thing that's ever happened to this family," said Greg.

"No, Regina's a fat-ass. I can take care of Dad way better than she can," my mom said, nearly ripping his trach out as she adjusted him in bed.

So we took a different approach. We realized my mom wasn't going to change her opinion, so we started convincing Regina that my mom was insane, that she had a head full of Fentanyl, that she should ignore any crazy-sounding utterances by her or Stana. Her focus was to be on taking care of my dad as best she could, and that's it.

A couple of nights later, to see if the strategy was working, I asked my mom how things were going with Regina. She answered, "Well, she doesn't seem to be listening to anything I tell her, so I just ignore her back."

"So you're cool with her?" I asked.

"Yeah. She's fine. I guess. She eats a lot, though, the fucking bitch," she said.

Success! Regina was now part of our crew. We finally had help. She was now on our team. She was in this adventure with us.

"You feeling better about all this?" I asked my dad one night as I poured some of the yellow Promote into his feeding tube. He looked so much happier, so much healthier.

"Regina is great," he said back. "You doing better?"

"Yeah, I'm finally sleeping, and I haven't touched your dick in a couple weeks," I said.

"That's a victory for both of us," he joked.

JESSICA IS NO SEEIN'
BRIGHT LIGHT OF FUTURE

By late February, things were looking a little brighter at home. Regina was around more—even some weekends now—and my dad seemed to be hitting some sort of plateau. His mental health was getting better. He was still walking a little, and trying really hard in speech and physical therapy. We were optimistic that he could last a long time with this disease. He'd be like his idol Vince Senior from his support group meetings.

My mom's health continued to improve. Her hair was even starting to come back in. She was still overusing the Fentanyl patches, though, and was out of it for portions of every day. One step at a time, I suppose. Greg was loving his new reporter job. He had put all the sleeping around he was doing in college on hold for a bit while things were chaotic at home, but now he was starting to rev back up the old fuck engines. Tiffany was still juggling school, a job, and BCB's big cock. I was even looking around for jobs in the Bay Area, thinking that maybe I could move back to California in time to save my relationship with Abby. We were starting to adjust to the situation and not let the disease ruin all of our lives.

Then shit got real again.

In early March, I went out to visit Abby in Berkeley. It had been a trying year for our relationship, but things were improving between us. There was some light at the end of the tunnel, and there was even some talk of us trying to find a place together in Berkeley. We were at least hanging and having a fun time.

But, one morning, while we were still in bed flirting with the idea of a second round of morning sex, I got a call from my crying mom. Nothing derails morning sex like a call from your crying mom. I figured she was calling to ask something about my dad's respirator, as I was practically a respiratory nurse by now. Jeff was so proud of me. My mom instead said, "Well, Jessica just dropped a bomb on us."

"Fuck," I said. I thought maybe Jessica had decided to drop out of school. She had turned eighteen in January and it was her decision at this point. She hadn't really been going to school anyway, despite Greg's and my best efforts to wake her in the morning and get her out the door. We were also finding her passed out from drinking more and more often in weirder and weirder places: the shower, her car, our trampoline, next to a plate of half-eaten lasagna, under a pinball machine. We had recently caught her in our basement drunkenly making out with some random kid from our rival high school. So I also thought that, because she was combining drinking and fooling around with boys, she had accidentally gotten pregnant.

"Jessica's dropping out of school so she can marry Todd. They just told us," my mom said.

"Todd, the lacrosse coach? Or some other Todd?" I asked.

"The lacrosse coach. Creepy Todd," she said. "God, I need another Fentanyl patch."

What the fuck? We'd thought that Creepy Todd was out of the picture. I'd thought that by coming home and acting like an overprotective parent, I had scared him away, but apparently it just made them more and more secretive about their relationship. They had still been hanging out behind our backs. And now Jessica was eighteen. She was legally an adult. She could do whatever the fuck she wanted, and she wanted to marry Creepy Todd. It was her decision.

I dropped the phone and started to cry. Not a soft cry either. It was a really, really hard cry—one of the hardest in my life. To me, this announcement meant that we had lost. Lou Gehrig's disease was getting my dad and turning our family into a muddled pile of white-trash shit. How could this happen? Why would this happen? Could we really handle another big piece of news like this?

I had these moments I called "if only" moments, where I'd think of the way things would be if only my dad didn't have Lou Gehrig's disease. If only my dad didn't have Lou Gehrig's disease, I'd still be working toward a normal life in California and have a functional relationship with the girl I love. If only my dad didn't have Lou Gehrig's disease, our house wouldn't be turning to a crumbling pile of shit that looked more like a hospital than a home. If only my dad didn't have Lou Gehrig's disease, my mom wouldn't be taking so many Fentanyl patches to numb the cancer and life pain. This felt like another "if only" moment. If only my dad didn't have Lou Gehrig's disease, Jessica wouldn't be marrying Creepy Todd. My dad wouldn't have let this happen if he were healthy.

But he wasn't, so it did.

The worst part of the announcement was that I could hear my dad crying in the background—a low and wobbly hum that sounded like a dying animal. Since his diagnosis, I had rarely heard my dad cry or complain. Complaining wasn't in his nature. To him, this announcement meant that he had lost control of his family. He was helpless and hopeless. He couldn't be the protective father he wanted to be anymore. He had to lie paralyzed in his hospital bed as all this bullshit happened around him. So he cried, and cried, and cried. Poor guy.

Abby couldn't believe it. She cried a little, too, and held me tightly. We had dinner with her parents that night, and I got absolutely shitfaced, because that seemed like the right thing to do.

I flew home after spending the rest of the weekend bawling in Abby's arms. As I left, I could sense that shit was officially getting too intense for her. She hadn't signed up for all this drama. Life in your mid-twenties was supposed to be fun and easy, not full of dying parents and insane family news. We were supposed to be off wine tasting in Napa, lying in the sun in Palm Desert, and trying every brunch spot in San Francisco's Marina.

When I got home, there was a palpable tension in the house. I could hear my dad crying the instant I opened the door. I ran upstairs. Jessica sat there holding his hand. "Don't say anything, Danny. I know you're pissed," she said.

"Why would I be pissed? You're only making a terrible decision that will add lots more grief and tragedy to our lives," I said back.

My dad cried even harder.

I finally had a chance to speak with him alone during a feeding.

"Well, this is totally fucked, isn't it?" I said as I watched the yellow Promote slowly drain into him. The smell of it was starting to make me nauseous. I hated it. I hated everything. Fuck Lou Gehrig's disease.

"How could this happen?" he managed to say in his respirator voice.

"I don't know. Jessica isn't thinking right now. Her head is all mixed up," I said.

194   DAN MARSHALL

"DJ, I feel like I failed as a father," he said, his wobbly hum-cry starting as he looked up to the ceiling, trying to hide his tears.

I rubbed his bony hand. "Nah, you've done all you can. You're a great dad," I said, starting to tear up a little as well.

"Not anymore," he said, officially bursting into his wobbly hum-cry. I wanted to punch that creepy son of a bitch for bringing so much added grief to this situation and making my dad doubt whether he was a good father.

At some point during this whole mess, Stana came up to me. She loved getting in the middle of our family drama. This Jessica news was a gold mine; it doesn't get much juicier than this. She said, "Danny, you is believin' this son of a bitch is marry Jessica?"

"I can't believe it, honestly. Of all the crazy shit to happen," I said.

"Jessica is tryin' replace Daddy with this old man, but Stana cuttin' penis off," she said, making scissors with her fingers.

"I'd love to see that," I said. "This whole mess is just too bad. It seems like Jessica has just given up on life."

Stana shook her head and said, "Danny, Jessica is no seein' bright light of future."

Stana always said things best, in broken English that seemed to make more sense than regular English. Jessica was in pain. She was struggling with school and it was making her feel like shit. To top it off, she was losing her dad—the one man who always stood up for her. It was hard to see the future as being bright instead of dark. She wanted an immediate fix to the problems right in front of her. Her solution was to create a new life with a new person.

It all makes sense now, but at the time we were fucking pissed. We were so pissed, in fact, that we tried to talk Jessica out of it. It was a big decision, because, in addition, she had decided that she would convert to Mormonism after dropping out of school. Now, in our family it's better to be a murderer than a Mormon. We had been subjected to Mormons' judgmental opinions of us throughout our lives. They always assumed we weren't good people because we drank and occasionally—okay, frequently—said "fuck." Plus, some of their core beliefs were just insane, like believing there were three heavens. We didn't even believe in one. We really didn't want one of us joining them. We explained to Jessica why she shouldn't go through with the marriage.

But Jessica wasn't listening. She had made up her mind. "I'm doing it, and you can't stop me," she said. She loved Todd, and Todd loved her. They were getting married. What a fucking fairy tale.

They were planning on running off to Vegas (because that's where all successful marriages begin). My mom, however, talked them into holding the ceremony in our living room so my dad could attend. Though at first my mom had been appalled by the idea, she became strangely supportive of Jessica's decision to marry Todd, despite our pleas. I'm not sure exactly what brought about the transformation. Maybe it was the Fentanyl. We were on her ass, constantly trying to get her to change her opinion and stop this wedding.

"I'm not going to call it off. Jessica is happy. We have to be happy for her," she explained to Greg and me, working on a yogurt.

"But Mom, this is so fucked up. We can't let this happen. You're her mom. Fucking do something," said Greg.

"This is no more fucked up than you coming out of the closet."

"Wow. That's the most screwed up thing anyone has ever told me. I'm going to try to pretend you didn't say that, because you're better than that," said Greg.

"And if I do something, they'll still get married. If we support it, then at least we get to go to the wedding," my mom said.

"Yeah, because I really want to go to a Mormon wedding," Greg said.

My mom was choosing to see this as good news instead of bad. She was excited to see one of her children get married, and thought it was sort of neat that Jessica was doing so while my dad was still alive to see it. She also thought that maybe if Jessica married Todd she'd stop drinking, which would potentially stop her from getting into harder drugs.

"Like Fentanyl?" I quipped like an asshole.

"Shut up. These are for my cancer pain. I need them," my mom said.

But she had a point. Maybe this marriage would at least put an end to the drinking and passing out. Greg and I were pretty sick of carrying Jessica to bed at night.

"Well, she's Todd's problem now. It's actually sort of a relief," said Greg.

Tiffany was taking the marriage news the worst. She and Jessica were relatively close, and it was hard to see something like this happen. She kept talking about cutting Creepy Todd's dick off. Everyone was after Creepy Todd's dick, it seemed. Tiff and I finally made peace over this situation. We were no longer at each other's throats. We realized that we were in this together, that it was us against the rest of the world. She even came over and had a glass of wine with me.

"I can't believe our family has gotten this ridiculous," she said. "We used to be this classy family, and now we're shit."

I agreed and said that things had gotten really out of control this year, and noted that none of our friends had to go through such intense family drama so early in life. "All those other fuckers are in graduate school. It doesn't seem fair, but fuck it. Oh well," I said. "At least we're still rich enough to afford wine."

"God, I really want to cut Todd's dick off," she said.

At the time, I was still the only person who knew how to make my dad's respirator portable. So my mom begged me to make him portable for the wedding. I told her to fuck off, that I wasn't going to do it, that she'd have to figure it out if she wanted to support this marriage. She tried to learn, but would get halfway through, break down, and begin crying as I watched her fumble around with the tubes, smiling like the devil. "I can't do it, Dan. It's too complicated. Just stop being a fucker and help me."

"Fuck off," I said back, the devil's horns growing out of my head.

I had started to truly resent her. She was losing her mind. She was letting her eighteen-year-old daughter marry a thirty-five-year-old. She was making a difficult situation more difficult. Couldn't we just be a family full of dying parents? Did we also have to have this creepy stuff happen?

The afternoon before the wedding, Regina came and found me being sad in our basement, playing pinball. I was playing a lot of pinball lately. It was nice to feel that I was able to control something. She said that my dad wanted to see me. I walked into his room, sat next to his bed. His cuff was deflated. He wanted to chat.

"DJ, I know you hate this whole situation and don't want any part of it. I don't either. But it's going to happen, so we might as well be there for Jessica. We have no choice but to support each other. We're still a family, even if we're broken down," he said, struggling to not cry. "So would you please make me portable for the wedding?"

I took a deep breath and said, "Nice speech, Dad, but I'm not doing it."

I started to head out of the room. He started to cry, sounding like a cow being kicked to death.

I turned back. "Ah, Jesus. If you want to support this marriage, I'll support you. I'll make you portable. But I'm doing this for you. Not for Jessica. Not for Mom. Not for Creepy Todd."

He smiled and thanked me, implying that I was a hero (of sorts) and the best son in the history of sons. "Thanks, Dan. We couldn't do this without you."

"Whatever, Dad. This horrible shit is ruining our lives."

The next day, in our family's living room, in front of the windows facing out on trusty, snow-capped Mount Olympus, we were to hold a ceremony with some friends and family from both sides.

To prepare, my friend Dom and I spent several hours getting drunk. I had asked Dom to film the event, since I thought it was so fucked up. Having a dead dad, Dom was used to tragedy, so he didn't mind hanging around. I was surprised the rest of my family members—minus my dad—weren't drinking. However, when Tiffany showed up, and I asked, "Why aren't you drinking?" she turned to me with a sly smile and said, "Oh, I had six beers before I came here." Tiffany wasn't a big drinker, so seeing her drunk was rare.

Minutes before the ceremony, Tiffany pulled Jessica into the basement to try to talk her out of the marriage. Jessica was already in her wedding dress.

"Jess, run as fast as you can," Tiffany said.

"Ha. Yeah right," said Jess.

"I'm serious. Run. You don't have to do this. Don't do it. Don't do it. Don't do it," Tiffany pleaded.

Jess didn't run. She went upstairs to get married.

"Fucking fucker," said Tiff. "I need another beer." So we all cracked open some fresh beers and chugged them into our tired, sad bodies.

The guests started to arrive.

Regina and I got my dad into his suit. I made his respirator portable. We got him into his chair and into the elevator, heading down to the main level where the wedding would take place. As I wheeled him into the kitchen, I saw a sea of Todd's Mormon relatives snacking and drinking caffeine-free sodas. It was what I imagined hell looking like. Once I got into the kitchen, I yelled, "Ladies and gentlemen! I present to you, the father of the bride!"

All heads turned to my poor, crippled father, trying to manage a smile, looking as sharp as a man with Lou Gehrig's disease glued to a wheelchair can look. Everyone was stunned—shocked into silence. Eventually, Greg started to applaud. "Oh, Daddy, you look so good!" he yelled sarcastically.

Everyone started clapping along with Greg. There were even a few hoots. My dad smiled. At least he'd get to see one of his kids get married.

I got my dad into the living room and situated him in the back. All the chairs were set up. We had a few family friends there, like Sam and Sue, but it was mainly Todd's massive Mormon family. They didn't know what to make of the marriage, either. One brother-in-law on his side said, "Well, this sure is a strange event."

"Yeah, it's like a really fucked-up Woody Allen movie starring stupid people instead of intellectuals," I said back, realizing as I said it that he was probably too much of a Mormon to ever watch a Woody Allen film.

My mom's friend Janet sang Beatles songs as she strummed away on her acoustic guitar. Todd and Jessica had brought in a Mormon bishop to marry them. I guess this was officially a Mormon wedding, in our childhood house. Fucking unreal.

Right before Jessica was about to walk down the mock-aisle and into Creepy Todd's arms, my dad looked over at me and motioned for me to deflate his cuff, allowing him to talk. I did.

"I want to walk her down the aisle," he said.

"Dad, you can't really walk, though, remember?"

"I can go a few feet. I know it. As long as you hold me up," he said.

"All right. I'll try," I said.

Jessica appeared in her beautiful dress. She looked great. She looked happy. She looked like she was excited to start a new life. It was her rebirth as much as it was her wedding.

Janet started playing "Here Comes the Sun," the same song my parents had walked down the aisle to some thirty years earlier. I wrapped the gait belt around my dad's bony rib cage and strapped the respirator around my fat shoulder, making sure not to step on any of the tubes dangling from the trach. I pulled him up out of his wheelchair and got him standing. I moved around so I could hold him up from behind. He looked over and smiled at Jessica. She smiled back. She slipped her hand into his. Everyone stood, and he started the walk down the aisle with his little girl, his fat son holding on to him from behind like he was Bernie from *Weekend at Bernie's*.

"I love you, Jess," he said as he passed her off to Todd. "Good luck."

After the ceremony, a very drunk Tiffany tossed Creepy Todd up against our garage and threatened to cut his dick off. Meanwhile, I sat drunk and naked in the hot tub with a few random non-Mormon wedding guests I was able to round up, because that seemed like the right thing to do.

SPA DAY

As this horrible Lou Gehrig's situation grew more and more intense, I started to expect more and more support and sympathy from family and friends. No one experienced my demanding wrath like Abby.

From my perspective, I thought Abby should have made my life easier by being more attentive and loving. After all, we had been together for five years now. I was initially understanding of her lack of empathy, but then it started to annoy me. She acted as though I wanted to go through this, as though I had a choice. I didn't. I couldn't leave my family to deal with my dad's disease alone. I was on Abby's ass to act as if she cared more. It's not that she didn't care. She really did. She loved my dad and me. She just didn't know how to handle everything. It wasn't her tragedy, and it was a little too intense for a cute blonde in her mid-twenties to go through if she didn't absolutely have to. So for her, the easiest thing was to ignore the situation, pretend it didn't exist, and hope her boyfriend came out of it relatively normal and well adjusted, so that we could continue living our happy, sunshine-and-Jäger-shots lives.

A couple of weeks after Jessica's wedding, Abby began to distance herself from me even more than she had over the past months. But I stuck with it. She was, in many ways, all I had going for me. I would often think, while feeding my dad through his gastrointestinal tube or cleaning shit out of his commode, At least I have Abby.

I loved my trips out to Berkeley to visit her. When I was there, I was still stressed and consumed by family stuff, but at least we were together and not talking over the phone. Now I can look back and say that if I could do those visits over, I would make them more fun and try my best to not bring up my family. But at the time, it just felt impossible not to talk about what was going on at home. It was the only thing going on in my life, and it was the most intense thing to ever happen to my spoiled fat ass.

In April, I called Abby one Saturday night when she was out with friends, and she didn't answer. I called a couple more times. No answer. She didn't call me back for a few days. I figured that she was having doubts about our relationship, and that her friends—who never liked me much and vice versa—were egging her on to break up with me.

Eventually she called.

She was crying. It was hard for her. She knew what bad timing all this was, but she also knew that she couldn't remain in a relationship that wasn't full of fun, but rather full of tragedy. She said, through her tears, that she needed some space—that I had gotten too depressing to be around. I told her that I was in Utah, and asked her how much fucking space she needed. She said that she needed more. No visits or phone calls for a while, until she figured things out and determined what she wanted.

So our slow and painful breakup began.

The agreement was that we'd take a "break." I didn't know what that meant, so I instantly reacted by fucking a few girls I had met through mutual friends. I think that's the first thing most people do in such circumstances: they fuck the lowest-hanging fruit. I'm sure she did the same.

This fucking of other people didn't help, but instead made me much, much lonelier. It didn't give me solace or closure. It just gave me shame—and fears of having contracted chlamydia (tested negative three times—no big deal). I missed Abby and wanted her back even more. You can't fuck away the feelings you have for someone else.

After a couple of weeks, Abby and I started talking again, and there was still some hope that we'd get back together, at least on my end. I tried to be funny and full of life during our phone calls. I tried not to talk about death and my parents and my little sister marrying a Mormon. I figured that maybe if I focused on the positive, she'd remember what an awesome person I was.

I'd then hang up the phone, slump back into my depressed self, and go sit next to my dad. My dad felt bad I was going through this breakup. He would look at me with pained eyes, wanting me to feel better.

"I'm sorry about all this, DJ," he said. "Abby is a really great girl."

"Yeah, well, she's not being so great now," I said.

"It'll work out if it's meant to be," he said. He'd shake his head and look up at the ceiling. "This fucking disease."

He couldn't help but feel that the whole mess was his fault. He felt guilty about everything—me, my mom acting crazy, Jessica—and I felt guilty that he felt guilty. It seemed like a turning point in the way he thought about his disease. Now it was clear how ALS was affecting all our lives.

My mom was a little more blunt about the situation. She liked Abby and had hopes that I'd marry her, but instantly turned on her when the breakup began. "You tell that little bitch to stop being a piece of shit," she said. "Do you want me to call her?" My mom would occasionally text or call Abby when she was out of her mind on Fentanyl.

"No, Mom, stay out of this one. It's none of your business," I pleaded.

"You're my Danny Boy. It is my business," she said. "I'll go out to Berkeley and shove that laser, or whatever the fuck she works on, right up her skinny little ass."

Even Stana decided to weigh in. "Danny, this girl, she is no good for you."

"I don't know, Stana. I think she's pretty good for me," I said.

"No, Danny. You have big heart, she have small heart. No big heart with small heart. Is no good match."

My dad and I both started to really focus on each other, trying our best to cheer each other up. Regina was around, but my dad needed as much help as he could get, so I continued to put everything I had into him for a while—hoping that it would take my mind off Abby—and he put everything he could give right back into me. The snow was finally starting to melt, so we'd go for long walks. We had a favorite route through our neighborhood. My dad even learned how to use his little remaining arm strength to steer the electric wheelchair himself. We'd talk about some of the best Jazz games we ever went to, or our favorite family vacations. Mine was when he took Greg and me to the 1992 NBA All-Star Game in Orlando—the one where Magic Johnson came back from HIV to win the MVP. We got to our Disney-themed hotel late at night, and the pool was closed. But my dad helped Greg and me break in. I remember thinking it was cool as shit that I had a dad who would break us into swimming pools. My dad's favorite vacation was when we drove our boat up to Camano to spend time with his mom and go crabbing. He really loved it up there.

But my unhappiness was apparent. When Tiffany, my mom, and I were unloading my dad from our van for a walk up at Red Butte Garden, I lost my shit. His chair had caught on a seat belt. I tried to unhook it, but couldn't, so I started tugging on the seat belt and screaming, "Motherfuckers!" as loud as I could. I followed up the "Motherfuckers!" with a string of expletives that would make the devil cringe. I think I actually flipped off the seat belt at one point and punched the floor of the van. I started to cry and melted to the ground. I was losing it.

Other garden-goers—who were undoubtedly expecting a pleasant break from the day-to-day bullshit—were horrified. I'm sure they thought, Should that unstable fat-ass really be caring for that dying man? I probably shouldn't have been. But what the fuck else was I supposed to do? I had a full-blown case of caregiver fatigue, combined with a splash of heartbreak.

Depression was consuming me. I was drinking alone in the basement while playing pinball, about a bottle of wine a night. On the plus side, I was getting pretty great at pinball.

I was darker and a little more morbid than usual. One afternoon, I was picking Chelsea up from school.

"How was your stupid day?" I asked Chelsea.

"Good," she said. "How was your stupid day?"

"It was shit. Everything is shit. Nothing matters anymore and everything turns to shit," I explained.

"Oh, okay." She nervously giggled. "Can we stop at 7-Eleven and get a Slurpee?"

"I don't see the point, but sure." So we got pointless Slurpees. I was too depressed to drink mine, so I dumped it in the sink.

I knew I'd officially lost it when I bare-knuckle-punched the respirator when it wouldn't stop beeping. After that, my dad suggested I go see their shrink, Robin. I did. Initially I didn't like her because I thought I was smarter than she was. But eventually she started to offer up some good advice.

"Why would you want to be with someone who doesn't give you support and love when you need it the most?" she asked.

"Because she's adorable. God, I miss her," I wanted to say, but instead said, "No, you're right. That's how I need to start to think about it. But I miss her."

"You sound depressed," she said.

"No shit, Sherlock," I wanted to say.

"Yeah, I know. Nothing a bunch of alcohol can't cure though, right?" I really said.

"Alcohol is actually a depressant. How much are you drinking?" she asked.

"Not that much. Maybe like a bottle of wine and a few beers a night," I said.

"That's over forty drinks a week," she said.

"Is that too many or too few?" I asked.

"Too many. Way too many." She prescribed me some Wellbutrin for the depression and advised I not mix it with alcohol.

I eventually decided that I could save my relationship with Abby if I really focused on it. I didn't want to lose the person I truly loved over this whole mess. I'm not the type who is built to fall out of love easily. I couldn't handle a full breakup right now. I asked Abby if I could come visit her in Berkeley so we could sort some stuff out face-to-face. I was tired of our relationship existing in this mysterious state. She agreed.

I booked a flight and planned our weekend. My goal was to win her back and get her to fall in love with me again. I made us reservations for Friday at a spa in San Francisco called the Nob Hill Spa. Here's what its Web site said about it:

> Retreat to an alluring sanctuary of indulgence and pampering at The Huntington Hotel—renowned among the best San Francisco spa hotels. Treat yourself to personalized service, rejuvenating massages and treatments, and captivating skyline views at our Nob Hill Spa. Follow a therapeutic steam or sauna with a refreshing swim in the mesmerizing infinity pool. Unwind in the fireside lounge, ideal for personal reflection. Select from a stellar complement of services . . . including massages, facials, body treatments, and manicures and pedicures. Let go of your stress and worry—and discover an incomparable oasis named by the *San Francisco Chronicle* as "one of the most luxurious spaces in the city."

It seemed like the sort of place that could help you win a girl back who didn't want to be with you anymore, or at least that's what I thought.

As the trip got closer and closer, I could tell Abby really didn't want me to come, but I didn't care. I had to see her. I remember telling everyone that I felt like I was flying off to my own execution—that I was setting myself up for something very painful and awful to happen. If this had been a slasher movie, you'd be going, "No, no. Don't do that. Don't go in there."

I still went. I landed in Oakland.

We had agreed that she would pick me up, so I was expecting her there at Oakland's awful airport in her shitty Volvo, but she was a no-show. She left me standing curbside with my sad little bags. I figured that I shouldn't go to her house, since she clearly didn't want to see me, so I called a few friends. They agreed that I could stay with them in San Francisco. I took BART into the city.

I called Abby a few times, but she didn't answer. I got drunk and went to bed around 9 p.m. And by "went to bed," I mean I passed out from too much alcohol.

The next morning, I awoke hungover, feeling like my soul and spirit were completely broken—I had hit a genuine rock bottom. I actually wanted to be back home with my dad. He was dying, but he still had a way of making me feel like everything was going to be all right. Instead, I was off in the Bay Area getting my heart all sorts of broken.

Abby was still not answering her phone. It was clear she didn't want to be reasonable or humane about this whole breaking-my-heart thing. She was off cowering in Berkeley, probably scared that I'd show up at her place. So what did I do? I decided to go out to Berkeley and show up at her place. Might as well make this painful for both of us. It wasn't fair that she got the easy way out.

Plus, I had this magical spa day planned. Remember? Today was the big day.

I started to justify my stupid behavior. Maybe her phone wasn't working. Maybe she couldn't find her charger. Maybe she had forgotten when my flight was landing. Maybe she loved me so much that she had planned an "I love you so much, Dan" surprise parade and party out in Berkeley, I thought.

I popped a Wellbutrin and headed to Berkeley. I got off the Berkeley BART only to realize that no "I love you so much, Dan" surprise parade was planned. I went to Abby's house. God, I felt like a stalker, or some sort of criminal. I felt dirty and trashy, like a loser. But I didn't know what to do or how to get some answers or conversation out of Abby, since she was clearly handling the breakup by just ignoring me.

I knocked on her door. She wasn't home. I called her, and she finally answered. She had been at the gym. I told her that surprise! I was in the neighborhood; that I wanted to talk to her. She agreed. We ran into each other on the street while still on the phone with each other. She was in her workout clothes. At least she hadn't lied about that.

The first thing she said to me was "You smell like booze."

"Thanks," I said. "Oh, and thanks for picking me up from the airport."

"Sorry, I had homework . . ." she said, avoiding eye contact.

I started to picture her side of the story as she sniffed the leftover booze on me. "So Dan just showed up, out of nowhere. He had clearly been drinking. Isn't he a weirdo stalker fuck?"

As we walked back to her place, Abby started yammering on and on and on about how she had gotten a B in one of her classes even though she had worked really, really, really hard. I wanted to tell her that I really didn't give a fuck about her B grade. I wanted to tell her to get a real problem, like the dying of a father or something. I tried to empathize with her and talk about how horrible it was that some evil professor would do that to her, but I was too distracted to not sound sarcastic and callous. I wanted to figure out what the fuck was up.

I pictured her side of the story, again. "I told Dan about my B— which I was really upset about—and he didn't even seem to care. He's such a selfish fuck."

We got back to her house. I honestly didn't know what to expect. She was still going on and on about her grade. She was clearly just delaying because she didn't want to have the hard and awkward breakup conversation.

We got into her room. I sat on her bed, half expecting sex. I finally interrupted her and asked, "So what's going on here?"

"With my B?" she asked.

"No, with us. I mean, I know you're upset about your grade, but can we talk about us for a minute? I flew out here because I thought we were going to figure this all out."

"Yeah, but I don't think there's anything for us to figure out. I'm not your girlfriend. We should date other people," she said, finally being blunt.

Boom. There it was. Until now, I had been holding out hope that we'd fix things and go back to the good life we had together. But it was official. We were done. The "break" had made way to the actual breakup.

Even though the logical part of me knew it was coming, everything hit all at once. Life was awful. Life was shit. I didn't know what to do or say, so I did something pretty awful. I turned into a crazy maniac. I grabbed her by the shoulders and pushed her onto the bed and held her there for a second. I then got up and thought about breaking her computer, but didn't.

I snapped out of it, thankfully.

I was instantly ashamed. I had lost control. To this day, I wish I could have that moment back. I didn't hurt her. It was just one of those moments when you want to grab someone who's not acting like themselves and shake them in hopes that they'll snap out of it and return to being who you knew them to be. But you just imagine doing that. I actually did it.

She was instantly terrified. I pictured her side of the story again. "Dan barged into my room and threw me around after I broke up with him. He's a violent and abusive motherfucker."

I had officially scared the shit out of her. She started to overreact. She was now crying and talking about calling the police. I imagined the police coming and me explaining what was happening from my perspective. "Well, Officer, first let me mention that my dad's dying back home in Utah. Abby and I had been dating for five years. She suddenly wanted space. We agreed on that. But she stopped answering my questions and never gave any sort of explanation as to what the status of our relationship was, to use a Facebook term. So I flew out here after she agreed to talk to me, and then she didn't pick me up at the airport, and I finally got here, and then she went on and on about some stupid-ass grade, then I asked her what was up with us, and she officially broke it off with me, so I sort of lost my shit for a half second and gently pushed her onto the bed."

"You're arrested, you crazy fuck," I imagined the police officer saying as he drew his gun.

I instantly apologized for scaring her and told her that I was just frustrated because I had flown all the way out here for information she could have given me over the phone. I was tired of being dicked around like this after a five-year relationship. I felt I deserved better. I was sorry. My pushing her remains a very shameful low point in my life.

I sat on her bed, still half expecting sex. She continued to cry and told me to get away from her. I did, but I still wanted to talk. She suggested that we go for a walk so we could be in public where I couldn't push her down on a bed.

We walked around Berkeley, our old stomping grounds—the location where we fell in love. I was absolutely devastated. I was in shock. We didn't really talk. When we did, I just tried to make her feel guilty and awful, which is a really great way to win a girl back.

Abby's father was really into Buddhism, and was one of the best people I've ever met—the type who would never do anything to deliberately hurt someone. I often used his perfect soul against Abby.

"So, what does your dad think about you dumping me while my dad's dying? Pretty disappointed in you?" I asked.

"Yep, really disappointed," Abby said, playing along.

"Yeah, I bet. He's a good person, so I bet he'd be disappointed by his own daughter doing something so heartless and shitty," I said, digging myself deeper and deeper.

"Yep, I'm a horrible person. I have no soul," she replied sarcastically.

I started to get emotional, almost crying. "Can't we just wait until my dad dies and then deal with this?" I pleaded. "The son of a bitch probably has like two more months. Can't you manage two more months of me being a miserable fuck?"

"I want to date other people now," she said wagging her perfect ass back and forth—an ass that I then imagined a bunch of cum-easy San Francisco yuppies enjoying. I knew that Abby would have an easy time finding someone else, whereas it would be a struggle for me. I mean, who would want to take on the responsibility of dating a fat, depressed budding alcoholic with an offbeat sense of humor? At least they probably wouldn't have to deal with in-laws, given the state of my dying parents.

As we walked around, I remembered that I had set up a spa day for us. I told her that I had ordered us surprise massages at the Nob Hill Spa, originally hoping they would be "Yay, we didn't break up" massages. We were supposed to be there by 2 p.m., but I guessed since we had just broken up that we weren't going. I took out my cell phone to cancel. "I got us nonrefundable massages, but I'm going to cancel," I said.

She stopped my dialing, the first time she had touched me since I started my crazy march on Berkeley. "Well, we can still go if you want," she said.

Still go? Are you fucking kidding me?

I didn't really know what to do, but I knew that I still wanted to ask her questions and spend time with her. I was still sort of in denial and holding out hope that she'd change her mind or something. Maybe the spa-day trick will actually work and she'll remember why she fell in love with me, I thought. God, I'm such a desperate and pathetic piece of shit, I also thought.

So I told her that we should still go, that we shouldn't let some stupid little breakup of a five-year-long relationship ruin our day.

We got into her car and headed into San Francisco, like some sort of happy couple. I didn't talk on the way there. I just stared out the window, fantasizing about jumping off the Bay Bridge. That'd be a good way to get her back, right? Jumping off a bridge? Boy, would she feel like shit if I did something that stupid and dramatic, right? As we drove she kept on saying that I was acting strange and sad.

"How the fuck am I supposed to act?" I wanted to say. Instead, I said nothing.

We arrived in the city, found some parking next to Grace Cathedral—one of those two-hour-time-limit spots—and walked to the Nob Hill Spa.

We arrived at their alluring sanctuary ready to be indulged and pampered. I gave the attendant our names and awkwardly mentioned that we just broke up, so we wanted masseuses who would be a bit easy on us. Our massages weren't for a little bit, so we were encouraged to enjoy the captivating skyline views or go for a refreshing swim. We did.

Breakups are weird because often the person getting broken up with starts basically acting insane, exhibiting horrible displays of self-pity and jealousy. Love is scary because of how crazy it can make you. It's totally irrational because it's not likely the other person's going to say, "Your insane behavior is making me feel like we're a perfect match! I really want to get back together with you!" It does the opposite. It pushes the other person further and further away and gives them more and more reasons to not be with you. "Hey, I just was thinking about slitting my wrists." "Oh, really. That's hot. I totally want to fuck you and have a family with you."

So, as we swam in Nob Hill Spa's mesmerizing infinity pool, I started acting like an insane person in order to get Abby back. I started loading water into my mouth and spraying it her way. Abby might be in control of this breakup, but she's at least going to get a little bit of pool water in her face, my crazy head thought, expecting her to say, "I love you," in return.

"Stop that," she really said.

A few weeks before my trip to Berkeley, I had gone out with some friends and met an attractive girl who I could tell wanted to hook up with me. But I decided against it because of how depressed empty sex was making me. Plus, Abby and I had started talking again. I loaded that bullet into my insanity gun and fired it.

"A few weeks ago I could have fucked a girl hotter than you, but I didn't," I said while doing the backstroke and squirting water up in the air, doing a perfect impression of a schizophrenic person who loved water and the backstroke. ·

"Who?" she asked, not really caring.

"I'm not telling you because you're a bitch," I said in a supersmooth tone—a real-life Don Juan.

Abby got out of the pool and went for a therapeutic steam in her locker room to hide from me. I decided to unwind in the fireside lounge, because apparently it was ideal for personal reflection, and I felt like a little personal reflection was necessary. While there, I decided that this was probably the worst day of my life. I pictured myself swan-diving off the spa's balcony and exploding into pieces on the hard pavement below. It was probably the first time in Nob Hill Spa's history that such things were thought by a person sitting in a nice robe in this meditative lounge.

It was time for our massages. We were supposed to have a couple's massage where we'd be in the same room so we could relax next to each other and maybe say "I love you" a couple thousand times while synchronizing our heartbeats. But, given the whole breakup mess, we decided to have our masseuses work on us in different rooms.

Normally, during a massage, I close my eyes and relax. I think about how everything will definitely be okay, and how the world is a peaceful, awesome place full of butterflies and rainbows and rainbows made of butterflies. But this time, my eyes were open and I could only think about how I would probably never see Abby ever again after this stupid spa bullshit. I thought about how much I loved her and how badly I wanted her to just love me back.

It's strange: when you've been with someone for a significant period of time, you start to paint this ideal picture of happiness, and that picture includes the other person. When a breakup occurs, it totally fucks that picture of happiness up, and it's stressful and awful to think about having to re-create the picture of happiness with someone else. It's also painful to think about the other person creating that picture of happiness with someone else, because you're fearful that that picture will end up looking just like the one you were hoping for, or better. You start to wonder whether your picture will ever even be achieved, and you start to feel like it was a miracle that you could even paint such a picture in the first place.

I also started to worry about Abby leaving me at this spa. The whole not-picking-me-up-at-the-airport bullshit had really hurt me, and I started to think that she'd probably weasel out of here as soon as her massage was over and leave me. I didn't want this to happen, because it would be too much grief and loneliness to take all at once. Loneliness is very, very painful when you're not used to it.

"Boy, you're really tense," my masseuse said.

"Yeah, I'm sorry. I'm just not relaxed today," I said.

"You okay?" she said.

"Yeah. Well. I don't know. My girlfriend just broke . . . My dad has . . . My mom is . . . My little sister just . . . Yeah, I'm fine," I said.

I then started to tear up. When someone asks if you're okay and you're not okay, it can open up a shitty floodgate. My eyes swelled up and a few tears hit the ground. This fucking sucks, I thought. I shouldn't have come here. I shouldn't have carried on with this stupid spa day. What the fuck was I thinking? The second Abby said, "We should date other people," I should have called her heartless, left, and never talked to her ever again. That's what I should have done, but that was the impossible thing to do. So here I was, crying while getting a massage, which is probably just about as pitiful as crying during sex.

I got up and told the masseuse that I was sorry and that I just couldn't do this right now, that it was me, it wasn't her, that she was great and would undoubtedly go on to give several great massages to more well-adjusted people, that I was the fucked-up one. I put on my robe and went to the locker room to cry a little bit more in the steam room.

I stayed in there for a long time, my tears blending with the steam. I wasn't just crying about Abby. I was slowly losing nearly everything that I loved. My dad was one of my favorite people and the rock in my life. And Abby had been the best thing to happen to me. She'd made me happier than anyone else ever had. I was going to have to figure out this world without two of the people most important to me. I was half expecting a call from a friend telling me that the Utah Jazz were being moved to Las Vegas or some shit.

I cried and cried. I wanted to go back to Utah to be with my dad.

Someone else finally entered the steam room, so I figured it was about time to get my shit together and start getting on with my life. I showered and dressed.

When I went out to the main spa area, Abby was nowhere to be found. I started to really panic. Did she leave? Was she already out there dating other people? Was that the last time I'd ever see her? Was my last interaction with the girl I loved going to be me floating around a pool squirting water in her face like an insane person?

I started asking around the spa. No one had seen her. I even had one of the female attendants go into the women's locker room and yell her name. She wasn't in there. She was gone. That was it. She had left me there. I was to be alone forever. I almost started to cry again.

Then she walked back into the spa, looking more beautiful than she ever had.

It felt like a miracle. I was so happy to see her that I finally cracked a smile on a day that was supposed to be smile free. I knew that she didn't want to be with me anymore and that love can't be forced. It was time to go our separate ways, but seeing her again—when I thought I never would—gave me some sort of hope in life, some sort of feeling that there would be ups after all the downs.

"I had to move my car. The two hours were up," she said, forcing a half smile.

"Oh, that's cool. Yeah, San Francisco parking is a bitch. I was just hanging out, enjoying the spa," I said, trying to hide the fact that I had just been casually crying and having panic attacks for the last two hours.

"How was your massage?" she asked.

"Oh, it was great. Yeah. Really relaxing. Deep. Sort of painful. But, you know, pretty great in the end," I lied, hoping the masseuse wouldn't come out just then and say, "There he is. There's the pathetic small-dicked bastard who cried during the massage. Let's get him."

"That's good," she said.

"Well, should we get the fuck out of this bubble of peace and relaxation? Get on with our lives?" I asked.

"Yeah, we've gotten all we can out of this thing," she said.

I smiled at her. "Yeah, I guess we have. Time to move on."

I was supposed to leave on Monday, but I decided to catch an earlier flight back. I got home and was greeted by Mazie and Berkeley, who jumped all over me and made me feel important. It was good to be back where I knew I'd be loved no matter what. I tossed my bag aside and ran upstairs to check on my dad.

"Hey, DJ!" he said as emphatically as the disease would allow him to. "How was your trip?"

"It was real garbage, Dad. We broke up. It's official," I told him. He got a little teary eyed and shook his head. He knew how much I loved Abby, what an important part of my life she was.

"That's too bad, DJ. But there will be other girls. Other fish in the sea," he said.

"I know, but I liked the fish I was fucking," I joked.

My dad laughed a little bit. "I know, DJ. I know. Seriously, you'll find someone even better than Abby, someone who deserves your love."

"Thanks, Dad," I said.

I believe that once you love someone that you always love that person a little bit, no matter the circumstances or the amount of time that's passed. The pain would lessen. I'd eventually move on. I'd meet someone else. I'd find someone who deserved my love. But I knew I'd always have some love for Abby.

"Bad timing, but I've got to take a shit," said my dad.

I helped him out of bed and onto the commode. It was like all the other shits he had taken before. But, for the first time, I could no longer say, "At least I have Abby."

THE DILDO SHOW

So I was back home trying to mend a broken heart. Nights were starting to get lonely, especially since I still wasn't very social. Sure, I'd go out every now and then, but I was mainly hanging around my dad. It sucks when you have a significant other you can talk to, and then suddenly don't. All the emotions build up, especially if you're spending your nights staring at your dying father.

Even though most of us don't admit to it, when you're in a relationship you keep a mental list of people you'd like to fuck if you were single—a little "fuck list," if you will. While I was with Abby, I certainly kept one. It consisted mainly of girls from college I wished I had hooked up with, and a few from high school. As I entered the lonely world of the single male loser in his mid-twenties, I did a quick mental scan of my fuck list and realized that most of the people either weren't in Utah or were in relationships.

But one who wasn't was Becca, my dad's best friend's daughter. Becca was also one of Greg's best pals. They had met in the first grade and had been close ever since. Most of Greg's friends were scared of me because of my bully ways, but Becca never was. Her parents were so focused on making her a good girl that she turned into a bad girl. She was sexy and wild. She had tattoos, she drank and smoked, and it was rumored that she had her clit pierced. A couple of Thanksgivings ago, she'd been giving me fuck-me eyes and trying to get me super drunk. I was with Abby then, so we didn't hook up. But I was single now, so I figured Becca might be interested in finally firing up a little fling.

But would it be shitty to make a play on one of my dad's friends' daughters? Would that secure me a place in hell? Would that make me some sort of filthy asshole with no chance of ever being a good person ever again?

Fuck it, I thought. I can't lose much more.

I decided to figure out how to contact her. Greg was always weird about me trying to hook up with his friends. So I used good old Facebook—the site started for creeps by our society's most successful creep, Mark Zuckerberg. I sent her a message saying that we should get a drink, catch up, hang out. She said that sounded nice. We set a time and arranged for a few other people to be there so it didn't seem like a date.

I picked her up, and we went to a bar in downtown Salt Lake. She was good at drinking. Probably even better than me. It's rare to see a girl who can really put it away. I was impressed. We flirted. I forgot how sweet she was. She had a big heart and a kind soul. I guess all the drinking and rebelling she had done over the years hadn't worn down that part of her. I was more and more into her as the night went on, and was thinking that it was looking pretty good. Fuck, she's pretty awesome. Maybe I should actually try to fall in love with her, I remember thinking.

However, after a few rounds, she started talking about a boyfriend. I hadn't realized she was in a relationship. She was going on and on about him. There's nothing worse than listening to someone you want to fuck talk about some other person who's actually fucking them. Once a girl starts talking about another guy, I assume it's over—a coded way of saying, "It's not going to happen, fat loser." So I just got drunk and cracked some jokes. Alcohol is always a nice silver medal to real intimacy.

After drinks and listening to boyfriend problems, I drove her home. She lived alone in a house by the University of Utah. Before she got out, she turned to me and said, "So, that boyfriend of mine, he's actually out of town at a weeklong bachelor party in New York."

"Oh," I said, thinking that there still might be a chance.

"You want to come in for a drink? I have Wii Bowling. It's fun," she said.

"Yeah, absolutely. Love Wii Bowling," I said, even though I had never played it.

Inside, she mixed up a couple of really strong drinks and fired up some Wii Bowling. We played a round. She was better than me. Drinking and Wii bowling: two things she was better at than me.

After the game, she set down the remote and hit me with a bit of a shocker. "Hey, have you ever tried ecstasy?"

"No, I haven't, actually," I said. Back in high school, the administration got word that ecstasy was really big with students at our school, so they made us all sit through several videos explaining how horrible ecstasy was for us. Though it was meant to scare us away from the drug, it made most of us want to try it. "I never even thought of doing it, but now I have to," I remember my friend Henry saying. One of the videos went into detail about how it puts holes in your brain. I'm not that smart, so I have to do everything I can to keep my brain intact. I decided then and there to never try it under any circumstance.

"Do you want to try some?" she asked.

"Nah, I told myself that I wouldn't ever do it. And putting holes in my brain isn't really my thing. I'm not that smart as is," I explained.

"Well, I want to do some. I don't mind the holes in my brain. I think it'd be fun," she said. "You sure?"

"Yeah. I'm sure. I shouldn't. But, by all means, you can do some. You have some here?"

She didn't, but her drug dealer was always up because he's a drug dealer. She called him. It was two in the morning, but he answered as if it was two in the afternoon. He said we could swing by and pick up a few pills. Becca hung up and said, "Let's go. I told him we'd need two of them, just in case you change your mind . . ."

I drove us around town trying to find this drug dealer. I shouldn't have been driving that drunk, but the chance of getting some action made it seem worth the risk. Becca had a vague recollection of where he lived, but we still drove around lost for about an hour. Finally, we got to the house and made the exchange. "Enjoy, kids," this loser said, assuming we were going to take them together and then probably fuck each other.

"Oh, I'm not taking any," I said.

"Yeah, right," he said and winked.

As I pulled back up to Becca's house, I got to thinking. I was so close to rock bottom that I was nearly at the center of the earth. My girlfriend had just left me because I was too sad. My dad was about to die. I didn't have a job. I lived in fucking Utah. The idea of taking a pill to make me artificially happy for a couple of hours sounded like an easy decision. Sure, it would put some holes in my brain and might ultimately make me a little sadder in the long run, and I'd be breaking a promise to myself . . . but sometimes you've got to live in the moment, as so many of those inspirational quotes and movies about being young teach us.

I said, "You know what? I think I'll live in the moment. Be young. So, I will have that pill of ecstasy. Sounds fun," I said. I felt like a nerdy accountant who decided that, after all these years, he was finally going to say fuck it all and cheat on his taxes.

"Great. All right. So a couple of ground rules. It's a very touchy-feely drug. We're going to want to touch each other."

"I'm cool with that," my horny, heartbroken ass said, not really caring that she had a boyfriend. I had never met this dude. We weren't friends. Fuck him.

"So we can do everything. We can kiss. You can grab at me and touch me. I can grab at you and touch you. We can even do a little oral if you're into that . . ."

"I'm into that," I interjected, sounding way too eager.

". . . But we can't have sex because I have a boyfriend."

The logic seemed a little off. Isn't kissing and grabbing and sucking at each other's bodies cheating? It is in my book. Guess everyone has a different definition.

"Yeah, of course. No sex. Wouldn't want to ruin a relationship," I said.

We shook on it. "It's a deal. Now let's do some drugs," I said, instantly realizing that that's probably not something people who actually do drugs say.

We went inside, crushed up the pills, cut them into lines, and snorted them into our bodies. Until then, I didn't know that you could snort ecstasy. You probably can't. I had tried weed and cocaine a couple of times, but wasn't a big drug user, aside from all the alcohol I was always drinking. But I figured that Becca knew what she was doing, since she had apparently done it a bunch.

"So what do we do now? Just dance around and suck on pacifiers until the sadness comes back?" I asked, already feeling like a crazy, drugged-out loser.

"Lie down on the carpet over there and I'll give you a back massage," said crazy, drugged-out Becca.

"That sounds perfect," said crazy, drugged-out Dan.

I took off my shirt and lay on the carpet. The carpet felt nice and soft and relaxing—like home before all the dying-parents nonsense. I loved the feel of it, and sort of wanted to roll myself up in it and live there for a couple of years.

Becca sat on my ass. She squirted a little lotion on my back. It felt as if the lotion was going to help make my skin be the best it could be. She started rubbing it in. And Jesus Christ. I'm not one to be like, "Hey, try drugs," but try this drug if you haven't. It's probably worth the brain damage. Because I don't know that I've ever felt better. It felt like a million blow jobs in the best part of heaven. It seemed, for a second, that everything was going to be okay. Sure, my dying dad was dying and my heart was smashed to shit, but I had ecstasy in my body and Becca's smooth hands working up and down my fat, naked back. Life couldn't really be that bad, right?

I reached back and started rubbing what I could reach of Becca. I think it was her leg. I rubbed that for a bit, then flipped over and we started making out as if we had to do it to survive. I got her naked. She got me naked. We were just two naked people on ecstasy, not saying a word, just exploring each other's bodies like it was our first time touching one.

Okay, put your dicks away. Let's not get too pornographic here.

Just kidding. Let's do.

I was so hard it felt like my cock was going to launch off my body and burst through the wall, then the neighbor's wall, then the neighbor's neighbor's wall, then it would continue on like that forever until it blew up a small mountain somewhere in China. I pressed it against her body. She pressed her body against it. It was as though we were trying to jam that thing into her by just pushing it against her, like we were two idiots who had never been taught how to properly fuck.

We rubbed and poked and licked around for a bit, then Becca suggested that we go to the bedroom. I thought that sounded like a great idea, so I said, "That sounds like a great idea. God, ecstasy is pretty awesome."

"Remember, no sex. I have a boyfriend."

"But my dirty tongue was just on your clit," I wanted to say.

I had heard some rumor that if you had an orgasm while on ecstasy it would feel so great that you wouldn't be able to have another orgasm ever again. That sounded pretty terrifying. My dad was about to die. The thought of never having another orgasm after tonight sounded like no way to live. I better not cum, I thought. Fuck, I'm so happy and everything will probably work out! I also thought.

We crawled up on her bed and plopped down on there like a couple about to make a sex tape that no one would want to watch because we're just a couple of okay-looking losers and my dick isn't that big.

As we made out and did everything but sex, I started to get a little light-headed. All the booze combined with all the ecstasy seemed to be catching up with me. I'm not going to be one of those assholes who accidentally overdoses, am I? I thought. Can you even overdose on ecstasy? I also thought, trying to remember all those warning tapes from high school.

"I need to take a break. I'm not feeling great," I told Becca as she rubbed one of her nipples along the tip of my cock.

She stopped. I had ruined the moment.

Becca grabbed me a glass of water and I chugged it like some sort of depraved prisoner. She refilled and I chugged again. I started to feel better. Becca curled up next to me and tried to do a little making out. I said that I just needed to lie here for a minute and focus on staying alive. She said, "Well, do you mind if I keep going?"

"Yeah, fine by me," I said.

Now, I didn't know what she meant by "keep going" at first, but then I knew right away when she pulled out a large pink dildo from her bedside dresser drawer. She gave it a lick like I'd seen in all those pornos I'd studied over the years, clicked on the vibrator switch, and pushed it against her.

I didn't know what to do, so I just watched and jerked myself off a little. We kissed. I eventually took over the controls of the dildo and glided it in and out of her until she came. Apparently she wasn't worried about the orgasm-on-ecstasy rule.

There was nothing left to do but cuddle.

We drank more water and started to recover a little bit. Though we had connected physically, we also started to connect emotionally. I realized that she was an exceptionally special person. We had been around each other throughout our lives. We had gone to the same schools. We had had Thanksgiving and Christmas dinners together. But in all that time, we had never really gotten to know each other.

"It's weird growing up alongside someone but never really knowing them," I said.

"Yeah, for sure. I guess we all need to be more aware of our surroundings instead of focusing on all the stupid little things," she said.

We clung to each other, getting sad when the other had to get up and go to the bathroom or grab more water. We were connected for that moment. It's rare to feel that way. And it's a great feeling. Like natural ecstasy, which feels even better when you're actually on ecstasy.

We kissed and talked. I said that I felt guilty about all this because I could tell that she cared about her boyfriend. She said not to feel guilty because it probably wouldn't work out between them. I guess he was an asshole who didn't treat her right. Guess if he treated her right she wouldn't be blowing lines of E and having her not-boyfriend rub his tiny cock up and down her and push a pink dildo in and out of her.

We started talking about our dads. I told her how much her dad meant to mine, and how I thought my dad had never had a true "best" friend until he came along. They had run thousands of miles by each other's side, talking about everything they could think to talk about along the way. Fuck, I bet they even felt as connected as Becca and I at the peak of our ecstasy binge, though I doubt they had ever lain next to each other masturbating. Maybe we were actually closer.

Becca said how sad the whole mess with my dad was. She wondered why bad things happen to good people. I said that I didn't know, and that not much seems to make sense when we think about the big questions. Maybe that's why we focus on those little things. They seem to make a little more sense than the randomness in our endlessly large universe.

We lay there all night. I had put on my boxers at some point, because I don't like people seeing my gross penis if I can avoid it. And she had slipped on some sexy black and red nightie, probably meant for her boyfriend to enjoy on Valentine's Day or something. We didn't sleep. We just rubbed each other and talked, breathed, lived. It was like a spiritual experience. Though I've never had one of those, so maybe it wasn't. But it felt like more than the usual day-to-day grind.

The sun came up and all the people who weren't up all night doing drugs and pushing sex toys into their bodies started their busy days filled with distractions. Becca's boyfriend called, asked what she was up to.

"Not much. Just getting up. Going to work soon," she said. Man, she was good at covering shit up. I had the urge to grab the phone and say, "I nearly fucked your girlfriend, but didn't, but will if you're not better to her." Instead, I just stayed quiet and let Becca be okay with her lies.

The ecstasy and alcohol had worn off, and I was just back to my tired old sad self. I needed to get home and get some sleep, or I was going to probably die. I dressed and kissed Becca good-bye. "What a night," I said.

"Yeah, I know. Exhausting, but fun," she said.

"It sure was," I said. "Really special. Thank you."

"Don't be a stranger anymore," she said.

"Our dads are best friends, and we did ecstasy together, so that's impossible."

I drove home, checked on my dad. He was still alive. Regina was already there, already taking care of him. I went to bed in the dark basement and dozed off with the image of dancing dildos in my head, not knowing what I had done, but knowing that it had really hit the spot.

FATHER'S DAY

How are you supposed to spend Father's Day with your dad when there's a good chance it will be his last? I didn't know. With my dad in his current state, every day was Father's Day. He was the main focus. What was I supposed to do? Wipe his ass better? Suction the secretions out of his lungs with more precision? Turn on the TV for him with more spunk?

I wanted this Father's Day to run smoothly. I envisioned a perfect day. My dad would no longer have Lou Gehrig's disease. He would be healthy and plump like a king. His hair would be brown and combed to the side—a style that symbolized that everything was in order. The Jazz would have just finished beating the Jordan-led Chicago Bulls in the finals and Scottie Pippen's head would have exploded in the process. My mom would accompany us with a full head of hair flowing well past her shoulders. She would look young and full of the charisma that made all her children such interesting, funny, modest people.

We would be in a Suburban driving up a canyon, which, despite it being June, decided to decorate itself in fall colors and turn the temperature to seventy-two. The windows would be down and the wind would flap through our hair. My dad would sit in the driver's seat. "Heaven," by Talking Heads, would blare. Our two golden retrievers would sit on my mom's lap and hang their heads out the passenger-side window, letting the acceleration of the car dictate the position of their tongues. Slobber would stream from their mouths and hit Greg—who would be sitting with his head out the window in the backseat—in the face. We would all laugh uproariously and Greg would wipe the slobber off, realizing that nothing matters but being together. Tiffany would laugh uncontrollably and tell us that she was laughing so hard that she might piss herself. Greg and I would egg on the laughter by singing, *"Don't go chasing waterfalls . . . please stick to the rivers and the lakes that you're used to."* The song would finally bring the piss out of Tiffany. Chelsea and Jessica would braid each other's hair in the back of the car and talk about how they would be friends forever, no matter what. My dad would have a fat smile on his fat face, knowing that he's done it, that he's created a functional family that will go on to create more functional families.

Cut back to reality. It's the morning of Father's Day. I'm walking through the Utah heat wearing a worn-out 1992 NBA All-Star T-shirt with caricatures of the ten starters that I took from my dad because what's he going to do? Stand up and hit me? My jeans have unintentional holes in the left knee and the back right pocket. I'm barely able to walk because I'm wearing white slippers I stole from the Four Seasons on a family vacation back when things were good. I haven't showered or combed my hair. The effects of gin and tonics stab my brain. I look like a criminal.

I shake my head in self-loathing, knowing that my dad has been expecting me to hang out with him and take him for a long walk up Millcreek Canyon—one of the few places he can still frequent in his 450-pound chair.

To top it all off, I'm fresh off sleeping with Becca. I hadn't seen her since our ecstasy adventure a couple weeks earlier, but she came over last night to hang with Greg. We all got drunk. We all went swimming. It just happened. She was still with her boyfriend. I felt guilty.

I had just driven Becca home in my mom's car. On my way back to my house, I ran out of gas. I had been driving the thing on empty all weekend, assuming that luxury vehicles don't ever run out of gas—that they run on being better than everyone else or something. I had a cell phone, but I had been too busy fucking Becca to think about charging it. It was deader than my dad was going to be. I was only about a mile or so from Becca's house, so I walked back to it.

I arrived. "My fat ass ran out of gas. I'm sure a dumb, unemployed motherfucker with a dick that most non-Asian girls would consider small. Well, you know. It was inside you last night," I wanted to say.

"I ran out of gas because I'm a big fat idiot," I really said.

She drove me to a gas station. I filled up and fed my thirsty car as sweat and apologies poured out of me. In the process, I accidentally poured some gas on my pants and hands. "I'm a fucking shithead," I said aloud.

Perfect way to start off Father's Day.

After filling up, I sped home, yelling at myself the whole way. "Dan, you're a fucking asshole. What were you thinking? That was pretty great sex, though, wasn't it? She's a real sweetheart. I think I actually like her."

I pulled into our driveway, having just done a number on my self-worth.

"Hey, Dad. Happy F. Day," I said, bursting into the room, hoping my mom wouldn't notice the combined stench of gasoline, sex, sweat, and self-defeat I radiated.

My tired mom—who had spent the night with our dad while Greg and I and our friends poured gin on our brains and puffed nicotine into our lungs—didn't take note of my appearance or tardiness but instead said, "Can you get him up so I can change his sheets?"

"Anything for my father on Father's Day," I said.

I walked over to his bed and pulled his limp body up to a sitting position.

"How are you doing?" I asked. His cuff was inflated. He couldn't talk. He just nodded and gave a shrug.

"Well, that's good. What you been up to?" I asked. He gave me a what-do-you-think-I've-been-up-to-given-the-fact-that-I-can't-move-my-own-body look.

I straightened the shirt that hung loosely from his bony shoulders and reached over to a nearby dresser to grab his gait belt. As I began to lift him from the bed and onto the recliner, my mom began peeling the wrinkly sheets from my dad's sticky hospital bed. She seemed too tired to give a shit about anything but getting those sheets off. I was thankful. Then it seemed to hit her.

"So, did you sleep with Becca last night?" she asked casually.

I was so shocked by the question that I lost strength in my arms and dropped my dad to the floor. Happy Father's Day! He lay there screaming in pain, but since he was on the trach no words came out. It was just a facial expression.

"That's none of your fucking business, Mom," I said.

"I know, but did you fuck her? We know she slept over," she said.

"Mom, stop. You're being nosy," I said.

"I'm just kidding," she said.

"Help me get Dad up. It's Father's Day and he's lying in pain on the floor," I said.

"But seriously, did you fuck her?" she asked again.

"Mom. Stop it," I said. I didn't want to get into this. I mean, my dad probably would've been fine with it, but I still didn't want to talk about it with him.

"I'm just joking," she said. "But did you?"

"Yeah, all right. I slept with her," I said, finally giving in. "Guilty as charged."

My mom smiled big, forced a high five onto me, and said, "Good, maybe you'll get over that bitch Abby faster."

My dad was still on the ground like a 130-pound sack of bones. He was too heavy for my mom and me to lift, so I told her to get Greg, who was fresh off fucking his new boyfriend down the hallway of our once normal house. He had started dating a Mormon named Kevin. They'd met on one of those fuck sites for gay people: manhunt.com, or gay.com, or Craigslist. Kevin had acted straight his whole life, even going as far as marrying a woman for a bit. He finally broke free and now found himself fucking the son of a dying man. In addition to being a gay Mormon, Kevin was also a chef and would cook for us. I was so sick of lasagna and Stana's potato salad by now that any new food was welcome. He made these croissants filled with ham and cheese that my fat ass loved. He was surprisingly comfortable around my dad, and would even help with some of his care. I liked Kevin.

"Greg, get your ass in here. This is an emergency," my mom piercingly yelled, using all the strength in her cancer-filled body.

Greg came stumbling in after five or six more yells, wearing a robe. "He better be on the brink of death for you to yell like that," he said.

Greg noticed that Dad was on the floor and finally reacted like it was an emergency. Dropping our dad on the ground was about the worst, most painful thing we could put him through at this stage. He looked as uncomfortable as I've ever seen him. His eyes were watery. Happy Father's Day!

As we were pulling him off the ground—which required that Greg, my mom, and I lift with all our strength—I began brainstorming ways we could prevent this in the future. "We absolutely need to have more people now. Dad's legs are weaker. He can't stand on his own," I said.

I knew the Hoyer lift was the next option. A Hoyer lift is a gallows-shaped device that patients can be harnessed into and lifted from bed to chair, from chair to bed, from bed to coffin, etc. But he didn't want to use one. When you have an illness that slowly starts destroying all the things you used to be able to do, you begin hanging on to whatever you have left. He had said good-bye to eating, to walking, to talking, to scratching his own nose, to turning on the TV and watching whatever he wanted, to fucking, to driving, to picking up his kids from school, to wearing boxers instead of diapers, to being treated like a father rather than a hospital patient. The Hoyer lift would symbolize that things had gotten about as bad as they would get, that the disease had won, that there wasn't any fight left in his dying body.

I didn't think I should mention it. I knew that it was Father's Day, and that that was the last thing he wanted to hear, especially since both of his sons reeked of sex. I mentioned it anyway. "We should start looking into getting you a Hoyer lift," I said. I looked over at my dad. He had defeat in his eyes.

"No way. If it's time for a Hoyer lift, it's time for you to go," Greg said. Greg was becoming more blunt, more callous as this situation evolved.

"Jesus, Greg. It's fucking Father's Day. Can we have one day where we don't talk about death?" I said.

"I know. What I meant to say was, 'I love you, Daddy, and don't want you to die. Not today, at least,'" Greg said, giving him a kiss on his forehead.

After we got my dad back into the chair—a position in which his face no longer grimaced—I turned on the TV. Tiger Woods was leading the U.S. Open and was playing with a hurt knee. Many of the highlights from the Saturday round showed Tiger crumpling to the ground in pain after smacking the ball three-hundred-some-odd yards. He had eagled the eighteenth hole and was three under par heading into the final eighteen at Torrey Pines. I turned to my dad.

"Goddamn. That Tiger is amazing. I can't believe what a fighter he is. I mean, to have a sore knee and still be winning one of the most prestigious tournaments on one of the hardest courses in the world. My God. He has gone through so much and still remains strong," I said.

My dad looked at me as if he had just watched a sample clip from the Biggest Asshole in the World awards ceremony.

Here my dad was—having been thrown the biggest curve ball of all, having gone from being a marathon runner to a permanent hospital patient, having gone from breathing on his own to not—and his son was marveling at Tiger Goddamn Woods's fucking golf performance.

And the winner for biggest asshole in the world is: Dan Marshall, for his Father's Day Tiger Woods rant!

Later in the day, Greg finally drove his boyfriend home. I showered the sex and gasoline smells off me. My mom went to sleep, curling up in her bed with our cat Brighton. Chelsea had left for a dance camp in Boise, Idaho, so she was gone for a while, but Tiffany came over, as did Jessica. She and Creepy Todd were now living together in Todd's parents' basement. She was about to leave for Thailand with him. They were trying to "bring lacrosse to the girls of Thailand because many of them don't get to exercise," in her new husband's words. If marrying her wasn't bad enough, he was now taking our Jessica halfway around the world to start a girls' lacrosse league. To top it off, Jessica had just announced that she was already pregnant. She was officially cementing herself into this shitty situation. And all my dad could do was watch.

Overall, it was a pretty dismal showing for what would probably be our dad's last Father's Day.

Eventually Greg, Tiff, and I decided to turn things around and drive my dad up Millcreek Canyon for the walk we had promised. Jessica decided not to come. She needed to rest since she had a Mormon growing inside of her now. She went back to her new home. Greg, Tiff, and I loaded my dad into the van. Greg was singing Disney songs to emphasize how nonchalantly we were approaching Father's Day this year.

Tiffany sat shotgun and I drove. Tiffany dove right in. "So I heard you slept with Becca last night," she said.

"Yeah, so what?" I said.

"I just think that's an interesting choice. I think she's into drugs, and doesn't she have her clit pierced or something?" Tiffany said.

"Those are rumors. Please, just leave me alone. And leave her alone. She's a sweet girl," I said, flashing back to our amazing ecstasy night.

"Was she good?" Tiffany asked, not letting it go.

"She fucks like a racehorse," I said as I adjusted the rearview mirror to see if my dad was catching all of this. He was.

"Fucks like a racehorse? What does that even mean?" asked Tiffany.

"I'm not really sure," I admitted.

Greg was a little uncomfortable with Becca and me hooking up. He knew Becca had a boyfriend and didn't want either of us to get involved in a sketchy situation. So he wasn't a proponent of Becca's and my budding relationship. Becca had apparently told him about the ecstasy night, so I was always on edge that he would bring it up anytime Becca was the subject of conversation. I didn't want my dad knowing that I had not only fucked her, but had also done illegal drugs with her.

"Becca's not really your type," Greg said.

"What do you mean?" I asked.

"She's not a blond bitch like Abby," he said.

"Listen, why don't you assholes just stay out of my life, okay?" I demanded.

We arrived at the parking lot at Millcreek Canyon. A handicap parking spot was available! We are so lucky sometimes, you guys! Several other families were also treating their fathers and grandfathers to some nice, fresh air. But all those families could go fuck themselves. That's right, go fuck yourselves, families—what with your fully functioning fathers, and your smiles, and your laughter, and your hiking boots, and your backpacks. The only thing hanging from our father was a thirty-pound breathing machine. But we loved him more than they loved their dads. We had proved that through the constant care we gave him: all the hospital visits, all the feedings, all of everything. We had poured our lives into keeping him going. We were way better kids than they were. Fuck those other families and fuck their stupid, shitty dads.

Toward the top of Millcreek, there is a road that's closed to cars. It's big and wide open. This is our family spot. During the previous summer, my mom and dad would walk our dogs up there every night. When I was growing up, we'd often celebrate Marshall family events by hiking in the canyon, enjoying the mountains, and letting Berkeley and Mazie run in and out of the swift-moving river. The dogs would shake off right in front of us and ensure we couldn't get mad by flashing us big smiles. Assholes.

We steered my dad's chair onto the road and began heading up. It wasn't the Suburban voyage up the canyon that I had been imagining, but it was nice to get some fresh air and to talk to Dad.

I envisioned us being treated to some words of poignant wisdom from our dad. I imagined him solving all our personal problems with a simple logical statement. I envisioned us all stopping in front of some shit-eating family and circling our dad for the world's longest and loudest "I love you, Dad" chant. I envisioned a lot of hugs, a lot of shoulder rubs. Fuck, maybe we'd get halfway up the mountain and it would turn out that the fresh air and togetherness was the perfect mixture needed to cure Lou Gehrig's disease. That's it. He was going to walk back down this mountain. We would push his chair into the river and, later on, he'd come walking up here with my mom and watch as the dogs ran into the river to play on the chair as if it were a toy instead of a device used to get my dad's limp body around town.

My daydream was interrupted by Tiffany's scream. "Fuck, you ran over my toe! Shit, that hurt." We stopped. My dad wanted to be deflated so he could talk. This was the start of the miraculous turnaround, I thought. He was going to give his triumphant speech. Tiffany deflated him, even with the hurt toe.

"The chair is running out of batteries fast. We should turn around and head back," my dad struggled to say. Fuck. We hadn't properly charged the chair, so it had run out of battery power. We had to turn back. We were epic shitheads, and on Father's Day. I had wanted to use the day to show how much we really did love and appreciate him. I wanted to show him that we didn't mind caring for our pal, because he had spent so much of his life caring for us. I wanted the day to be a reflection of how great we were capable of being, instead of how shitty the situation had made us. Oh well.

We got my dad back home and charged the wheelchair battery. We then took him outside to our gazebo. The gazebo had always been my dad's favorite spot on our property. It was surrounded by cottonwood trees and flowers, providing a perfect home for chirping birds during the day and crickets at night. It was where my dad had his grill, where he'd sip wine, watch the dogs play around in the yard, and think about his day while cooking food for his selfish family. During the summer, we'd eat just about every dinner out there. Dinners were important to my dad, the one time we were all together, free from distraction. My dad missed these dinners, not for the food—though I'm sure he would've loved taking down a steak—but for the unity and order they brought us.

My mom woke from her nap and joined us out on the gazebo. She always made a big deal of every holiday, even silly ones like Father's Day. Usually they were filled with gifts and cakes, but she only had the energy for a card this year. We all signed the card. It had a picture of a bear on it and it read, "Hi Daddy, Can you guess who's my hero? I'll give you a clue—He's strong and he's brave." *[Open card to reveal another, taller bear wearing a cape.]* "He's the best Daddy—you. Happy Father's Day." I thought it was weird as fuck. It was clear my mom had picked it out when she was wandering around high on Fentanyl. Our selfish asses should've gone to pick out the card instead of sending our poor mom to do it.

But the card was true. He was brave. He was strong. And he was a hero. This had been the worst year of our lives (so far). We were all tired and on edge and sick of thinking about death. We wanted our old lives back. We wanted to be brought together by dinner around the gazebo table instead of by a terminal illness. But had my dad not been brave enough to go on the respirator, he'd be gone. His heroic act gave us the gift of time together. Had he elected to not extend his life, I would've been in Los Angeles or San Francisco. Greg would've been in Chicago. Tiff probably would've been in Maine with BCB. But we were here, circled around our dad, spending time with him and with each other. Sure, most of that time was spent taking little digs at each other about the people we were fucking or the life decisions we were making, but time is time, regardless of how it's spent.

After reading the card, my dad smiled at all of us. He asked to be deflated so he could talk.

"Thanks. You've all been the best kids I could ask for. This hasn't been an easy year, but it's been so nice spending time with each of you," my dad managed to say in his respirator voice. We smiled back at him. Tiff took one hand. Greg took the other. I stood behind him and rubbed his shoulders. My mom ate yogurt.

It was a nice moment.

I didn't know what to say, so I said, "Pretty weird Greg's fucking a gay Mormon, am I right?"

"At least I'm not doing ecstasy and fucking a girl with a boyfriend," said Greg.

My dad smiled, enjoying his time with his family. Our imperfect Father's Day was perfect.

THE END OF THE
HOPE CAMPAIGN

By early July, we were nearly eight months into life with the respirator. We were living out the hope campaign, the full never-give-up package my mom had outlined at the Marshall Family Christmas Summit—a night that now seemed as if it had happened twenty years ago. As the summer progressed, my mom really stepped up. Sure, she'd have moments of panic where she'd break down and cry and talk about how she couldn't do this anymore, how she missed how things used to be before my dad got sick. And sure, she'd have glimmers of insanity, like when the respiratory nurse, Jeff, was joking about how fat he was and my mom said, "You want to see fat, look at this," and proceeded to pull her pants down, flashing her ass to the poor kindhearted Mormon. And sure, she was addicted to her Fentanyl patches the way a heroin junkie's addicted to the needle. But her hair was back. She'd learned how to work the respirator. She was active all day. She slept next to my dad every night, meaning Greg or I didn't have to do nighttime Daddy Duty anymore. Her spirits were up. She was doing pretty well.

This had been her plan all along—to get healthy enough to take care of my dad for a long, long time. But my siblings and I were starting to wonder how realistic this vision was. My dad was still getting a little worse every day. Unlike Vince Senior from the support group, my dad didn't seem to be plateauing. And even if he did eventually, how long were we going to do this? Was I destined to become Vince Junior? Vince Junior was, like, forty and still taking care of his father. Was this going to last another fifteen years?

Greg and I didn't know if we should start thinking about our futures or if this was a long-term situation. We felt that our lives were on pause for now—that we couldn't fully focus on ourselves until this nightmare was completely over. Everything was centered around my dad's health. Lou Gehrig's disease was still in the driver's seat.

Greg and I would hang out in the basement talking about all this, Greg with a cup of OJ and me with a glass of wine. Our basement was full of hobo spiders during the summer, so I'd kill a few as we talked. Greg was terrified of spiders, so he'd sit on the stairs and point them out.

"How long do you think Dad's going to do this for?" I asked as I whacked a defenseless spider with a pool cue.

"Oh my God, that was a big one," he said.

"That's what he said," I said.

"Not funny, and I don't know how long he's going to do this. Dad might outlive us . . . Oh my God, look at that one in the corner." I walked over and crushed another poor spider.

"It certainly seems that way," I said.

"We're going to be forty and still caring for him, like Vince Junior," he said.

"You're probably right. We'll have kids by then who'll help us change his diaper."

"Yeah, oh man . . . Holy shit, another one!" screamed Greg.

My mom was optimistic that she and my dad were both going to live a long, long time. "I'm great doing this for the next twenty years," she said.

But that's not what my dad seemed to want. He was starting to lose hope. He was aware of the reality that he wasn't getting any better, that, in fact, he was only getting worse. There are winners and losers in every battle, and so far, Lou Gehrig's disease is undefeated. My dad knew this, even if my mom was trying to convince him otherwise. She'd try to push optimism down his trachea like fresh air.

"At least you can still talk," she'd say. But his speech was becoming more and more labored, and he was harder and harder to understand.

"At least you can still stand for a couple of seconds." But his trusty legs were too weak to hold him up. We'd gotten the Hoyer lift to get him in and out of bed.

"At least you have your communication device." But his communication device was a piece of shit. The technology just wasn't there yet, and my dad seemed to have no real interest in trying to learn how to control the thing with a silver dot on his forehead, especially since he could still talk. It mainly functioned as a tool I used to tell blow job jokes to visitors.

"At least we can make your respirator portable so you can go outside occasionally." But it was such a hassle, and it's hard to adjust to life being that difficult when going outside used to be as simple as twisting a doorknob.

"At least you have a comfortable wheelchair to get around in." Good point. He couldn't argue with that one. That wheelchair did kick some major ass. What a dream!

Dad was also wearing down mentally. He had never been a consistent crier. He had always had a positive, "Life is so great. Let's make the most of it" attitude, but this situation had finally gotten to him. He was now either crying or on the brink of it almost all the time.

"Oh, come on, Dad. Let's not resort to being a baby about this," I would joke as he cried. "So you can't move your body. Boo-fucking-hoo."

But my dad wasn't amused. It wasn't funny anymore. It was the first time in my life I had actually seen him depressed. His shrink, Robin, was now making house calls. I wouldn't sit in on these sessions, but I could hear them talking through the door. I'd stand there like an asshole listening in. He would cry to her and tell her that he didn't know how much longer he could do this. She would console him and tell him how brave he was.

"I'm not brave. I don't know how much longer I want to live," I heard him say. Poor guy couldn't handle the hopelessness of Lou Gehrig's. He wanted the pain to end.

It was a Sunday. Regina hadn't been around that weekend, which meant that we had to do all the care. My mom was still having issues with Regina. She was convinced that Regina—having a broken heart from her divorce—had fallen in love with my dad. She probably had. My dad's pretty lovable. She would sit next to my dad holding his hand and talking about all her relationship problems. My dad was a great listener, mainly because he couldn't go anywhere. My mom was jealous and hated everything about Regina. I thought it was sort of adorable that my mom was still protective of her husband, even though he was glued to a hospital bed and near death—I took it as a sign of true love.

"That fat bitch Regina isn't here, so what do you want to do today?" my mom asked my dad. He just shrugged. He didn't give a fuck. He looked like a mountain of miserable sadness lying in a pile of grief and hopelessness.

Eventually, Greg, Chelsea, my mom, and I decided to get my dad out of the house and go up to our Park City condo. Jessica was in Thailand with Creepy Todd, and Tiffany was vacationing with BCB.

We figured we'd lie out by the pool and let ourselves be distracted enough to not think about death for an afternoon. You know, act like rich people without a care in the world, ignoring all tragedy to focus on relaxing. Making sure we applied enough sunscreen to preserve our white skin would be our biggest concern. It would be like nothing bad had ever happened to us, or was ever going to.

We made the thirty-minute drive up Parley's Canyon to Park City and got situated in the condo. We hung inside for a few minutes, mainly to just marvel at how nice it was. I slipped on a robe, feeling like the king of some castle I didn't deserve.

"I love being a rich asshole," my rich asshole ass said.

We eventually made our way outside to the communal pool. I brought a few beers and stuffed them in the robe pockets, because that seemed like the thing normal, carefree rich people would do. Greg brought a book and lounged in the sun close to my dad. Chelsea brought some of those pool noodles that look like giant cocks. We sword-fought with them on the pool's edge.

We got my dad all set up in the shade. I downed a beer and dove into the pool, trying to be active and full of life. My mom sat at my dad's side, gulping down yogurt. They watched me splash around like a degenerate alcoholic with his brain turned to mush by wealth. Chelsea jumped in the water with me. I smacked her in the face with a pool noodle. She giggled and then went to sit in the hot tub, trying to put some distance between herself and her bully.

I got out and sat in a chair near my dad, letting the warmth from the sun and the light mountain breeze dry me. I popped open a fresh beer. I felt great.

"What a dream it is up here," I said, looking around. "Glad you rich assholes bought this place for your rich asshole kids to enjoy."

I glanced over to my dad to watch his reaction, as I do after most attempts to make people laugh. He usually forced a supportive smile, but this time he looked like he could win a contest for being the sad-dest person on earth.

"Shit, Dad, you look like you're going to explode with sadness," I said, taking a slug from my beer, looking like I was going to explode from alcohol.

"Bob, what's the matter?" my mom said, also taking notice.

My dad's cuff was inflated, so he couldn't talk.

"Answer me, Bob," my mom yelled.

"His cuff is inflated. He can't talk," I said.

"Oh, shit. Sorry," my mom said.

He mouthed a few words. We tried to read his lips, but that never really worked, so we deflated his cuff. Air began to pass over his vocal cords.

As he cleared his throat, my mom said, "What do you want, Bob? Can I get you something?"

"I . . . want . . . to . . . die," he said.

And there it was.

All the work, all the energy, all the attempts to still make life man-ageable, had led to this conclusion. He wanted to die.

Every life ends in death. There's not one that hasn't. We knew it was coming, but still, to hear the words gave it a reality that was previously incomprehensible.

"I want to die," he repeated, this time with more assurance. The respirator hummed and the hot tub churned out bubbles. Greg set down his book. Chelsea got out of the hot tub. We all circled around him. My dad's eyes watered up, and a couple of tears found their way out.

"You don't mean that," my mom cried. Being such an advocate of hope all these years, she had never heard these words uttered, or probably even thought them. In my mom's mind, it wasn't supposed to happen like this. This story wasn't supposed to end with my dad's giving up. It was supposed to be a fight to the very last moment, to the moment when there was absolutely nothing more to fight with.

"I do mean it. I want to die," he said. "I can't do this anymore."

"Well, it's about time," said Greg, trying to make a joke of the situa-tion.

"I'll care for you for the rest of my life, Bob. Don't do this," said my frantic mom.

"It's time. I want to die."

"Fuck you, Bob. You can't give up," my mom said, already looking as though someone had hit the crazy-widow switch. Tears streamed from her eyes, causing her makeup to run down her cheeks. "You've got to keep fighting. We've all worked so hard to keep you alive. You're not a quitter. You've got to have hope. Bob, you just can't leave me."

"I know, but I still want to die. It's time," my dad said.

"Well, when? When do you want to die? Now?" my mom managed through the crying.

"September 22," said my dad stoically.

"Wow, already have the date picked out? Fuuuuuuuuck," I said.

My dad nodded. He meant it. This was clearly something he had been thinking about. It wasn't just a spur-of-the-moment decision. He didn't wake up and casually think, Say, what should I do today? Oh, I know, I'll decide to die. He couldn't fight this losing battle any longer. He didn't want to sit in a wheelchair trapped in his own body. He didn't want people wiping his ass. He didn't want to eat through a tube in his stomach. He didn't want to lie there and watch his family slowly wear down and go insane while they cared for him. He couldn't. He had no hope. This wasn't going to get better. It was time to finally give up.

I didn't really know how to feel. I had listened in on his conversation with Robin, so I wasn't super surprised. Part of me was relieved. My dad's death would be incredibly sad, but it would also liberate me. I could unpause my life. I felt guilty for thinking this way, but I was tired of all this, just like he was. I didn't want to become Vince Junior. I wanted to live in my own apartment in some other city working some job doing something else.

It had been outrageously difficult watching my dad slip into this debilitated state. He had transformed from seeming invincible to being crippled—he was a shell of his former self. This wasn't how I wanted to remember him. I wanted to remember him as the sturdy rock in our lives, that dependable source of love and comfort who bought me popcorn and beer at Jazz games. The Lou Gehrig's was threatening to forever change the image I had of my father, and I wanted its destruction of that image to stop.

He was also in pain—so, so much pain. Back in college at Berkeley, a friend and I once took a study break outside the Moffitt

Library. There was a dying pigeon flailing about on the polluted, cigarette-butt-covered pavement. Many of the hippie Berkeley students looked on, concerned, wanting to do something to help. There was even talk of calling some sort of animal support unit to try to save this thing's life. My friend had grown up on a farm and was totally comfortable with the reality of death. He looked at me and said, "I really want to stomp that thing to death, put it out of its misery." He obviously didn't, because Berkeley's student body would've executed him. But it made sense. End the pain. End the spectacle of death.

My dad's not a pigeon, but still, having that metaphorical foot stomp him to death seemed more humane than watching him suffer any longer.

"But Bob, what about never giving up? You're not going to just let this thing win, right?" my mom cried. My dad just shrugged. He was ready to go.

"Well, I think that's really shitty, Bob. Really shitty. You can't just leave us like this," my mom said.

"It's time," my dad said. "It's time. Please understand."

"I think this is the bravest decision any of us has ever made," said Greg.

"Shut up, Greg. Don't be an asshole," said my mom.

Chelsea just sat there stunned. I'm sure not too many of her classmates spent their summers watching their father slowly melt away and eventually announce his own death date. I imagined how Chelsea would describe her vacation to her friends when school resumed.

"How was your summer, Chelsea?" a classmate would ask.

"Good. How was yours?"

"Great. My parents took me to California. What'd you do?"

"I danced and went swimming and my dad decided to die."

I looked around at our surroundings: the sparkling, perfectly clear blue pool water, the rustling aspen leaves powerfully green in the heart of summer, the stillness of a peaceful mountain town. This place was meant for reflection. Maybe that's why my dad had chosen to make this proclamation here.

"You're probably the only person who will ever announce their death next to this fabulous pool," I said.

"You're probably right," my dad managed.

I did the math in my head. September 22 was roughly seventy-five days away. I grabbed another beer, popped off the top, and extended it to my dad. "You want a beer? Might as well live it up a little before you die."

He smiled and tried to move his hands to reach for it, but couldn't.

"Well, if you're not going to drink it, I will," I said, and started chugging it, hoping it would instantly numb me forever.

Though my mom was still crying, my dad looked relieved, surprisingly calm, as if a weight had been lifted off his shrunken shoulders. Must have been nice to know there was an end to all this. He must have been struggling with the "to be or not to be" question for some time now.

I finished off the beer and dove into the pool, hiding beneath its wavy surface for as long as my breath allowed.

We had seventy-five more days with my dad.

THE OFFICIAL LETTER
AND SOME SUBSEQUENT
QUESTIONS

A week after my dad made his poolside death announcement, we took him to meet with his neurologist, Dr. Bromberg, up at the University of Utah, to talk to him about my dad's decision to be taken off the respirator on September 22, 2008. Dr. Bromberg wrote this letter to my dad's general practitioner:

Dear Dr. Wood:

Bob Marshall, accompanied by his wife, his son Dan, and his caregiver Regina, was seen in the Motor Neuron Disease Clinic on 16 July 2008. He is a 55-year-old gentleman being followed for ALS and was last seen 4 July 2008.

History of Present Illness: Mr. Marshall has been on full-time artificial ventilation since November 2007. Prior to his being placed on a ventilator, he had episodes of shortness of breath. We had talked about ventilatory support prior to his going on the ventilator, including the fact that his weakness will progress, and at one point, he will likely make a decision to be taken off the ventilator. Since November, Mr. Marshall has become progressively weaker. This includes difficulty with speech, such that one could understand with great care and repetition, no arm movements, and inability to walk and now can only shift positions with his legs. He, therefore, needs full-time care. He has been receiving excellent care, and there have been no medical complications.

On today's visit, Mr. Marshall wanted to talk about when to be removed from the ventilator. He clearly stated that he has been thinking about this essentially full-time. He is very frustrated and does not

240 DAN MARSHALL

want to be totally dependent upon other people, even though they express their willingness to care for him. He, therefore, has decided that he wanted to be taken off the ventilator sometime during the fall.

I explained to him how the process would be accomplished. We would likely enlist the services of hospice. He would be given sedating medication in high dose, such as benzodiazepam, and given morphine for any potential painful components. He would, therefore, be fully sedated and covered for any pain, and then the ventilator would be turned off. I would predict that he would pass away within minutes in comfort. Mr. Marshall acknowledged that he fully understood the process.

There was, understandably, a degree of reluctance on the part of his wife for Mr. Marshall to pass away. I emphasized that this should be his decision, and it represented a very courageous decision. His wife has a serious medical condition, and I reminded her that in the past, that if she had wanted to discontinue her therapy that he would have understood, and that I hope that she will understand if he wants to discontinue the ventilator.

Mr. Marshall also asked about organ donation. I had looked into this previously, and with respect to organ donation, the only organ he could donate ethically on the part of the hospital would be a kidney; if he were to do that, he would come in and donate one kidney and then go home, and then pass away as a separate issue. He could more easily donate cornea, skin, bone and tendon after he has passed away.

At the end of the discussion, I told Mr. Marshall and his wife that I would contact hospice and determine the procedure in clear detail. I would also contact the Transplant Service and determine how the above superficial organs could be obtained. I would also be happy to see him in the clinic at any time or make a home visit.

I tried to make some suggestions for Mrs. Marshall as how she might manage her feelings and those of their children.

Overall, more than 70 minutes were spent, all of it in counseling and coordination of care.

Mark B. Bromberg, M.D., Ph.D.
Professor of Neurology

The night after my dad's announcement, I couldn't sleep. I was too restless. I had too many questions. Usually when I can't sleep, I turn on the TV and let it lull my active brain to rest, or I masturbate. Masturbation is the original sleeping pill, after all. But even those tactics didn't work. So I got up and sat at the basement bar. I cracked open a beer and grabbed a pen. I had some questions on my mind. I took a big gulp of my beer and wrote away. Here's what I wanted to figure out:

How is one supposed to take the news of another's death? Isn't it strange to know the day someone you love is going to die? What do I say? Can I still tell cock jokes? Should I just curl up into a ball and cry? Can I go to a local titty bar and redeem this tragic news for a free lap dance? Should I run through the streets yelling it so everyone knows? Should I start calling my dad "Captain Un-Hook"? Should I write a bunch of rambling questions about it?

Should I film his last month? Is that too invasive? Would that be cool? What would I film? Would I just film my dad lying there counting down the days? Should I ask him life questions and try to extract all the knowledge I can from him while I can? Or would I just end up holding the camera and trying to steal the show by making shitty wisecracks that ruin everything?

How will my mom handle this all? Will she go even more batshit crazy? Will she be too sensitive to handle me calling her batshit crazy? Will she even be able to speak or will she be crying too much? After my dad dies, will she remarry? Who will she remarry? Do others still find her attractive despite the cancer? Will she still love yogurt? Will she call me up in the middle of the night and request that I move home? Will she overdose on Fentanyl? Will she continue living in our family house or move out? Will she travel and see the world? Will each kid have to take turns letting her live with us? Will we pass her around like an abandoned orphan? Will we have a calendar? Will one of us take her more than others? Will this cause fights and make us yell things like, "I had her all of November, asshole," and create resentment toward her and each other? Or will my mom move on and write a book about her life and go on Oprah and have the world rally around her and cheer for her?

And how will my siblings handle this news? Will Tiffany manage to stay calm in a world without her ski pal? Or will she have that nervous breakdown that always seems to be on the horizon? Will Greg find someone who will advise and inspire him the way my dad did? Will Jessica get back into drinking despite being pregnant? Will all of this finally hit Chelsea? Will she, mid-dance-practice, break down and cry her skinny face off? Will we all forever be painted with a tragic brush? Will the Lou Gehrig's disease haunt us forever? Or will we bounce back and move on? Will we learn to live in a dadless world?

How many people will attend the funeral? Will friends from out of state come? Will it be one of those things where I don't say but feel, Well, this is shitty, but gosh, it was nice seeing Cousin Jonathan again? Will I be drunk? Aren't you always drunk these days? Shouldn't you get help for that? Will everyone know I'm drunk? What will I say when people say the whole "I'm sorry" bullshit? Should I be a dick about it? Should I look them in the eye and say, "Well, you should be because this is all your fault," or "Sorry isn't going to bring my father back, now is it?" or "Yeah, it sucks, but I get his Lexus," and start dancing around like I won a game show? Or should I just stare at the person and change the subject, saying things like "Feel how smooth my hair is"?

Should I get a new suit? Will everyone cry at the funeral? If people don't cry, should I look at them with a wet, red face and yell, "Why aren't you crying, asshole?" Should I poke people in the eye so it looks like they're crying? Should I laugh at the people crying and say, "There's no crying in baseball"?

Will I be asked to deliver a speech? If I do speak, what will I say? Should I purposely try to make people cry? Should I show a slideshow that starts off with pictures of my dad when he didn't have Lou Gehrig's disease and ends with pictures of him lying helplessly in a hospital bed to the song "Do You Realize" by the Flaming Lips? That would get everyone to cry for sure, right? Should I read some passage out of the Bible that doesn't really make sense and seems so out of place that people turn to each other and ask, "What the fuck?" Should I write my speech as though I'm running for high school president instead of laying my father to rest?

Or should I give a real speech that accurately reflects what a kind and caring and loving person my dad was? Should I not talk about his experience with Lou Gehrig's disease, instead focusing on his life before? Should I talk about how he met my mom and how he started his own successful business or how he traveled to a remote area in Austria called Hallstatt, which he considers the most beautiful place on earth? Should I suggest that he's going to a better place, maybe even

Hallstatt? Should I talk about how he taught me how to play basketball and encouraged me to do what makes me happy? Should I then reveal that the only thing that makes me happy anymore is masturbation? Should I talk about how he would wake up at five in the morning to drive me to John Stockton's basketball camp? Or how he used to take me to all the Jazz games and give me the first stab at the popcorn?

Could I swear in a church? Is *ass* okay? *Fuck? Shit? Fart? Bitch? Bastard?* Could I give a whole fucking speech without using one shit-eating bad word?

Is God going to play some sick trick on us where he cures Lou Gehrig's disease the day after the funeral and comes down to earth and yells, "That's for all the shit you talk on me," and then ascends back into heaven to pick on the next family? Does my dad believe in God and heaven? Wouldn't things be so much easier if he did, if we all did? Did the Mormons get it right? Have you ever seen a depressed Mormon sitting in a coffee shop writing about death and how awful the world is? Is the reason why you haven't seen that simply because the Mormons aren't allowed to drink coffee? Should we have converted when we had the chance? When discussing religion with a Mormon friend should I have asked, "How do I join?" instead of "How do you believe some of this bullshit?" Is the only saved soul in my family going to be my sister Jessica, because she converted after marrying Creepy Todd?

When does college football start?

What is going through my dad's head right now? Is he happy with this decision? Does he really want to die? Why does he want to die? What was the breaking point? Was it when, in a burst of tiredness and anger and frustration, I yelled, "How long are we going to do this shit?" while struggling to get him out of the van? Did I kill him? Was that the breaking point? Or was it when the Lakers eliminated the Jazz from the playoffs and I responded by throwing my phone across the room and breaking it? Or was it when his legs stopped working? Was that it? Was that the point when he realized he wasn't going to be getting better, that, in fact, things were only going to get worse? Was it when Jessica married Creepy Todd and then got impregnated by him? Did Dad just grow tired of my batshit crazy mom sitting by his side crying? Was it when we stopped doing all the care and instead hired Regina? Was it when I brought home those chicken fingers from the Wing Coop and ate them in front of him? Was it when people outside the family stopped being able to understand him? Was it when we stopped being able to move him out of bed with ease, dropping him on his bony ass several times? Or was all this blended into one giant, shit-filled smoothie that was just too shitty and sad and awful for him to stomach anymore?

What should I do with my remaining time with him? Am I supposed to sit at his side and rub his arm and say, "Doesn't that feel nice?" until he's gone? Should I show him all the best movies and let him listen to all the best music? What are the best movies? *Life Is Beautiful* was pretty fucking good, wasn't it? What about *Home Alone*? Isn't *Forrest Gump* his favorite? Can anyone recall a time when you were watching a movie with him and he remarked, "Wow, that was a great movie. If I'm on my deathbed, I would love to watch it"? Should I massage his body? Should I read him David Sedaris? Should I find a way to sneak him into a hot tub? Should I stand at the base of his bed and say, "I love you. I love you. I love you," over and over again? Should I help him make a bucket list and hope "Walk again and move my body" isn't one of his listed items but that "Watch *The Bucket List*" is? Should I take him on a shopping spree? Should we go get pedicures?

Should I be mad at him for making us put in all this work just to watch him give up in the end? Should I remind him that I quit my job and lost my girlfriend over this whole mess? When he asks me to do something for him, should I say, "What's the point? You're going to die anyway"? Should I take a bat to his wheelchair? Should I resent him?

Or should I organize a living funeral that he can attend where we all dress up and honor him and say nice things about him and give great speeches that are funny because he hasn't died yet? Who should I invite? Do we all talk? Do we all cry? Do I really have to dress up? Should everyone bring a gift for the family? Would everyone just bring lasagna? Should I have fireworks and dancers and circus performers? Do I know anyone who juggles? What food would we serve? Should I request that we all have a Promote, which is the only thing we put into his feeding tube? Should we all clap for him? Which motherfucking Hilton should we do this shit at?

Or should I not make a big deal of this all and just kiss him on the forehead and say, "I respect your decision and will always love you"?

Should I thank him for all he's done for me? Should I tell him what a great dad he's been over the years?

And what about me? Should I sit around and mope? Should I call Becca up and do a bunch of ecstasy with her again? Should I lower my standards and pathetically say, "I'll fuck anything with or without a pulse," as I sip on my second forty of the morning? Should I get to the point where I can say, "I know her. She's a stripper"? Should I start getting in fights with everyone, including my best friends? Should I always remind everyone of this all the time? Should I hate myself for not doing enough? Should I disappear and not tell anyone where I am?

Or should I just try to do all that I can and never question whether it was enough? Should I try to move on with my life, get an M.B.A. or something? Should I forever remember that all this happened but not let it affect the rest of my life? Should I walk up to the next pretty girl I see and give her a kiss on the lips? Should I order the best steak dinner in town? Should I go to a Taco Tuesday party and eat so many tacos that observers look at me and say, "Wow, he is having the time of his life!"? Should I go on a roller coaster and purposely piss my pants? Should I see the world? Should I buy myself a nice car and a nice watch and nice clothes? Should I go to Vegas and get the motherfucking *Rain Man* suite? Should I move to Paris and fall in love with something that's not a baguette? Should I learn how to cook gourmet meals for myself? Should I live in a place with a view? Should I start sitting in more hot tubs and eating more cheese?

When does college football start again?

I set down the pen and looked over the mess of questions. It's going to be an interesting little stretch of life here, I thought. I went back to my room and clicked on the TV, finally ready to get some rest.

I'LL BLOW YOU
TILL THE END

My dad only had a handful of days left. He was reminded of this every morning when I would come into his room and say something to the effect of "Fifty-five more days until you're dead, Daddy-O." He'd raise his eyebrows and attempt a smile, his version of *sounds good, you sick son of a bitch*. He was used to my morbid jokes by now.

I asked him what he wanted to do with his last few weeks. "Go running, and skiing, and eat a nice big steak dinner." I laughed. What a jokester.

"Oh, good one, silly, crippled, dying Dad. But seriously, what do you want to do? You're gonna be dead soon here," I joked back.

He got serious. "I'd like to go for walks in my chair, and say good-bye to people, and spend time with all of you," he managed to say. I guess when we're about to die we drop all the other distractions and go back to the basics: family, peaceful walks, spending time with loved ones. Fuck the rest.

"Maybe you can go on a cocaine, stripper, and heroin binge, too?" I suggested, figuring that he might as well fade out on a high note. He sort of laughed.

"I'd also like to go to Snowbird one last time," he said.

"So, was that a yes or a no to the cocaine-stripper binge?" I asked.

My dad was actually excited about the upcoming farewell and weirdly looking forward to the end of all this. He was in pain. It was time to die and let his family try to live. His decision was tough, but admirable and rooted in selflessness. He figured that he had lived a very fulfilling life already. After all, he didn't have Lou Gehrig's disease for fifty-three years of it, and those had been good, happy, and healthy years full of skiing, running, and drinking wine with his family and friends in his gazebo.

In a way, his announcement affected all of us more than him. From his perspective, he was out of here soon, riding off into heaven's sunset on some sort of flying blow job machine while Alice Cooper's "School's Out" blasted on a boom box. Meanwhile, the rest of us still had to continue to exist in the world without him, having to mop up this mess and rebuild our lives, trying our best to fill the giant hole his absence would leave behind. If it had been up to him, I think he would've just pulled the plug right when he made his announcement, but he knew that we weren't entirely ready for him to go. We still needed closure, and hopefully this extra time would allow for that.

Greg and I were fairly relaxed about the announcement. We had put the most work into caring for him, so we were the most burned out. We knew it was going to suck to lose our dad, but we also knew living like this wasn't sustainable—mentally or physically. Tiffany was pretty freaked out, though. Now that there was a ticking clock on the situation, she pushed school, work, and BCB to the side so that she could spend more time with our dad. Jessica returned from Thailand with Creepy Todd and was around more. She seemed to be doing a lot better since the marriage. Maybe it was actually a good thing for her. Chelsea wouldn't talk about the situation outright, but she'd occasionally come sit next to my dad and cry uncontrollably without saying a word.

As usual, Stana put it best: "It is be sad house when there is no more Daddy."

Regina was rather upset by the announcement. She had grown close to my dad, and because this situation had helped her to get over her failed marriage, losing my dad meant she wasn't just losing her job, but also her sense of order and balance in the world.

My mom was handling the news the worst. Instead of accepting my dad's death, she'd taken to constantly pleading with him to not do it.

"Please don't do this," she'd say. "How could you leave me like this?" She felt as if she were returning to her life as an orphan. She was terrified about having to manage on her own, especially all the little things that my dad always took care of, like the family finances.

I had taken over managing the finances because I'm a hero (of sorts) who is able to easily handle the weight of the world on my shoulders. Mainly, I paid the bills and dealt with the insurance cocksuckers. I sat down with my mom to try to teach her a thing or two.

"I set up bill-pay stuff online, so every time you have a bill, you just log into WellsFargo.com, go to 'Bill Pay,' find the company's name, and enter the amount."

"This is too fucking hard," she'd cry, instantly dissolving into tears, not even looking at the computer screen. "Bob, don't do this. Don't die. You can't leave me with this fucking mess. Everyone thinks you're such a nice guy, but you're really an asshole."

I looked at my concerned dad and said, "You're lucky you're getting out of here." He raised his eyebrows and attempted a smile, his version of *yeah, I know.*

Robin came by to chat with my dad and mom. They wanted to discuss how to manage the remaining time we had left with him. The goal with my mom was to try to get her to settle the fuck down and actually enjoy the time she still had with her husband instead of worrying about what life would be like after his death.

"This is hard. Loss is hard, but let's think of some ways to live more in the now and enjoy your time with Bob," suggested Robin.

"How about you just don't die? How does that sound?" said my mom. She wanted to feel that she was still taken care of—that someone was still looking after her. Eventually, my dad and Robin came up with an idea.

"Okay, so how about this. After Bob passes, every time you find a penny—whether it be on the sidewalk, on your kitchen counter, or in your car—that's Bob looking after you. So, even when he's gone, he's still there for you," Robin said. My mom nodded, buying into that.

"I love that," she said. I personally thought it was a load of shit, but hey, if it calmed my mom down, I was all for it.

With my mom slightly more relaxed, Robin also came up with the idea that we each pick an activity that we'd routinely do with my dad as September 22 approached. I liked that idea much more than the penny nonsense.

"Dad's got fifty-one days left, so we all need to pick activities to do with him before he goes," I told the family. Everyone agreed and picked activities.

Greg decided he would sit next to my dad's bed, asking him all sorts of questions about his life on his fancy recording device he had bought for his reporter job. Greg had always had dreams of being a

Charlie Rose–type figure. He even did a deep, intellectual-sounding voice when he asked questions.

"Let's talk childhood. What was growing up in Pocatello like?" Greg asked in his intellectual voice, as if he were talking to George Clooney instead of a man in a diaper.

"It was nice. We had a nice house and lived close to everything," my dad managed to explain in his Lou Gehrig's voice. I was a little jealous Greg had come up with the idea of interviewing my dad, so I would try to sabotage these interviews.

"Who gave you your first hand job?" I interjected.

"Don't listen to him, Daddy. Danny has his mind in the gutter, right next to his penis." Greg collected himself. "Now, your family had a ranch. What was a typical day on the ranch like?"

"Oh, come on. Who gives a fuck? He's got forty-seven days left. Ask some real questions. Who gave you your first hand job?"

"Caroline Summers, after a football game," my dad said with a smile.

"See, my questions are much better than yours," I said to Greg.

Jessica was starting to look more and more pregnant, her Native American belly poking out of the UC Berkeley sweater she had stolen from me, which I assumed she wore ironically since she was now a high school dropout.

"We're all picking activities to do with Dad before he dies in forty-four days," I explained to Jessica. "You need to pick something. And make it fun, since you already broke his heart by marrying Creepy Todd."

"Friends," she said, sticking to her usual short answers.

"What the fuck are you talking about?" I asked her.

"The TV show," she said. "I'll watch *Friends* with him."

"That's dumb. Your kid is going to be so dumb," I said.

"Fuck you," she said while pushing a *Friends* DVD into the player.

Jessica and I hadn't gotten along since her marriage to Creepy Todd. It was really hard for me to not go into full Dickhead Dan mode around her. I still hadn't accepted her poor decision, even if she was doing better. Seeing the baby bump on her just made me feel angry and sad. We had lost Jessica. The Mormons had won.

"Back off her, DJ," my dad said.

"Whatever you want, Daddy-O," I said as I left the room so they could spend time together without me there being an asshole. The sound of canned laughter from the *Friends* DVD started up. It was weird hearing laughter from my dad's room. It sort of sounded like we were all part of a shitty sitcom. "Next on ABC Family, *The Marshall Family Tragedy*. In this episode Bob announces he wants to kill himself while Debi gets addicted to pain pills." *[Canned laughter.]*

Tiffany would come over in the morning before work with a cup of coffee and read my dad the paper, then come back over for an evening walk around the neighborhood. My relationship with Tiffany had completely changed. I hadn't called her a bitch in months, and she hadn't called me an asshole. We had a silent truce going—an understanding that we'd no longer verbally assault each other. It was great. I suddenly found myself with a new sibling, a new friend. We'd grab a glass of wine and sit in the gazebo talking after my dad was asleep.

"What are you going to do after this all ends?" Tiffany asked, making it sound like we were being released from prison or war or hell.

"Not totally sure. I'll finally get another job and apply to graduate school, I guess," I said.

"For business or for what?" she asked.

"I don't know. Maybe business. I might see if I can get into a screen-writing school," I said. I had always had a desire to try something completely different. I loved movies and loved writing. Why not combine the two? While all this was going on, I had started writing down what was happening and posting our stories and unusual conversations on a blog. Surprisingly, people enjoyed reading about our tragedy, even though the writing was crude and sloppy. I never had the balls to risk everything and focus on writing as a real career. But since I now had nothing, I figured maybe I'd give it a shot. Why not?

"What about you?" I asked.

"Finish my M.B.A., then probably move to Maine to be with Brian." I called him BCB so much, I had forgotten his real name was Brian. "Maine's about as far from here as I can get."

"Yeah, it'll be nice to get away. Fuck, can you believe we were eating family dinners out here with Dad just over a year ago?" I said.

"I know. How the fuck did all this happen so fast?"

"I don't know. I really don't know." I poured us both a fresh glass of wine to the brim.

For her activity with Dad, Chelsea decided that she would practice some of her dance moves around his bed.

"I figured you'd want to just come in here and fart," I said.

"I can do that, too," she said mid-plié, and then pushed out a perfectly timed fart.

"Get out of here. Dad has thirty-nine days left, and he's in enough pain without smelling your farts," I said. Chelsea giggled her giggle and danced out of the room.

I had spent more time with my dad over the last year than any of the rest of my siblings, so I sort of felt like we had done everything already. But we'd go on a walk a day, and at night, I'd bring a bottle of wine up to his room and pour us both a glass. I set his on the stand next to his bed.

"You don't want any of yours?" I asked.

"I still can't drink," he said.

"Well, more for me," I said, swooping up his glass and gulping down the contents like a fat alcoholic. My dad and I didn't really need to talk. We just liked being around each other. It was as if we had crammed all the hanging out we were supposed to do over the next twenty-five years into this single year. I'm sure he got sick of me always being there, always being a smart-ass. But maybe not. Who knows?

As I was hanging with my dad one afternoon, my mom stumbled in and sat in the chair next to the bed. Her eyes were half closed, meaning she was in Fentanyl Land. She looked as if she was about to drop into a grave.

"Mom, so everyone's doing their special little activity with dad before he dies in thirty-four days. Why aren't you?" I asked.

"I am," she said.

"Sitting next to him eating yogurt and almost dying isn't much of an activity."

"For your information, I'm giving him a blow job a day until he's dead," she proudly said, like she was donating to charity or feeding the homeless.

"A blow job a day? That's a lot of blow jobs," I said. "Good thing you're such a blow job machine."

"Oh, shut up, you little shit-eater. One day you're not going to have a mother to treat like shit," she said. "And for the record, I'm really good at them. He loves them."

I looked to my dad to see his reaction to all this. "This true, Dad?" I asked. "Are you getting a blow job a day?" He raised his eyebrows and attempted a smile, his version of *it's none of your business, but yes, I am!*

It was a little weird—my mom blowing my dad until the end of his life—but also really compassionate. I never liked to picture my parents fucking, believe it or not, but I assumed they had a regular sex life. My dad, more than my mom, liked to joke about sex. With any joke comes a little bit of truth and desire. But once my dad got sick, I figured the sex-related activities had slowed down, then disappeared completely. But I guess they hadn't.

"That's cool. I just hope I never walk in on that," I said. "Be horrific to see my mom's mouth full of my dad's cock and cum."

"DANNY," my dad managed to say in as angry a tone as he could muster. "Let's not be so disgusting all the time."

"I'm not the one getting my dick sucked by a cancer patient," I said.

My mom was beyond proud of the blow-job-a-day goal she had set for herself. I don't know if it was because she was all fucked up on Fentanyl or what, but she seemed to bring it up any chance she got, and to anyone who would listen.

"A blow job a day. Not a bad deal," I heard her explain to a visitor. "You wouldn't think it, but his penis is still strong," I heard her explain to another.

"God, that rich-bitch sister of his is finally coming," my mom told me toward the end of August. My dad's family had been a little reluctant to visit because of the mutual hatred between them and my mom. They simply couldn't stand each other. Of everyone in my dad's family, my mom disliked Aunt Sarah the most. They used to be friends. In fact, Aunt Sarah actually introduced my mom and dad to each other. Sarah and my mom grew apart over the years, and eventually they started absolutely hating each other. Getting them together was like putting two betta fish in the same bowl.

"The best part of him dying is that I'll never have to see any of those assholes ever again."

"They probably feel the same way about you. And, this is about Dad, not you," I told her. I would defend my dad's family. I liked them, even if my mom didn't, and I knew my dad wanted to spend time with them. So I'd try to play peacemaker.

"When she's here, just sit quietly and let Dad have some time with her. She was his sister before you were his wife," I said.

"I won't say a word for Dad's sake," she said. "But still, fuck her."

My mom was true to her promise. She mostly got out of the way, but one afternoon, the two betta fish found their way into my dad's room. Aunt Sarah sat bedside, holding her brother's bony hand as they talked about their childhood, while Mom sat off in the corner like a kid on time-out, silently spooning yogurt into her face.

"So, we've all decided a few things we're going to do with my dad before he dies in twenty-nine days," I told my aunt. "Greg is interviewing him. Chelsea is dancing for him. Tiffany is reading him the morning paper. Jessica's watching old episodes of *Friends* with him. I'm having a glass, or bottle, of wine a night with him. I was thinking that you should come up with something as well."

"Oh, that's a great idea," said Aunt Sarah. She thought for a minute. "Oh, how about I call every day I'm not here with a memory or a story?"

"Great idea," I said. "He'll love that. Won't you, Dad?"

"Yeah, that'll be nice," he said. We all exchanged smiles. What a nice family moment.

Then my mom interjected from her corner. "I'm giving him a blow job a day for the rest of his life," she proudly said.

Sarah looked at my mom and said, "Boy, I didn't need to hear that."

"But your story thing is good, too," she said with a smirk.

"It's not a competition," Aunt Sarah said.

"No. It's not. But if it was, I'd win." My mom finished off her yogurt and dropped the empty in the trash as she left.

I'm not entirely sure if the blow-job-a-day thing actually happened. Who knows. My mom says it did, and my dad seemed awfully happy during this stretch. Maybe because he was finally going to die. Or maybe because he was getting a blow job a day for the rest of his life. What was important was that he was getting to spend time with everyone he loved. Oh, and we did take him to Snowbird.

FUNERAL PLANNING
WITH CHELSEA

Funerals are uncomfortable—and not just because you have to sit on a hard bench in a cold church with snot and tears pouring out of you. Planning a funeral for a person who's still alive is even more uncomfortable. A lot of times people put words in the dead person's dead mouth, saying things like "Well, Grandpa would have wanted us to have a cocktail party," or a former friend might say, "He would have wanted me to fuck his widowed wife just after his funeral."

If there was one silver lining in my dad's situation, it was that he had the ability to sit in on the planning, which gave him some control over something—though my mom basically monopolized all the decision making. We had one such planning session as the September 22 date approached, attended by everyone in my family: Tiffany, Greg, Jessica, Chelsea, my mom, my dad, me, and our two panting golden retrievers, who I wanted to slam over the head with a shovel for being so happy in the middle of this Greek tragedy. Even a couple of our horrible cats lounged around the room.

My mom was in charge of the meeting, the old red notebook she'd had from the beginning sitting on her lap. She had a list of everything she wanted to plan: who would speak, what songs would be played, where we'd do the reception.

My mom suggested that we each do a speech. I had delivered a speech at Grandma Rosie's funeral a few years back that got a few chuckles, so I figured I could do the same at my dad's funeral. I didn't want to turn it into a stand-up comedy routine—"What's the deal with my dad dying twenty-five years earlier than I thought he would?"—but I had already scribbled down a few jokes and anecdotes for it. I figured all the other speeches would be sad and sentimental, so I wanted to make one that focused on how great my dad's life was before he got Lou Gehrig's. I wanted to try to get people to re-member him without the disease. I wanted them to think of him as the happy guy who made every situation better through his mere presence—not as a crippled mess lying around shitting into diapers while hooked to a breathing machine.

"Do I have to do a speech?" asked Jessica.

"Only if you love Dad. If not, don't worry about it," I said. Jessica would hardly talk during a one-on-one conversation, so I was sort of excited to see her speak in front of a giant collection of people. I won-dered what the fuck she would even say.

"I don't want to speak," she said.

"Then I guess you don't love Dad," I said.

"Todd will speak for me," she said.

"Creepy Todd isn't speaking at Dad's fucking funeral," Greg said.

"Yeah, Jess, that's insane. Family only," I said.

"That fucker shouldn't even be allowed at the funeral," Tiffany said. "I wish I'd cut his dick off before he got you pregnant."

"Bob, what do you think?" my mom asked. He just shrugged. He didn't care. He wasn't even going to be there. Well, I guess he'd be there, but he'd be sitting in the blue, cloud-covered urn we had pur-chased for his ashes a couple of weeks earlier.

"Okay, so Todd will speak for Jessica," my mom said, scribbling down a note. The rest of us shook our heads in disbelief. Not only had this weirdo infiltrated our family and impregnated our defenseless, emotionally fragile little sister, but now he was speaking at my dad's funeral? Fuck that. Fuck that hard.

For music, my mom was getting her friends Craig and Janet to sing. Janet had sung and played the guitar at Jessica's wedding. She was like our hired musician for all our tragic events. I bet when she got into music she was hoping for better gigs. My mom kept insisting that she perform "Over the Rainbow" instead of something my dad actually liked.

"Okay, so we're going to have Janet sing 'Over the Rainbow,'" my mom said.

"Why? Dad doesn't even like that song," Greg said.

"Yes, he does. There's a new version out," my mom said.

"We're not fucking playing 'Over the Rainbow.' Let's have her play something he likes by the Beatles or James Taylor or Paul Simon," said Greg.

"I agree with Greg. We're not playing 'Over the Rainbow,'" I said. "Dad doesn't even like rainbows, probably hates them since his life has become the opposite of one."

"This is really about Dad," said Tiffany. "What do you think, Dad?" He just shrugged again.

"Okay, I'll think about it," my mom said.

My mom mentioned that the pastor would be a woman named Erin, and that she would give a brief introduction. Chelsea, who had been a silent observer, picking fur balls off our cat Pierre, finally interjected.

"No, Mom. We're not having Erin do it," said Chelsea.

"Why?" asked my mom.

"Because Erin is a slut," Chelsea said.

"She's a pastor. How is she a slut? Please explain," I said with a smirk. Chelsea's weird comments always amused me. Part of me thought she'd say weird shit just for my entertainment.

"She thinks she knows God personally and talks to him and we don't know if there is a God," said Chelsea.

"So that makes her a slut?" I asked, trying to see where this logic was coming from.

"Yeah, that makes her a slut," Chelsea explained. She then began laughing uncontrollably, so I'm not sure how serious she was, but I was proud of her for being skeptical of God and for blindly attaching the word *slut* to a near stranger—it was a very Marshall thing to do. Chelsea's handling of the whole Lou Gehrig's shitshow had been really bizarre. She'd cry without warning sometimes, and then at others she'd just make these odd jokes. Whenever I'd ask her what she thought of anything related to Lou Gehrig's disease and what our dad was going through, she would just pinch my arm, say, "He'll be fine," and change the subject. I think she was just trying to block everything out. Made sense.

We started discussing what to do after the funeral. I suggested that we all stand out in the parking lot smoking cigarettes and kicking the gravel while talking about how dark and horrible life had gotten. My dad finally piped in with a suggestion.

"It shouldn't be sad, but rather a celebration," he said.

"I think it's going to be pretty fucking sad, Bob," my mom said.

"No, everyone should get drunk and be happy," my dad said. He was tired of his disease bumming everyone out. He wanted his death and his funeral to be a turning point back toward the good life. He didn't want to pull us through any more shit.

I was all for a celebration after the funeral. This had been a hard year. The thought of getting shit-faced while friends and family comforted me and told me how great my dad was sounded like a dream. No one can judge you if you're in mourning. You have the ultimate trump card. So I could get as drunk as I wanted to.

"You probably shouldn't have any more," a guest might tell me after my tenth drink.

"Fuck you, my dad just died," I'd tell them as I chugged from a jug of wine like some sort of drunken pirate.

Chelsea offered her own suggestion on what we should do after the funeral. "How about we do a campout?" she said.

There was a long pause in the room, the in-out of the respirator the only noise. "A fucking campout, Chelsea?" I said, finally breaking the silence.

"Yeah, up Millcreek Canyon," she said.

"That's about as weird as calling a pastor you've never met a slut," I said.

"Erin is a slut. She thinks she can talk to God," she said.

"Chelsea, now's not the time to act weird," Tiffany said.

"Yeah, Chelsea, shut up," Jessica said.

"At least I'm not pregnant like a loser," Chelsea said.

"So we're going to play 'Over the Rainbow,' right?" my mom said.

"Mom, we're not playing 'Over the fucking Rainbow,' so just drop it," Greg said.

"But there's a new version out. Have you even heard it?" my mom said.

"Don't you think a campout would be fun?" Chelsea said.

I thought about the campout for a minute—us going up into a canyon and grilling hot dogs after celebrating my father's life. It might be fun. Janet could strum on her guitar and sing songs, and everyone could drink cheap beer, and piss in the river, and make s'mores. It might be worth doing just so we could see the expressions on everyone's faces. I pictured a husband slapping a mosquito on his arm and saying, "This is fucking weird. A campout after a funeral?"

"Yeah, really bizarre. But they've been through a lot, so maybe they just weren't thinking," his wife would say.

Then I'd approach and say, "Hey, thanks for coming. Did you guys get enough s'mores?" Then I'd look around and take a deep breath of mountain air. "This is great, isn't it? What a dream. My dad would love it up here. Sure wish he wasn't dead."

When night approached—just before taking off to our separate tents—we could tell ghost stories and spook one funeral-goer so bad her parents would decide it was best that they not spend the night, that they better get little Katie home to bed.

"Fuck little Katie. We don't need her anyway," someone might say. "We got a funeral/campout to enjoy."

We could wake with the sun and fish in the river. I hope there aren't any bears up there, but if a bear did eat one of us, the headline in the morning paper would be pretty classic: "Funeral-goer Eaten by Bear." A big "ha ha" would fill the world.

We'd need insect repellent.

I loved the idea. The whole thing would be close to priceless. "I think we should do the campout," I said.

"Okay, so Todd's going to speak for Jessica, we'll play 'Over the Rainbow,' and we'll think about the campout idea," my mom said as she scribbled a note into her notebook, presumably about the campout. My dad rolled his eyes, probably wishing he were already in that cloud-covered urn.

THE GOOD-BYE PARADE

My dad's death was very unusual because he had a set date for it. It wasn't a fatal car crash. Everyone knew exactly when he was going to go, right down to the hour (4 p.m. on September 22). Consequently, family, friends, neighbors, and total strangers all wanted to see him before he was to be unhooked from his respirator—an event that I started calling "The Big Unhook." In fact, so many people wanted to say good-bye to my dad that there was actually a line in front of our house. He was like a celebrity.

"Wow, Dad, you're super popular," Tiffany said as she looked out the window at the line of people waiting to say good-bye.

"God, I wish all these fuckers would just leave us alone," Greg said.

"Every person is lovin' Daddy," Stana said.

Chelsea asked me what all these people were doing at her house. "They're saying good-bye to Dad," I told her.

"I know, but can't they just, like, send him an e-mail or something?" she joked. "I mean, I'm trying to study here." Chelsea was starting her junior year of high school and was taking several AP classes. She had a near 4.0 GPA and didn't want to fuck that up. And, though she was book smart, socializing was very difficult for her. So suddenly having a house full of people made her feel really uncomfortable.

"Go into his room and fart. Bet that'd scare everyone away," I joked. She giggled and ran off to her room. Poor Chelsea. I spent my junior year of high school taking Accutane, masturbating, and trying to feel comfortable enough with my body to talk to a girl. I couldn't imagine losing my dad at the same time.

We set Saturday, September 20, as the last day for visitors, so that we would have a little time to say good-bye to the dying fucker, too, but the days before the twentieth were a seemingly endless parade of good-byes.

The visitors ranged from really good friends and close family members to absolute strangers. A few Mormon neighbors and religious nuts also wandered in so they could preach to my dad. The religious people would say their "You're going to a better place" or "Everything happens for a reason" bullshit. After they left, my dad would look at me and say, "Who was that?" and I'd tell him that I didn't know. "Probably just some asshole who used you to feel like they did their good deed of the day."

My dad wasn't religious, so he didn't like the pious visitors. He had grown up going to church, but religion didn't stick with him and was never a definitive part of his life. He believed that when someone dies, his or her spirit melds with all the other spirits of the people they knew and loved. He believed that your spirit is comprised of your experiences, your personality, the lessons you have learned, your traits, and your ideas. After a person dies, he or she passes on certain aspects of their spirit to people and it combines with the spirits of those others. The exact same piece will not be passed on to everyone. Each is customized. He didn't believe that there was a heaven or a hell. In his mind, a dead person was not sitting with God and eight supermodel virgins deciding which one to screw that night, but rather was alive in the people they cared about, guiding them through difficult times.

But people didn't bother to ask what my dad believed. Instead, they assumed he held the same beliefs they did. So they'd transform him into whatever religion they were. If they were Mormon, my dad was Mormon. If they were Catholic, my dad was Catholic. If they were Jewish, my dad was Jewish. Since Mormons believe that you become a god of your own kingdom upon death, they treat the whole dying thing like it's a positive instead of a negative. So Mormon visitors were especially perky, wearing these creepy smiles. While they labored on about God, and heaven, and kingdoms, and reuniting with dead relatives, and going to a better place, my dad just had to sit there. It wasn't like he could stand up and walk out of the room.

He also didn't think praying did anything, other than making the person praying feel slightly better. One religious woman who we didn't know came over and gave our family a little decorative brass sign that read, WHEN LIFE GIVES YOU MORE THAN YOU CAN HANDLE: PRAY.

After the woman left, I looked over at my dad. "We really fucked this up, Dad. Instead of doing the respirator, feeding tube, suction machine, cans of Promote, and wheelchair, we just needed to drop to our knees and pray."

He smiled and said, "Who are these crazy people?"

"I don't know, but I can't wait for them to leave us alone."

The visits with actual friends and family members were always heart-felt. Lots of crying. Lots of holding hands. Lots of hugs. Lots of sharing favorite memories. Lots of wishing this wasn't happening. These were hard to watch. It seemed like everyone who had ever known my dad showed up. Hell, Ralph even came over from across the street and cried a little. I didn't think I'd ever see him cry, since he had such a tough-guy attitude. I showed Ralph—who also thought religion was bullshit—the WHEN LIFE GIVES YOU MORE THAN YOU CAN HANDLE: PRAY thing. He shook his head and said, "Could you imagine if you actually believed that shit?"

His closest friends would do something special when they came to say good-bye. Sam was coming over for the Big Unhook, so he was waiting until then to say his good-byes. But when my dad's other running partners, Donna and Paula, came over, they asked for some time alone with my dad. "Okay, but my mom's already giving him a blow job a day," I told them as I closed the doors to his room, giving them some privacy. They were in there for a couple of minutes, then walked out with smiles on their faces. I went in and asked my dad what that was all about. He smiled and said, "They flashed me."

"Oh, fuck, yeah, Dad. See, there are some perks to Lou Gehrig's disease," I said, forcing a high five on him.

His drinking and ski buddies all came over one evening with beer and wine and threw my dad a party on our house's main level. They all got shit-faced. I actually asked Dr. Bromberg if I could put a small amount of alcohol into my dad's feeding tube, and he okayed it. But my dad didn't want to. More for the rest of us.

We even got visitors from out of town. My dad's business partner, Kris, came to say good-bye. Kris lived up in the Pacific Northwest near a couple of the newspapers they owned. Since they'd sold their company, Kris had retired and started walking all the borders of all the states, beginning with Colorado because it was easiest, being square shaped and all. I guess we all need a hobby once we retire or we'll just end up sitting around thinking about death.

"It's a little bizarre, I know," said Kris. "But it's something to do. And I'm going to write a blog about it." My dad nodded, always too polite to call people out for being fucking weirdos.

Robin stopped by the house to have a final discussion with my dad and make sure he was approaching the Big Unhook with a positive attitude. I sat in on this one instead of listening from outside the room. My dad basically said he was ready to go and knew it was time, and that it was good that he had a chance to say good-bye to everyone. I was so emotionally burned out at this point that I just sat there, not really listening, but instead just thinking about all the free time I was going to have after this son of a bitch finally croaked. Maybe I'd find a job and make some money. Maybe I'd buy a home and start a garden. Maybe I'd meet a cute girl and fall in love again. The possibilities were endless.

After Robin's last session with my dad, I walked her out of the house to her car. We chatted like pals. She was a friend by now. She asked if I was doing okay. I smiled, shrugged, and said, "Yeah, I'm doing great, actually. I was thinking about getting a house with a garden, or some shit like that." She then started to cry. She hugged me and said, "I don't know how you're so calm and stable during all this. I can't handle it."

"There, there," I said, patting her back, thinking that it was bizarre that I was comforting her, instead of the other way around. "It's all going to be fine. Life goes on. Maybe you should start a garden."

"I wish I had your strength," she said.

"Nah, I'm a weak little pussy under it all. I'm just numb and tired," I said. She gave me one last hug and got in her car, still crying.

Regina wanted to say good-bye as well. My mom was getting meaner and meaner to Regina because she was more and more convinced that she was in love with my dad. She would take any chance she got to cut her down.

"I want to say good-bye, too," said Regina.

"These good-byes are more for family and friends," said my mom.

"But I'm a friend," said Regina.

"No, you're his hired aide—an employee," said my mom.

I stepped in and told Regina that she was more than an aide, that she had become a family friend, and that of course she could say good-bye to my dad. Her presence on the scene had kept us all from burning out and had probably prevented our murdering each other, so I valued her a great deal, as did my dad. I also felt sorry for her, as her divorce was hitting her hard. I was getting groceries one night at the local Albertsons and noticed her green Ford Explorer. I walked over to it and she was sitting there gripping the wheel and crying. I knocked on the window.

"Regina, what the fuck are you doing here?" I asked.

"Nothing. Just grocery shopping," she said.

"Really? Most people don't cry when they grocery shop," I said. She started crying even harder. She told me how mean her ex was being to her. She had come all the way from Brazil to marry the bastard and now she was completely alone.

I convinced my mom that it was okay for Regina to be around during the last couple of days. "Fine, but that fat bitch better not try anything with Dad," she said, protective of her dying husband right down to the final days.

My dad's family started visiting more, despite their ongoing hatred for my mom. Aunt Sarah had actually been spending most weekends with us, helping out and sharing stories with my dad. She even got comfortable enough to spend a night on Daddy Duty, which we all appreciated. I went out with my friends Aria and Henry that night. Jessica drove me down to the bars, since I had pre-gamed so aggressively at home and was already too drunk to drive myself. Now that she was pregnant, she was turning into my DD. I got so drunk, I woke up the next morning with a strange girl in my bed—so I was especially thankful to Sarah for doing Daddy Duty. My bed had been a lonely place for some time now. Aunt Sarah, Uncle Jack, and Aunt Ellen even rented a house in Salt Lake for a couple of weeks so they could be in town for the death and the funeral.

My dad's family requested that none of us be in the room when they said good-bye, especially my mom. They wanted some time alone with him, at last. So I'm not sure what they said to him. I'm sure they called my mom a bitch a couple more times. Their hatred for her was at an all-time high. My mom would certainly get her wish of never seeing them again. But I'm sure they also recounted the great life my dad had lived and promised to keep him alive in their memories. He would be part of their spirits now.

"Well, I'm glad they came," I told my dad after they all left, rubbing tears from their eyes. My dad was crying the hardest I'd seen him cry during all the good-byes.

"Yeah, me, too," he said. "I love them."

"So, how many times did they call mom a bitch?" I asked. My dad just smiled.

My pilled-up mom mainly hung in my dad's room during the good-byes. She insisted that after each good-bye was said, the visitors and my dad listen to the Beatles' "I'll Follow the Sun" so they could take some extra time to reflect on the meaning of it all. I really didn't like this whole idea, even though I really liked the song.

"That's so stupid, Mom. Do we really have to listen to this silly, faux-sentimental bullshit?" I argued.

"We need the song. Dad loves it. Don't you, Bob?" my mom said. My dad just shrugged his shoulders as usual.

"See. He loves it. We're playing the fucking song," my mom said.

So, at the end of the visit, after the good-byes, we'd all link hands, stand in a circle, and listen to that fucking song. I probably heard it about a hundred times.

The good-byes were always harder for the visitors than they were for my dad. It made sense. The people saying good-bye hadn't watched this disease slowly take everything from him. The last time most of them had seen him was when he was an active runner sipping a glass of wine. To transform from that to a skeleton on the brink of death was extremely startling. My dad's outlook was a lot cheerier than the visitors' as well. In the weeks leading up to his death, he had accepted and embraced that this was inevitable. He was totally Zen about it. He seemed surprisingly happy. He had been through a lot and was ready to go. He knew that there wasn't anything else he could do. He was freeing himself from his cocksucking terminal illness, and also freeing us from the burden of caring for him. Dying with dignity in full effect.

As more and more visitors came through, my dad seemed to be desensitized to it all. He couldn't match their emotional intensity. Shit, another person's coming in to tell me how special I am and how sad they are about my disease and untimely death. Blah, blah, blah, he probably thought as they cried and cried. He would often end up consoling the visitors, instead of the other way around, as I had done with Robin.

Most visitors' good-byes were pretty forgettable, to me at least. The typical visitor would come in already teary eyed, a little tentative and awkward. They'd smile and try to be cheerful. They'd sit right next to my dad's hospital bed. Some would take his hand or place a hand on his shoulder. Others would just sit there.

They'd start with small talk. "How you doing today?" or "How you feeling?" or "How about this weather? Fall is beautiful around here." My dad would answer, but he was almost impossible to understand at this point, so we had to translate for him. I loved fucking with people as I did these translations.

"Thanks for coming. It's good to see you," my dad would say after clearing his throat. The visitors would stare blankly at me, waiting for the translation.

"He said that it's good to see you," I'd say.

"Oh, thanks, Bob. Good to see you, too," they'd loudly say, like my dad was deaf instead of terminally ill.

"What's new with you?" my dad would ask. More blank stares from the visitors.

"He said that he wants you to get me a spicy chicken burrito from Del Taco," I'd say.

"Oh. Is there one around here?" they'd ask.

"I'm just kidding. He asked you what's new with you," I'd say.

"Oh. Ha ha. Nothing. Things are really good . . . So, wait, do I need to get you that burrito?" they'd say.

Eventually, the conversation would turn a little more serious. They'd apologize for Bob's misfortune, as if it was their fault. They'd tell him that he was a good friend, a good husband, a good father, a good person, and that they'd miss him. My dad would then pay them back a compliment and maybe give a little life advice, usually about something specific in their lives: a child getting married, a new grandchild, a new job, a new house.

"Thanks for being a good friend. You're a great person. And good luck with your new granddaughter. Spend as much time with her as you can," my dad would say. They'd look over to me to translate again.

"He said that he was never that great of friends with you and he wants you to leave so we can chill out, maybe watch *Forrest Gump* before he dies," I wanted to translate.

"He said thanks for being a good friend, and wished you luck with your new granddaughter. He suggests that you spend as much time with her as you can. I think he's saying that because he's dying and won't ever see any of his grandchildren, whereas you're living and will. Live it up and cherish every moment, in other words," I'd actually say, tacking on my own interpretation at the end.

"Oh, thanks, Bob. You're so special to us. Thanks for being so great. I know you're going to a better place," they'd say.

"Okay, well, thanks for coming. Love you," my dad would say. They'd wait for the translation again.

"He wants you to leave," I wanted to say.

"He said thanks for coming and that he loves you," I'd actually say.

"Love you, too, Bob. We'll pray for you," they'd say.

"Don't bother. We think praying is bullshit," I wanted to say.

"Great! Thank you so much!" I'd actually say.

The visitors would usually then cry a little bit. My dad—depending on how close he was to the person—would sometimes cry, too. But he was mostly all cried out. The visitors would then linger around, not sure exactly how to exit, probably thinking, This would be easier if it were just a car accident. They'd eventually give my dad one last hug and say, "Well, I'm going to go now. Great knowing you," but then still hang around for a few more minutes, thinking they had to do or say more. It was awkward and uncomfortable for everyone. I wanted to tell people that they'd done everything they could and that they were good people for caring so much, but also to get the fuck out so the people who mattered more in his life could get more time with him.

As visitors were about to leave, my mom would remember the Beatles song. She'd say, "Oh, we've got to play the song," and then fumble around with the CD player remote until she figured out how to work it.

"Okay, you guys ready?" my mom would ask. "Hold hands. It works better that way." Everyone in the room would link sweaty hands. Most didn't know each other, but they knew that they loved my dad, so they would go along with it.

"Okay, here we go," my mom would say, after finally finding the right button.

All would hang their heads, like they were in a deep state of thought, even though they were probably thinking, Okay, this is fucking strange. And I think I'm holding hands with Jessica's creepy husband.

CLICK. The song would play. My mom would close her eyes. My dad's would remain open, looking around at all the love he was getting.

After the song finished, everyone would look up, nodding to each other, acknowledging that it was nice. Maybe the song wasn't such a horrible idea. My mom's eyes would remain closed for about a minute after the song ended. People probably thought she was praying, or meditating, or crying, but I think she was probably just zoning out because of the Fentanyl. She had also gotten her cancer hands on some Klonopin, so she was even more out of it than usual.

Eventually, the visitors would hug us all and leave. "Stay strong," they'd say. "Love you so much, Bob," they'd add.

Friends and family were so terrific during all this. All these visits really showcased what a great man my dad was and how much love he brought in. He had truly influenced a lot of lives in a positive way, which is all you can really hope for when you die: that the memory people have of you is a good one. Sure, these visits were hard and tedious and repetitive for me. But they also gave everyone, especially my dad, a lot of closure. People got to say what they wanted to say to him, and he got to say what he wanted to them. Regret is probably the worst feeling you can die with, and it was nice to know that my dad didn't have to die with any. Instead, he would die filled with love, thinking that he was special and great and had had a positive impact on the lives of his friends and family. This is how everyone should go. Or, at least, those who lived a good life, like my dad.

It soon became Saturday, September 20. The house started to clear out. The line out front vanished to nothing. The doorbell stopped ringing. My dad had said all his good-byes. Visitors were no longer allowed. It was our turn to bid adieu to the old man.

THE DAY BEFORE
THE DAY OF

I was having a hard time sleeping during the nights leading up to my dad's death. When in bed, I felt like I was wasting time I should've been spending with him. I could lie down in the basement watching HBO anytime, but I only had a handful of hours left with my dad. So I'd wake up in the middle of the night and go sit in his room. My mom was always already in there, curled up alongside him in bed, clinging to him like her favorite childhood stuffed animal. Tiffany had also started spending the night. Must have been weird for her, because my dad's hospital room used to be her bedroom. My siblings and I used to sleep in her room on Christmas Eve. But all the happy memories we'd accrued in there would soon be trumped by the memory of the death of our father.

I'd just sit, listening to my dad's respirator, watching him sleep as peacefully as a man about to die can sleep. I took comfort in this. Though he wasn't the man he used to be, he was still my dad. He was still my road map. He was still alive.

I'd eventually crawl back into the basement with the other spiders.

The cats had officially won the battle over my room. They were using it as their primary litter box. I guess they were getting back at me for wanting to get rid of them. Maybe they were collectively trying to drive me out of there for good. The room's sheets and wallpaper were yellow, so an optimistic interior decorator could say, "Well, the piss matches the room's color scheme, so that's good."

But I'd say, "My God, what am I doing? I just turned twenty-six years old. I'm unemployed. I'm not going to school. And to put some shit-filled icing on the cake, I'm sleeping in a bed that reeks of cat urine. It's been a long, hard tumble to rock bottom for old, fat Dan. Good thing we have HBO."

When I did sleep, I would dream about not actually pulling the plug and my dad walking again. I dreamed about us watching a Jazz game together. High fives were easy. We didn't have to use our feet. LG stood for "Life is Good," not "Lou Gehrig's." I was safe and protected from all the spiders and trash of the world. You know when you have a dream where you fuck someone you've wanted to fuck, and then wake up and realize that you didn't fuck that person, but instead had ground your privates against the hard mattress? My dad-related dreams those nights were sort of like that, making waking up torturous, especially when combined with the pungent smell of cat piss.

I also had one dream wherein I was balding, perhaps a sign that I'm aware of aging and death—or a sign that maybe I was actually balding. I woke up relieved, feeling my full head of amazing hair. I might not have a father in a couple of days, but I'm guaranteed to have this beautiful hair, I thought, hoping it wouldn't start falling out in handfuls just to ensure I was really at rock bottom.

On the morning before the big day, I woke up at seven. I couldn't sleep later than that. I figured the best way to start today would be to eat a really hearty breakfast: eggs mixed with ham, perhaps, and a banana, washed down with a glass of orange juice. That would give me energy and maybe start a trend wherein I would start taking better care of myself by doing things like eating hearty breakfasts. Fuck, maybe I should go for a run through the neighborhood, I thought.

Don't get ahead of yourself, fat Dan, I counterargued.

I showered. I brushed my teeth. I put my contacts in. I dressed.

I walked out of my room to find Stana. She didn't have a broom, vacuum, duster, any sprays, mops, or trash bags. It was just her. Sometimes during those days, I'd catch her aimlessly wandering through our house, not doing anything. This was what she was doing at seven thirty that morning—just wandering, maybe looking at pictures, thinking about shit. Who knows.

"Danny, you is huggin' me. I is sad today. Tomorrow is Daddy's, how you say, good-bye," Stana reminded me as I brought her in for a more-loving-than-usual hug. "Danny, you is be man of the house now. Daddy is no more. You is need be as kind and carin' and lovin' like Daddy."

"I don't think so, Stana. I'll never be a true man and good person like him . . . Hey, have you noticed that my bed smells like cat piss?" I asked.

"Yes, Danny, I is smellin'. Once Daddy be gone and Mommy be gone, you is takin' kitty and . . ." Stana lifted her thumb up to her neck and quickly brought it across her throat, as to imply that once my dad and mom were dead, I should start my new "kind" and "carin' " and "lovin' " postparent era by slitting a cat's throat.

"We'll worry about that later, but could you wash the sheets?"

"Danny, I washin' and if I is seein' kitty, I is kickin' in head," Stana said while pumping her left leg forward in a kicking motion. "I is sad about Daddy. He is such, how say, nice man, but I is hatin' kitty."

I trooped upstairs from the basement and headed straight for the fridge to begin cooking my hearty egg and ham breakfast. I reached into the back of the fridge to the egg basket and dug my hand deep, only to find that we didn't have any eggs. I opened the meat drawer. No ham. The fruit and vegetable bin. No bananas. I opened the orange juice and found that someone had played that joke where the person drinks all of something and then puts the empty carton back in the fridge. The only thing I could find was a giant potato salad Stana had made and some leftover lasagna.

Stana walked upstairs holding all the sheets in her tiny, Holocaust-surviving arms. It looked as though she were hugging a giant bear draped in cat piss–stained sheets. I should have helped her. My dad would have taken all the sheets and washed them while Stana kicked up her old feet and had an Arnold Palmer. But instead I said, "Stana, are we out of eggs?"

"Stana is usin' eggs and makin' potato salad and puttin' in fridge. You have that."

So, I reluctantly made myself a plate of potato salad with a side of lasagna and started the day. So much for the hearty breakfast.

I walked around the house to see what everyone else was up to. Greg was still asleep. Greg was a big sleeper these days. He was exhausted from our long year and crankier than ever. He, more than the rest of us, just wanted this to be over so we could move on. His sharp tongue had gotten even sharper and he had become terrifyingly blunt. He had gotten the week off from his reporter job. The poor gay goof had to spend his one week of vacation time watching his dad die and then attending his funeral. He probably would have rather gone to Costa Rica, like all those spoiled yuppies with no real problems.

Tiffany was returning from getting coffee. She had brought me one, just to ensure that I would have diarrhea throughout the day, especially when combined with the potato salad. She, too, had taken the week off work. She, more than the rest of us, really had her shit together. She was a real adult. She had a job, was getting her M.B.A., and had a boyfriend with a large cock who was on his way to becoming a lawyer. She was set. Somehow ALS hadn't ruined her life, but instead made it stronger. Conversely, I was a wandering soul—a reflection of an aimless and spoiled generation pulling America into a downward spiral.

Chelsea gòt up. We told her that she had to miss the whole upcoming week of school because her dad was dying. She was pretty upset with that—not because her dad was dying, but because she didn't want to get behind in her AP classes. She was consequently running around the house trying to get all her homework done.

"Relax, Chelsea. Take it easy. Your dad's dying tomorrow. That's more important than school," I told her.

"Nothing's more important than school," she argued back.

"What if they offered a class on your dad dying? Then would you give a shit about all this?" I asked.

"If it were an AP," she replied.

Jessica arrived. She was almost five months pregnant now. She just plopped down on the bed next to my dad's bed. She looked sad and tired.

"You look like you need a drink," I said.

"Yeah, but I can't because of the baby," she said rubbing her belly.

"One more reason to not get fucked and impregnated by your lacrosse coach, I guess," I said. God, what's the matter with me?

My mom then woke up, peeled her sweaty body off Dad's, and started her day by popping a few Klonopins. "My doctor told me to take these," she assured us. "I need them."

My dad lay in his bed, awake. He always seemed to be awake in the mornings. I can't ever remember a time when I caught him sleeping past eight. I was greeted by his beautiful and calming smile. It was going to be hard to lose that smile. Life would always be a little sadder. Knowing that, just like me, he didn't want to make this day into a sad one, I said, "Last full day. You ready for this?"

He nodded his head, as much as he could.

"Good. You look like complete shit, by the way," I joked. He smiled.

Greg finally woke up and wandered into the room. We were now all there, ready for the last full day with our dad. He looked around at his tired family. He had lost everything in this battle, but he still had us. We pledged that today was going to be great.

"Should we start by playing the song?" my mom asked, referring to the Beatles song she had been blasting on repeat over the last few days.

"God. Please, no. That song might make my head explode," I said.

"If you turn on that song, I'll turn off Dad's respirator right now," Greg said.

"Yeah, I'm pretty tired of the song, too," my dad managed to say.

"Fine, but we've got to play it at some point," my mom said. We all rolled our eyes.

I had been filming the last couple of weeks of my dad's life. My pal Dom was into film and had suggested I get a camera because this situation was so unique, so I did. Since I had started filming, I had been directing a lot of the drama. Like, if someone said something dramatic and poignant, and I wasn't rolling, I'd make them repeat the line as if it was original. Today, I decided that I'd set up the camera on a tripod and just let it sit there in my dad's room while the day played out.

First things first, my mom wanted to talk about the logistics of the big day tomorrow. She had compiled a list in her red notebook of all the people who were supposed to be in the room when my dad officially went off the respirator. I really didn't want to be in the room for it. I figured that we'd seen enough, that we'd watched him get closer and closer to death over the last year, and that we didn't need to watch him *actually* die. I just knew that I didn't want my last memory of him to be one in which I had to watch his life drain from his body. I brought this up.

"I'm not sure we should be in the room with Dad when he dies," I suggested.

"We're going to be in the room. You don't have to be if you don't want to be, but the rest of us are all going to be here," my mom said.

"Yeah, Dan, it's important to Dad," Tiffany said.

"Fuck, well, I don't want to be the one asshole who's not in the room. Dad, do you want all of us with you? It's really up to you," I said, looking over at my dad.

"I'd like you all to be there," he said.

Fuck. I'd be in the room.

My mom started assembling the exclusive list like she was the bouncer at some shitty nightclub. Besides us, the others to be in the room were my mom's best friend Kelly, Dr. Buys, Sam, our family friend Gary Neuenschwander, Stana, Creepy Todd, Dr. Bromberg, a nurse named Sunny from hospice, and Regina. No one else was to be let in.

"I can't believe Creepy Todd is going to be in the room," said Greg. "He's practically responsible for killing Dad."

"Fuck you, Greg," said Jessica. "Get used to him."

"God, has anyone seen my calculator?" said Chelsea. She had her pre-calculus book opened and was getting some studying in while we sorted out all this shit. We ignored her.

The big debate was over whether my dad's siblings would be in the room.

"Those fuckers can't just show up at the last minute and expect to get to spend all this time with him at the very end," my mom said. "Plus, they probably have some bullshit golf game planned before they go off and get all fucked up and drunk," she added, looking pretty fucked up herself from all the Klonopin.

I felt that my dad should have his siblings with him when he passed. I know I will want to have my siblings around me when I die from liver disease in a few years. So I argued on their behalf. But my mom insisted that they not be allowed in the room. At least they had gotten some time alone with him so they could say good-bye.

In addition to the list, my mom—with the help of Creepy Todd— had organized this incredibly tacky send-off where all the children of the neighborhood would be given a balloon. On the day of the Big Unhook, my dad would be wheeled to the upstairs window over-looking the driveway and look down at the children. He would some-how wave, and then be wheeled to his room to be taken off the respirator, having spent his last moments saluting a bunch of Mormon strangers. He would die. Then we would run to the window to alert these incredibly important neighborhood children—most of whom had never even met my dad—that he was dead. We would symbolically close the blinds shut, and they would all release the balloons, carrying his spirit to a heaven that he didn't believe existed.

"Okay, so who's going to pick up the balloons?" she asked.

"Can we drop the balloons and focus on Dad?" I yelled. "We haven't focused on him at all and it's his last full day. You need to stop flipping out about shit that doesn't matter," I said.

"Yeah, Mom, you need to turn the crazy down a couple notches today," Greg said.

"I'm sorry that I'm losing my husband and I'm upset about it," she cried back, popping another Klonopin.

"We're losing our father, so it's hard for us, too, but we want to spend the time we have with him, and not worry about lists and releasing a bunch of bullshit balloons," I said.

"Yeah, Mom, just shut up for two seconds," Chelsea said, looking up from her math book to get in on this mom-bashing session.

"Why are you all being mean to me?" she asked.

"Because you're insane. Take some more Klonopin and relax," I said. I walked over to the TV and began clicking around HBO On Demand. "Here, I'm going to find us a nice soft-core porn and it's going to chill us all out."

I finally found *Y tu mamá también*, which opens with a nice fuck scene that made me hope no one I've loved was presently having wild sex in Mexico. It took about three or four moans combined with thrusts before the room consensus deemed it inappropriate and made me turn it off.

"I hope Abby isn't fucking someone in Mexico," I quietly murmured to myself while clicking off the TV.

My mom eventually decided Creepy Todd would take over the whole balloon-release extravaganza. He would pick the balloons up in the morning. We could finally focus on hanging out with our dad.

"What should we do?" I asked.

"I might go back to sleep," said Greg.

"Greg, come on. We can sleep when this is over," said Tiffany.

"I swear someone took my calculator. People keep moving all my shit around and I'm getting really sick of it. I need my fucking calculator," said Chelsea.

"I know exactly where it is, Chelsea. I buried it thirty feet below the earth's core last night," I said.

"Really?" she asked.

"No, Chelsea, I have no fucking idea where your calculator is. You need to keep track of your own shit. You're seventeen years old," I said.

"You're seventeen years old," she giggled back.

"Let's go for a walk," said my dad, finally cutting in.

"Sounds good to me," I said.

"No, not yet. I want to spend some time alone with your dad," my mom said.

"Can't we all spend time with him?" I asked.

"Yes, but I want to give him his daily blow job first," she said, while washing a Klonopin down with a spoonful of yogurt.

"Jesus, Mom. That's fucking gross," I said.

"Todd's going to pick up the balloons in the morning. Did I mention that? One less thing to worry about," she said, dropping the blow job momentarily.

"Oh, great. What a load off. I was super stressed about the balloons," I said.

"Yeah, me, too," said my mom, not picking up on the sarcasm. "Okay, everyone out of the room. I need some time with Dad. It shouldn't take too long," she added with an air of confidence.

We all shook our heads in disbelief and exited the room, not wanting to stick around to watch our dying parents do oral.

My mom and my dad had been married for thirty years. They had a really loving relationship. Life is all about accumulating people who love you no matter what, and they loved each other no matter what. He had stood by her through all the cancer. Through all the battles she had with his family. Through the deaths of her parents. Through the deaths of her many cancer friends. And now she had stood by him through all this. Their love for each other really came through during my dad's last year, even if my dad was crippled and my mom was zonked out for most of it. They would do anything for each other. Fuck, my mom was even giving him blow jobs right up to the last minute . . .

"Oh, fuck!" I yelled to Greg. "My camera is in there. Fuck. Fuck. Fuck."

I had to get it out of there. I really didn't want to be the owner of some amateur porno of a cancer patient blowing a terminally ill man about to die from Lou Gehrig's disease as they both cried. "I've got to get that thing back," I said.

I knocked on the door. Nothing. It's pretty hard to talk when you have Lou Gehrig's disease, or if you have a dick in your mouth. I knocked again. Nothing. What should I do? If I thought the image of my dad dying tomorrow was going to be haunting, imagine having the image of my mom blowing my dad imprinted onto my brain forever. It'd be too much. I'd have to check straight into an insane asylum. Should I risk it? Should I swing open the door? Should I send Stana in there? Should I just go in there with my ears and eyes covered?

"Fuck it, I'm going in," I said.

I swung open the door with my eyes covered, trying to go straight for the camera. But, as I entered, I didn't hear the sounds of someone getting blown, but rather an in-love couple gently weeping and whispering "I love you," over and over. I took my hands off my eyes. My mom was curled up next to my dad, holding him tightly. My dad was crying.

"Don't go, Bob. I can't lose you. You're the love of my life. I can't live in a world without you," my mom bawled.

"It will be okay, Deb. You're stronger than I am. You'll be just fine," my dad said.

"Sorry to interrupt. I just didn't want the, you know, camera on during the blow job, or whatever," I said, picking up the camera and turning it off.

"Tell him not to go. Tell him that we'll continue to take care of him. Tell him that everything will get better," my mom cried.

I took a deep breath. "Well, it's his decision, and he's made it. So I think we've got to accept it. We've fought this disease long enough," I said, getting a little weepy. "Fuck, that was a great moment. We really should have gotten it on camera. Can we reshoot that?" I asked.

"I'll have no one," my mom said, ignoring my question.

"You'll have us kids. We're not Dad, but we'll help you out," I said, while giving a reassuring nod toward my dad, finally feeling like the man of the house for once. I walked over and wrapped my arms around them both. I pulled out of it. "I'll leave you two to it. Just wanted to grab the camera."

After my parents had done whatever it was that they did in their time alone, the whole family went on a walk through our neighborhood. When we got home, we read some letters from friends and loved ones to my dad. He loved listening to those. The letters combined with all the good-byes made him feel like the most loved person on earth.

As night hit, we were all in my dad's room, not really saying much, just enjoying the comfort of being a complete family for one last night. I read my dad some of my writing. I was expecting him to laugh and cry and love it, but he just noted that he didn't know I masturbated so much. "I do," I reassured him.

It was finally time for bed. Jessica, my mom, Tiffany, and Chelsea were all sleeping in Dad's room, so there was no room for Greg or me. Oh well. We got to spend a lot of time with him over the last year, more than the rest. I felt fulfilled.

I said good night to my dad for the last time and headed out. As I was about out of the room, my mom yelled after me. "Wait!" I was half expecting to turn back and see my dad standing up, smiling, not having Lou Gehrig's disease, holding my laughing mom. "We just played the most epic prank of all time on you. We're fine. We just wanted to see if you truly cared about us. It was a test, a way for us to get you to become an adult and experience some real-life shit. You passed. You proved your love. Everything will go back to normal starting now," I expected them to say as everything faded back to normal. A WELCOME HOME DAN THE MAN sign would drop from the ceiling. My dad would hand me a glass of wine. My mom's hair would shoot out of her head, growing into the beautiful, curly delight it had been before cancer got to her. We'd dance around the room and laugh and sing and promise to be happy forever.

Instead, my mom shot out of bed, fumbled around for the CD player remote, and said, "We've got to listen to the song one last time." My dad rolled his eyes as "I'll Follow the Sun" started to play.

I finally got to bed. The sheets still smelled like cat piss.

THE DAY OF

M y dad picked September 22 as the last day of his life because it was the first official day of autumn, his favorite time of the year. When fall hits in Utah, the leaves begin to change, making the mountainside as colorful as a box of crayons. The weather hangs around the seventies—never too hot, never too cold. It's the last warm gasp of fresh air before the snowplows and salt cover our icy roads.

Just as the season began to change, so, too, would our lives. We were about to lose our leader, our teacher, our father, our friend. The suffering would be over, but the mourning would begin. I wasn't sure if that was a good or a bad thing. Sure, my dad wouldn't be in pain anymore, and I'd get my life back. But my dad, my pal, wouldn't be around.

On the day of, I woke up around seven and lay in bed thinking about how I wanted today to be the perfect send-off for my dad. I wanted it to be a magical day full of love, heartfelt good-byes, and reminders of what a great guy he was. I wanted him to feel good about his decision to end this. I wanted him to realize that he lived a meaningful and complete life, even if it was cut short by a shitty disease. I wanted him to know how much he meant to me, to us all.

I got out of bed and did my whole showering, dressing, brushing my teeth, judging myself in the mirror for getting so fat routine, then started the last day of my dad's life.

I timed my steps with the audible in/out air pumping from the rhythmic respirator as I ascended the stairs to his room. I had grown to love the sound of the respirator, even though I'd initially hated it. Sure, it would beep, and it was heavy, and I would occasionally bare-knuckle-punch it and talk shit to it. But its noises had come to be the heartbeat of the whole household. In a few hours, we would no longer hear its sounds, and that scared the shit out of me. A silence would fall over this house as though it was Pompeii after the volcano. Would we all be left covered in ashes and blackened until someone dug us out? Would we be frozen in this moment and become a tragic tourist destination?

"Dad, wake up. Wake up," I said as I wiggled his big toe dangling off the end of his home hospital bed. He was still asleep, amazingly. He looked as peaceful as I'd ever seen him. He even had a little smirk on his face. He was content.

My mom was curled up in bed with him, a frown on her face. She was not content. She didn't want him to go. She was clinging to him so hard that it looked as if she wanted to follow him to the grave. Maybe that'd be for the best: the two of them going at once. Maybe we could get a discount on the funerals, some sort of fucked-up two-for-one deal.

"Wake up, Dad," I said again. "I made you a big breakfast."

My dad slowly blinked awake. Last day on earth and he had to wake up to his fat son hovering over him, rubbing in the fact that he couldn't eat real food. "Made you eggs Benedict with a side of extra-greasy bacon and a big glass of freshly squeezed OJ," I joked as I grabbed some cans of Promote and set them bedside for his last meal.

Tiffany, who had slept on the floor of her old room, appeared with her morning Starbucks. Jessica and Chelsea had slept in the bed next to my dad's. Greg wandered into the room in his morning robe. We were all there.

My mom slowly woke up as well. She had been completely knocked out by the Klonopin. The short hair that had managed to grow back in after the chemo was standing straight up. Her face was glossy from her body trying to sweat out all the toxins. She looked like the Grinch.

"You look like the Grinch," I told her. "The Chemo Grinch."

"Did you really make him breakfast?" asked the Chemo Grinch.

"No, it was just a stupid joke because he can't eat," I explained.

"Well, I'm just going to have yogurt for breakfast," she said.

"Changing it up a little. I like it," I said.

I looked outside for the first time. It was rainy and gray. "Oh, perfect," I muttered to myself. We had planned on taking my dad up Millcreek Canyon for one last family stroll alongside the river. But, with the rain, that plan was ruined.

"Fuck, I lost my rosary," the Chemo Grinch said. "Fuck, fuck, fuck, fuck, fuck. I need that goddamn thing if I'm going to get through this." The rosary was my grandpa Joe's, one of his only possessions through several years in a Japanese POW camp during World War II. She figured if it could get him through that, it could get her through this. She shot out of bed. "Quick, everyone look for my rosary. I need it. How am I going to get through all this without it? There is no way."

"Well, there is no God, if that helps at all," I callously said.

"Danny, I need that fucking rosary," the Chemo Grinch said as she dropped to the ground to look for it.

As usual, I was being a real asshole. And my poor dad had to watch my awful display of behavior. But I was upset with my mom. Sure, I felt sorry for her, but I was angry that she had spent the last few weeks completely numbed out by drugs. I understood how hard it was, but still, I wished she would put her own needs aside for just today so that we could all focus on my dad.

"We'll find it. It's here somewhere," Tiffany said. She wasn't in the mood to joke around. She got on the floor and started to look for the rosary with my mom. Tiff was always the leader—the one who took things seriously while Greg and I dicked around and made stupid jokes.

"Oh, here it is," I said.

"Where?" my frantic mom said.

"Just kidding," I said. "Oh, wait, here it is."

"You found it?" said my mom.

"Just kidding," I said, really racking up my asshole points for the day. What's the matter with me? Fucking with my mom on my dad's last day. We were supposed to have a very peaceful day that left my dad thinking that we'd be all right after he left us.

"Please. Stop that. This is very serious. I can't deal with today if I don't have some comfort," she explained.

"Okay, I won't fuck with you anymore," I said. "Oh, here it is. I'm not kidding this time."

"Really," she said.

"Just kidding," I said.

Tiffany finally found my mom's rosary beneath my dad's hospital bed. My mom started to calm down instantly. I guess religion can provide some comfort, if nothing else. I told her to go take a shower and chase down a Klonopin with some yogurt to relax, so we could proceed with my dad's last day. She agreed.

* * *

Today wasn't all fun and games. Sunny from hospice was due to arrive at our house around 1 p.m. She would start my dad on a low morphine drip that would slowly leave him unconscious and unable to feel pain, or anything for that matter. Dr. Bromberg would arrive around two thirty. He would start turning down the respirator when my dad was officially deemed unconscious via the morphine. He would gradually die via loss of oxygen to the body, around four o'clock. Then we'd run to the window and we'd signal to the neighborhood kids to release the balloons. Creepy Todd had that all organized. That was his job.

The other people who were going to be in the room would arrive around noon. However, we got some bad news from Sam. He was supposed to spend the day with us, but, in an extra hard slap to the face by God's callused hand, Sam's father had passed away the previous Wednesday. So he was in Florida laying his dad to rest as we prepared to do the same back at home. He left a nice message on my phone that I played for my dad:

> Hi, Dan. This is Sam calling from Florida. I know this is going to be really hard for you all the next couple of days. Tell your dad that I really wish I could be there. I'm so sorry that it didn't work out. Let him know that I'm thinking about him. I love him so dearly. I probably have two really close friends in the world and today I'm losing one of them. I'll miss him greatly. He'll always be with me. Yesterday I had a great run on Clearwater Beach. I thought about him. I don't think I'll have a run in the future without thinking about him.

It would have been great for Sam to have been there. It would have, at least, made my dad feel better about everything he was going through. Sam had been everything you could ask a best friend to be. The two ran six marathons together, and when my dad got ALS, instead of running the other way, Sam stood by his side. They didn't finish every race together—there was the occasional cramp or pulled muscle or bathroom break that separated the two—but I wish my dad had been able to finish this one with Sam by his side.

"You know I slept with Sam's daughter, Becca, right?" I asked.

My dad smiled and nodded. "You've told me several times."

My mom came back in with a smile on her Grinch face.

"You take that Klonopin?" I asked.

"I did," she said, forcing a high five on me. She looked really out of it. She clearly wasn't going to remember anything from today. She spoke in a soft voice that could hardly be heard, her speech now muddled by the drugs. Her eyes could barely stay open. "Could you read me the will? I'm not sure I trust it," she asked.

"Are you serious?" I asked.

"Yes, please. I don't want Dad's family fucking me out of money. It'll make me feel better," she said, handing me the will.

She thought that there was some trick in my dad's will that would give all his money away to people she didn't like. I opened it up and read it aloud to put her mind at ease. She was too out of it to hear a word I was saying, but I read it anyway while she spooned yogurt into her mouth, her eyes closed. She looked like a child being lulled to sleep by a bedtime story.

The rain stopped and the clouds began to clear, letting the sun suck up all the fallen precipitation like a giant invisible straw. The sky turned a perfect blue to match my dad's eyes. Things were looking up.

Regina arrived and helped get my dad ready as my mom dozed off in the chair next to his bed. He looked great: clean-shaven, his graying hair slicked from left to right, the way he always wore it. He wanted to wear his marathon-running gear on his last day. So we slipped the orange hat on his head and the blue shirt over his bony shoulders. We needed some sun to gleam off my dad's still-alive face one more time, so we decided to head outside for a walk around the neighborhood.

"No man should die without a sunburn," I said to him, taking off his hat and ruffling up his combed hair. "Come on, let's load this fucker into his wheelchair," I said to Regina and Greg.

Meanwhile, my mom shot back awake with a sudden burst of energy. She looked at Regina, Greg, and me as we started to transfer my dad to his chair.

"Where the fuck are you going?" she asked.

"We're going outside," Greg said.

"Well, I have some questions to ask your dad," she said.

She opened up her red notebook. She was trying to learn everything that she had to do once my dad died. She wasn't in the state of mind to really absorb anything, but she fired off a set of questions:

"How do I change the filters in the furnace?"

"How do I balance a checkbook?"

"Should we sell the van?"

"How do I fix the pool cover if it breaks?"

"What do I do if we need to cut down some trees in the yard?"

"Are your siblings going to fuck us out of money?"

"Can we read the will again?"

I interrupted, ignoring my frantic mother. "We're going outside now."

We all swarmed around my dad as if he were some sort of celebrity. We argued over who was going to drive him to the nearby elevator. As everyone pleaded their case, I grabbed the wheelchair controls and drove away.

"Fuck you all. I'm driving him," I said, middle finger raised. I had been the first in the family to learn how to run his stupid respirator. I had programmed his stupid communication device and helped him learn how to use his stupid wheelchair. I was the first to change his stupid diapers while he remained in his stupid hospital bed. I was the last to walk him up a stupid flight of stairs and the first to call his stupid suction machine a bad word. I had his neurologist's stupid phone number memorized and knew more about stupid Lou Gehrig's disease than stupid Lou Gehrig himself. I had earned the opportunity to drive him to the stupid elevator.

I got my dad into the elevator. We had had very few moments alone lately. Someone was always around. The elevator only fits him and one other person, so we got a lot of our intimate, one-on-one conversations done during these short rides. The last day of Dad's life was no exception.

"Can you believe today is the day?" I asked.

"No, I really can't," he managed to say.

"Seems like I was heading back from California just yesterday," I said. I had, in fact, been home for exactly 366 days.

"I know. I could walk back then," he said.

"What a wild, fucked-up year," I said.

"Thanks for being here for it," he said.

"Wouldn't have missed it. I love you, Dad," I said.

"I love you, too, DJ," he said.

The accordion elevator door swooshed open before we could get too emotional and sappy. Greg was standing in the garage with a bottle of water in his hand. It was just him. Everyone else had disappeared.

"Where's Mom?" I asked.

"I don't know. She's worrying about something pointless," Greg replied.

"So she's not coming on the walk?" I asked. "Jesus, we really need her around. This is the worst day in the world for her to pull her wacko shit."

Greg took a big pull from his water. "I know this is fucked up to say, but I feel like we're losing the wrong parent. I mean, we're stuck with her now? Things would be so much better if she were the one dying and you were the one living," Greg said, while gently stroking my dad's hair to one side.

Tiffany, Regina, Jessica, Chelsea, and Creepy Todd finally came out the front door. We all stood on our cracked driveway in front of our tired home. My mom was still inside. We waited for a minute, all our eyes trained on the front door, hoping that she would emerge.

I finally said, "Let's go. She can catch up if she wants to do this." We all turned our backs to the door and walked away, like disappointed children realizing that their parents didn't love them anymore, realizing that there was no one left to help them fight their fights, realizing that they were all alone.

We began our push down Briarcreek Drive, our street for nearly eighteen years. Just as our backs were good and turned, we heard our mom's familiar voice. "Sorry." We all excitedly turned toward her. She was running out of the front door. She caught up with us. "I thought I was going to shit my pants," she explained.

"Glad you decided to come," I said as I smacked her on her back.

"Not so hard. I just put on a fresh Fentanyl patch," she said with a coy smile and an attempted wink.

As we began to walk—our mom with a fresh dose of pain medication being sucked into her back—things started to sink in. This was it. This was actually the last walk with my dad. This was actually the last time the neighbors had the chance to look out the windows, look at my dad, and say, "That poor, poor man. To be stuck with both that awful disease and that awful family. My lord." This quiet, physically disabled man was the life vest that held this family afloat, even as Lou Gehrig's washed over the person he once was. We only had him for another hour. We needed to take advantage of this and ask all of life's important questions.

"Okay, so let's each ask dad one last question," I suggested.

"What's your favorite color?" my pilled-up mom asked.

"If you were a zoo animal, which one would you be?" Chelsea asked with a giggle.

"Daddy, who are you the proudest of? Keep in mind that Danny doesn't have a job," Greg joked.

"What's your favorite mountain to ski?" Tiffany asked.

"What's your favorite episode of *Friends*?" Jessica asked.

"I meant things that matter, like 'What's the meaning of life?' or 'What's the key to happiness in ten words or less?'" I shot back at them.

"No one knows that sort of shit, Danny. And the ones who claim they do are the biggest idiots of all, since we're all different, and we're all just trying to get through the day," said my druggy mom, displaying a remarkable flash of coherence.

We pushed forward. Regina kept trying to hold my dad's hand, but my mom kept shooing her away. "This is family time," my mom told her. Poor Regina—searching for love in all the wrong places. I pulled out the video camera and tried to capture the towering Wasatch Mountains in the background to remind us that the universe is huge and we are all merely parasites shit here by luck. I thought looking at the mountains would help dwarf our problems, but it didn't. My dad was still dying. Our problems were still as big as ever.

We were approaching a street named Keddington. When we first moved to Utah some twenty years before, we'd lived on this street. It was a modest tree-filled neighborhood full of happy families and old couples who I always thought would die before my dad.

We were silent. There really wasn't much else to say. The important thing was that we were all together. In a fucked-up way, my dad getting sick was good for this reason. Tiffany and I had never gotten along, but we had gone from being at war to being war buddies who had bonded over a real shit situation. Greg and I had rekindled our roles as each other's best friend, and we had spent many nights talking about life. I knew we'd have each other forever. Chelsea and I had been given the chance to make each other laugh. And though I was critical of Jessica, I made it clear it was because I loved her and felt protective of her. We knew we could turn to each other if we ever really needed something. Before she married Creepy Todd, she had asked me for help getting a prenuptial agreement drafted, and I had turned to her when I was too drunk to drive but still really wanted to go to the bars to try to sloppily hit on girls. And my mom and I—well, we'd sort things out after this mess. I had faith that she'd turn it around again and keep on fighting, keep on being our resilient, spirited mom cheering us on no matter what. We were a family. A nice big fucked-up family that was certainly cursed with some misfortune, but we were still a family. We looked after each other. We had to. No one else would.

Our walk came to an end. We rolled back into the driveway of our home. We took my dad out to our backyard gazebo area looking out at the mountains. Creepy Todd left to get the balloons for the balloon-release shenanigans.

We were all circled around my dad as if he was a fire keeping us warm. I couldn't believe this was actually it. I looked over at my tired dad, and he looked at me, at his whole family. He looked like he wanted to say more, do more. But he couldn't. This fucking disease.

And just then, the sun hit his face as though he was the only person on earth it was lighting up. All the chirping birds in our backyard shut up. In fact, they stood and began to salute my father with their little bird wings. His respirator, hanging on the back of his chair, turned itself off, finally shutting the fuck up. My dad lifted up his arm and unhooked himself from the device. The hole in his trach filled itself in. He took a big gulp of fresh mountain air on his own accord. He cleared his throat and, just like that, his voice returned back to normal, just as it had been before the disease launched its game-winning attack.

"There, that's better, and just in time to say good-bye," he said with clarity.

We looked to the gazebo table and it was suddenly set for a family dinner, just like old times. Steaks, potatoes, asparagus, salad, and wine to wash it all down. My dad gestured to it, and we all took our seats in front of this giant feast, him, of course, at the head of the table.

He looked at his youngest daughter, Chelsea. Her unexposed emotions finally started to kick in as she uncurled his brittle, skinny fingers and squeezed his hand with her own brittle, skinny fingers. She

stopped thinking about school and realized this was an opportunity
to learn a more important life lesson. My dad looked deep into her
eyes and said, "Chelsea, you are a great kid. You are very smart and
attractive. You will make a difference in the world. Keep your mom
company and never forget that I'm still here for you, even if I'm not.
Keep up the dancing. Keep up the interest in school. Good luck learning to drive and good luck turning into a woman; both events I wish I
could witness. You are uniquely you. Never change that." Chelsea cried
and said, "You're not really going to do this, are you?" flashing her
signature blend of optimism and denial. My dad nodded his head
and said that he was. Chelsea understood and released his hand.

My dad looked at Jessica. She was already crying. And not a soft
weeping, but a hard and painful expression of misery that was difficult
for all of us to watch. Her body trembled with powerful sobs, her
emotions banging against her rib cage. She got up from her seat, gave
my dad a two-armed hug, and watered his shoulder with her tears. My
dad said, "Jessica, I wish you the best of luck. Good luck with your
marriage. Good luck with your pregnancy. Good luck with everything.
Kiss your children for me. Go back to school when you're ready. You
are smarter than you think. You are a very gentle and kind person
with a bigger heart than any of us. I love you very much. Good luck."

My dad looked at Greg with a gleam of serenity and poise. Greg was
the strongest of all of us. He started to cry and thanked my dad for
going on the respirator so he got to spend an extra ten months with
his number-one conversation buddy. My dad said, "Greg, you are the
new rock. You react with both emotion and logic, making you a rare
commodity. You are the easiest person in the world to talk to, and a
great listener. You will use those skills to achieve more than the rest
of us. I hope you always cherish the time we spent together: the U.S.
Open in New York, the trip to France, the countless times we battled
it out on the tennis court. You have shown bravery and honesty in
your life and I am proud of you for who you are. I love you." Greg's
crying intensified. He didn't want to lose his dad. He didn't want any
of this to happen. But he understood and didn't try to talk him out of
his decision.

My dad turned toward me, his oldest son. I thanked him for all that
he had given me and taught me. I reminded him how a silly sport like
basketball had brought us together and thanked him for always letting me beat him to build my confidence. He said, "Get a fucking job

and lose twenty pounds, you bum, and then look after Mom and help her as much as she needs. I know you think she's crazy, but also realize that she's your mother and you are half her. You have given me a lot over the last year and let go of a lot along the way, but I want you to move forward without resentment toward me for putting us all through this, toward Abby for moving on with her life, and toward your mother for putting so much on your shoulders. I think in the long run you will look back at this and think it was all worth it because I'm your fucking father and it was your duty to care for me when I needed you the most. I'm sorry it happened when you were only twenty-five. It is now time to get on with your life and push forward as an adult without any excuses." I reached over and pinched his nipples and messed up his hair. I looked at him with a loving smile and said, "Don't watch me masturbate from heaven."

My dad looked at Tiffany. Tiffany tried very hard to not cry. The intense effort reddened her face, which she covered with her hand. She finally broke down and exploded into moans. Her rare expression of intense emotion caused us all to cry, even the saluting birds in the trees. My dad said to her, "Tiffany, some of my best days in life were spent on the mountain with you, watching you carve through the snow with grace and ease. I always loved the mountains, and of all my kids, you were the only one who loved them as much as I did. You will do great things in life and end up exactly where you want to be, even if you doubt yourself right now. Know that I'm always looking after you. You are beautiful and I love you." Tiffany cried and promised to think of him every time she was about to descend into a fresh batch of powder, beating all the tourists and wannabes to the punch.

Finally, my dad looked at my mom, his wife. Her mouth was a perfect upside down U, and her eyes were darkened by a genuine sadness. My mom said, "Don't do this, Bob. Please. Please. Don't leave me." My dad said, "Deb, I love you so much. I did from the second I met you. You are an inspiration to us all. Don't give up the fight even though you now have to battle it for both of us. I know you were the sick one, the one with cancer who was supposed to go before me, but it didn't work that way. I'm sorry to leave you, but I hope you understand and accept my decision without being angry. You now inherit the family that we created together, and that family will be there for you and help you through this. Hold our grandchildren for the both of us, and spoil the shit out of them. Remarry if you must. I understand.

Take your mind off me. Start eating things other than yogurt; you'll need the strength to keep up the fight. Buy yourself anything you want. Don't feel alone. Your kids, our kids, will look after you because they have inherited kindness from both of us. Clean up your language so you don't pass on your bad habit to others, like you did with that shithead, tit-fucker Danny. You are the bravest, strongest, feistiest woman I have ever known, but most important, you are a survivor who has never given up. Don't give up now. I love you with all my heart." My mom burst into tears and squeezed my dad's shoulder. They looked at each other, having cleared their eyes of the blurring tears, and thanked each other for making thirty years of marriage so easy.

We were all silent for a moment to take it all in, to feel the sadness but also the joy of being together one last time.

Suddenly, just as we were finishing our last family meal, Sam appeared out of nowhere, also in his running gear. He shook his head in disbelief. "Man, Bob, this all seems so surreal." My dad agreed. Then, my dad stood up, his bones creaking and popping back to life. He stretched his arms and legs, and just like that, he was back on his trusty old feet.

He looked over at Sam and said, "How about one last run, my old friend?"

"You got it, buddy," Sam said.

They ran out of our backyard and through Salt Lake City, up Millcreek Canyon along the river, down by the Delta Center where we used to go to Jazz games and talk about life, then back along the base of Mount Olympus. Sam laughed the whole way.

Suddenly, the surroundings started to change, and my dad and Sam were no longer running through Salt Lake, but rather through my dad's whole life. First they ran through his childhood in Pocatello. They ran down the elm-tree-lined streets, packed with kids full of youth and life. They ran past my dad's family sitting at the dinner table, all of his siblings passing plates around and discussing the day's events. They ran past my dad's dependable father, who always arrived at home right around five o'clock to emphasize the important balance between work life and family life.

My dad and Sam continued their run, now through my dad's adolescence. They ran past my dad talking to his brother Jack on the back patio in Camano. They ran past my dad beginning to take an interest in women, and even getting his first hand job from Caroline Summers. They ran past my dad and Jack working long hours at their family's nearby ranch, where they learned, "Your work is not done until the last bale of hay is in the barn." They then ran past my dad's family waving him off to Drake University.

My dad and Sam continued through his adulthood. There was a blur of random and formative events: college. The fuzz surrounding college disappeared and they ran past my dad asking my mom's hand in marriage on her parents' back porch. She said "yes" as a tear of joy rolled down her cheek and onto her lip, which he promptly kissed. They ran past all his children being born and growing more and more capable. They then ran past my dad helping his children whenever they needed it the most, but allowing them to fight through their own trials and tribulations. And finally, they ran past my dad and my mom watching their kids leave the house to begin to build their own lives.

Then, finally, my dad and Sam ended their epic run and returned to our neighborhood and back to the gazebo. My dad looked over all he had done over the years and realized that he'd lived a very good life.

"That was a great run, Sam," my dad said.

"It sure was, Bob. The best yet."

Just as they were catching their breaths, everyone who my dad had ever loved and who had ever loved my dad appeared out of nowhere and started filling all the empty space around us. People even climbed to our rooftop because it was the only available vantage point. My dad yelled, "I'm not done yet!" Everyone clapped and screamed. "We love you, Bob!" people shouted at the top of their lungs. He threw both of his arms up in the air and spun around until he was dizzy, as confetti streamed from the clouds above and fireworks lit up the sky. He ran onto our tennis court, which was also surrounded by people he had loved and influenced over the course of his life, and back-flipped onto the net after serving up an ace that Roger Federer and Rafael Nadal's child couldn't have touched with a tennis racket the size of a fishing boat. My dad began tightrope walking across the net while juggling all sorts of poisonous animals. He stopped tightrope walking and began a set of one-armed push-ups on the net. One spectator said, "Bob is amazing. He can truly do anything." Another yelled, "I hope this never ends." He then back-flipped off the tennis court net and stuck the landing so well that the judges in the crowd had no score available for his one-step-above-perfection performance.

He then ran out to the crowd of friends and family, now a thousand fans deep. He maneuvered through the people and kissed everyone on their forehead and reminded them that they could make a difference in the world. He told jokes and shook hands in a way that would be remembered forever. He pulled all the sadness out of everyone's hearts and wadded it up into a soccer-ball-shaped object, then kicked it into outer space with his powerful leg.

Eventually, his triumphant performance had to come to an end. He told everyone that they had made a positive difference in his life and that he hoped he had done the same in theirs. They started to chant, "You have!" and "We'll miss you, Bob!" He reminded them all that his spirit would live on in theirs, and that life is about the relationships you form with other people and not about collecting material things to fill the void. He encouraged each and every person to turn to their neighbor and hug him or her. Everyone performed this request and then agreed that it was nice.

He thanked everyone for the love and support they had shown him, blowing kisses their way. He then looked at his watch and said, "Shit, I really have to go." Everyone understood as they watched him walk back to his wheelchair, take a deep breath, and back-flip into it. The hole in his trach reappeared. He hooked himself back to the respirator. His body went limp again. Everyone, even Sam, slowly faded away. The birds started chirping again.

"BEEP. BEEP. BEEP," said the respirator. "It's time to face reality. It's time for your dad, your pal, to finally die."

Sunny from hospice showed up and brought with her a chilly set of clouds. She carried a little black backpack full of all the chemicals that would be used to numb my dad so the respirator could be shut off.

It was time to go back inside.

We wheeled my dad around to the front of the house, past all the children who were collecting outside for the balloon release, back into the garage, then finally into the elevator. I got in with him. The accordion door closed. It was just Dad and me again, the last moment we'd spend alone together. He looked up at me and said, "Thank you," as he does every time we return from an outing.

I'm usually a smug asshole and say, "Oh, you're welcome. I know

I'm fantastic, a hero of sorts," but this time I just said, "No, thank you."

I started to feel a little sappy, so I decided to steal the last line he had uttered to his mom on her deathbed. "I'm glad you were my dad," I said.

"I'm glad you were my son," he said.

I rolled him through his bedroom. He took one last look out the window at colorful Mount Olympus looming above our house, the changing leaves reminding him that it was fall, the start of his favorite time of the year.

We entered his room and transferred him out of his wheelchair and back into his bed for the last time. The whole family was there, plus Gary, my mom's friend Kelly, Dr. Buys, Stana, Regina, Sunny from hospice, and Dr. Bromberg.

"Okay, so, Bob, we're going to start the morphine drip. You're going to start to feel numb and will slowly fade out of consciousness. Then Dr. Bromberg will turn down the respirator and you will, well, you will pass on," said Sunny.

We all took turns hugging and saying good-bye to my dad. It was hard. It was really hard. I wished he could talk so he could impart some last words of wisdom to each of us. Instead, we mostly just said, "I love you," and he looked at us with his warm, generous, big, wet eyes. We had said everything we wanted to say to him before this moment, so we didn't have to cram it all in now. He knew how much we loved him.

My mom finally accepted what was happening. She snuggled up to my dad as close as physically possible, then said, "I love you, Bob. You are so strong and we all understand this decision. Thank you for such a wonderful life. You always were my marathon man, even before you ran marathons. It's okay for you to go. It's okay for you to go now." She started to cry. We all did. "It's okay for you to go."

Jessica and Chelsea both piled into bed with my dad as they cried. Each of us touched a part of him, whatever part we could get to. Tiffany grabbed a finger. Greg touched his head. Regina had a hairy calf. I grabbed a big toe. Stana had the other big toe. Dr. Buys, Kelly, and Gary all stood in the background watching.

Sunny hooked up all the chemical pouches and the morphine began to drip.

My dad looked over his battle-tested family one last time. Better people have been through worse, but we had finally finished going through this. It had been a bumpy road, but the struggle made us stronger. We treasured our dad more than anything. He had given us so much love, laughter, and life. We would never forget all that he had done for us, all that he had taught us, all the happiness he had brought us. But it was time to finally let him go.

Soon, my dad was unconscious. Dr. Bromberg looked us all over with sad eyes. This was the worst part of his job, but it had to be done. He started turning off the respirator. Its rhythmic sound began to slow—the time between artificial breaths getting longer and longer.

"It's okay for you to go," my mom said one last time.

The respirator pushed its last breath into my wonderful dad, then stopped. The children released the balloons into the blue sky.

EPILOGUE

G oddamn it, Mom. This is so embarrassing," I barked as we struggled to keep up with a pack of prospective writing students
marching through the University of Southern California rich-bitch
campus—the endless Los Angeles sun beating down on our tired
souls. I had applied and been accepted to their Master of Fine Arts
screenwriting program. We were at an orientation day, checking out
the school to see if it was a good fit for me.

"I'm trying my best," she said back. She was a mess, carrying her
shoe and limping. "I just had surgery to remove cancer from my leg,
you little shit," she noted.

"Well, I told you not to come. But you insisted," I said as I strutted
well ahead of her, trying to catch up to my potential classmates.

"I'm sorry," she yelled.

I looked back at her—a frail, widowed woman just trying to cling
onto a little morsel of happiness and support her son's minor achieve-
ment. I walked back and helped her walk. "Come on. I don't want
to miss the speech from Dean Daley," I said as she placed her hand on
my shoulder for support and limped toward the group.

We had had a rough couple of years, dumping everything into caring
for my dad. After his peaceful death, a strange silence settled over
our house. We had been so used to hearing the hum of all the medical devices keeping him alive, and now everything was shut off. The
traffic of visitors stampeding in and out of our house had stopped.
Neighbors no longer brought over lasagnas. Regina's cheerful laugh
had faded away. It was just us. Alone. Looking over the damage Lou
Gehrig's disease had caused to our home, our lives, our world. Stana
put it best: "Home is so, so quiet now Daddy is no more."

We were tired. There were bags under our eyes. Our shoulders were slumped. We needed to sleep for the rest of our lives. We walked around our house as if it had been burned to the ground, inspecting all the damage. Our carpets were stained with cat piss. The yard was littered with leaves and dog shit. We had a raccoon problem. Balls of unswept animal hair passed over our feet like tumbleweeds in an endless desert. Boxes of unused medical supplies cluttered up rooms already full of commodes, cans of Promote, and wheelchairs. Our sad, confused dogs wandered the house, not sure what had happened, wondering why no one was petting them. It was as though everyone and everything had aged ten years. It had become a dilapidated museum of our once prosperous life.

We had to rebuild everything with our tired hands. It wasn't going to be easy, but we had to move on. We had to awake from this nightmare and start our new lives.

My mom was in a state of absolute panic and depression. She now had to learn how to do everything on her own, without the help of my dad. Despite her best efforts, she was unable to learn the family finances, as her head was too mixed up on pain pills. I tried to help her as much as I could, but I was so exhausted and angry. I couldn't help the family anymore. I had nothing more to give. I had to worry about fat Dan's big, fat, stupid life. My mom was still overusing her Fentanyl patches. Anytime we'd go out to dinner, she'd fall asleep at the table, leaving her food completely untouched. When she was home, she'd grab a couple of yogurts and cuddle up in her bed with Brighton, her chemo kitty. She was nearly as dead as my dad.

I was a confused mess in the weeks following my dad's death. I felt like I was waking up from a coma or returning to a neighborhood swept away by a tornado. I had nothing. I was living in my mom's basement, where I got drunk and played pinball alone—chasing after any feeling of pleasure. I was the poster boy for loser. Years ago, my grandparents' house had burned down after my grandpa Joe left his electric blanket on during the night. The ensuing fire took just about everything, but left their living room and TV. When we went to visit them in Twin Falls, we found them sitting in the smoky living room—its walls blackened, everything in shambles—eating soup and watching TV. That's how I felt—like my home had been destroyed, but I was still hanging around.

I didn't want to be at home anymore, but I was stuck. I had no outs, nowhere to go. Abby was already dating someone else in San Francisco, proving that cute, happy girls can move on a lot faster after a breakup than dumpy, depressed dudes. She posted a picture on Facebook of herself in a swimsuit standing on a beach next to her shirtless new boyfriend, drinks in their hands. They were living the good life I had wanted to be living with her. I had officially been replaced. I cried as hard as I've ever cried when I saw that picture. Fuck Facebook.

I was also worried about the strange gap on my résumé.

"Looks like you weren't employed for the last year?" I expected any potential employer to ask.

"Oh, yeah, sorry. I was just taking care of my dying father. Lou Gehrig's disease. I'm pretty sad and lonely and beat up over it. I might now be dead inside forever. Anyway, you'll notice that I got my business and psychology degree from Berkeley . . ." I'd say back, wishing I had stayed in bed that morning.

After a few months of moping around, I got a job helping a friend write copy for his motivational Web site. He was building programs to help inspire people to work harder and build the lives they dreamed of having. It was a good job, and my boss was incredibly generous, but I should've been going through the program myself instead of helping to write it. I was completely depressed and didn't have a positive thing to say about the world, or aspirations, or dreams. I was a cynical asshole with a "What's the point? We're all going to die anyway" attitude. "If I learned one thing from my dad's death it's that we all die," I repeated to anyone who would listen.

I was mainly consumed with trying to move on and meet a new girl. Becca was on-again, off-again with her boyfriend, so I decided to leave that alone. It was too messy. I started going out a lot and drinking with my friends. Dom and I were closer than ever now that I was an official member of the Dead Dad Club. I rented a loft in downtown Salt Lake. It was nice to get away from the cat piss smell and to be out on my own again. It was just too much to live in our broken-down house. I turned into quite a party animal, making up for my lack of a social life while my dad was dying. My work hours were flexible, so I didn't have to worry too much about hangovers. So I started a year of living it up a little. Loft parties. Late-night drinking. Lots of dicking around and dead dad jokes. That sort of stuff.

Somewhere in the middle of this sloppy year, I pulled it together enough to apply to some screenwriting M.F.A. programs. This whole situation had given me a restart button at twenty-six. I had liked my old job in Los Angeles, but the business world now seemed so artificial to me—a bunch of slaves giving away their lives for a paycheck and an attempt to buy happiness. To become great at something, you truly have to love it. Over the course of caring for my dad and dealing with his death, I had grown to love writing and movies. They were an escape. So I figured I'd actually give screenwriting a go. I owed it to myself to at least chase after my unrealistic dreams a little. I applied to USC, NYU, Columbia, Austin, Miami, and UCLA, and waited.

Meanwhile, my other siblings were getting on with their lives. Tiffany was still dating Big Cock Brian, who was still out in Maine at law school. Tiffany finished up her M.B.A. at Westminster College the next spring. I went to her graduation drunk and whooped it up louder than anyone when they called her name. Afterward, she moved to Maine and started working an event-planner job, then she and BCB moved back to Park City, where they now live with their adorable golden retriever, Lilly. The year had made us closer than ever. Now we knew we had to have each other's backs. We had lost a lot, but we had finally gained a solid relationship with each other.

Greg continued working for *The Park Record* in Park City. The winter after my dad's death, he got to cover the Sundance Film Festival. Somewhere along the way, he ended up with my dad's Lexus. I always thought it was funny that he was supposed to be some poor reporter grinding it out in a small mountain town, all while driving a $60,000 Lexus. He had my dad's easygoing temperament and approach to life, so he seemed to move on pretty fast and not dwell on the death. Greg went on to study fiction writing at Austin's Michener Center on a full-ride scholarship. He just finished a memoir about his childhood called *Long-Term Side Effects of Accutane*. I'm endlessly proud of him.

Jessica got busy building a new life with Todd. I got to know Todd a lot better and stopped calling him Creepy Todd once I discovered that he was a pretty good guy. I still thought the timing of their marriage was horrible. It seemed to be the event that marked my dad's downward turn. But Jessica was happy, and Todd was doing a great job of taking care of her. She decided that school wasn't for her. It's not for everyone. So she focused on creating a family. On February 2, 2009, she had her first child. She's a terrific mother.

Chelsea continued dancing her skinny ass off. God, she loves dance so much. We eventually taught her how to drive, and she passed her driving test on the first try. It took me three tries. Once she got a car, she proudly placed an I LOVE DANCE sticker on the back windshield. Every time I borrow her car, I have to act like I really love dance. Chelsea was clearly affected by my dad's death, though she didn't show it. She spent most of her time at the funeral shaking her head and saying, "I can't believe we got that slut Erin to be the pastor for this." Her silly jokes kept me sane while everything else was crumpling to shit. I continued to try to step in as her horrible father figure. I'd ask her, "So, Chelsea, now that Dad's officially dead, who's your father figure?" She'd usually say, "Probably Greg, or our dog Berkeley," then giggle. She went on to graduate with honors from the University of Utah with a degree in psychology, then moved to New York City to attend the Joffrey School of Ballet.

As the year after my dad's death marched on, I continued working on motivating people and getting too drunk. The drinking started to become a problem. I was always the last man standing at the end of the night, which is a depressing party position to hold. It's lonely when everyone is gone and you're still going after it. Most of my college friends were a few years into working a corporate job, or were about finished with law or medical school. And here I was, stuck in Utah, moping around and trying to rebuild my life by drinking alone in a loft and writing "You can do it" bullshit for fat housewives.

I look back on the situation and realize I was a little angry. I was angry that I had dumped so much of myself into the tragedy. I was angry that I had let myself be so affected by it. I was angry that my siblings hadn't given up as much as I had. I was angry my dad went on the respirator, thus extending his life, and putting us through all that. I was angry that Abby had moved on so fast. I was angry my mom had placed so much guilt on my shoulders.

But eventually the clouds started to clear.

My mom's cancer was in check again, for the most part. She still needed IVIG and the occasional chemo or surgery, but she wasn't being bombed. Her hair had even grown back, down to her shoulders. However, she was still struggling with the Fentanyl addiction. One night she found my blog and read all the horrible, but true, things I had written about her. She was furious. She called me at 5 a.m., threatening to sue me for character defamation.

"How could you write such horrible things about me? I'm your mother."

"Because they're true, Mom. You were insane," I explained.

"No, I wasn't," she sniffled. "Was I?"

"Yeah, you were," I said. "Everything I wrote happened."

"Oh. Well, still, fuck you," she said. "Stop writing about me, you little shit-eater."

But it was a wake-up call for her. She seemed to realize that she couldn't put us through anything else. She realized that having one parent was better than having no parents at all. For a while, she was convinced that we would have been better off if she had died instead of my dad. "It's not a fucking trade, Mom," I explained. "We want you both alive." So she decided—as she had when she was first diagnosed with cancer in 1992—that she had to continue to survive so we could continue to have a mom.

It wasn't easy, but she quit all the pain pills cold turkey, all by herself. With no help. Oh, fuck, yeah! Fuck you, Lou Gehrig's disease! You didn't get our mom, too!

She started to slowly move on. She had to clear all the pictures of my dad out of the house because they made her too sad. She also started going by Frankie, the name that her parents had originally wanted to give her so long ago. I asked her how she was able to turn it around, how she was able to cope so well with the loss of Dad. "Remember how Robin said that every time I found a penny, it was your dad looking after me?" She lifted up a jar of pennies filled to the brim. "Well, apparently he is."

Everything was looking up for everyone while I was still struggling.

In the spring of 2009, I was sitting in a coffee shop, Salt Lake Roasting Company, in downtown Salt Lake, trying to blend in with the other patrons attempting to publicly appear busy and interesting, when my mom called.

"You got a letter from USC," she said with excitement.

"Oh, man. Okay. This is it," I said, suddenly nervous. "Is it a big or small envelope?" I asked.

"It's small, like a regular envelope," she replied.

"Fuck me," I said. Small envelopes from schools—undergraduate or graduate—usually mean rejection.

"Do you want me to open it?" she said.

I thought for a second, then said, "Yeah. Fuck it. Why not? Open it up." I took a sip from my disgusting Americano. I was expecting another punch to the gut.

My mom screamed.

"What? What does it say?" I yelled.

She started crying. "Stop fucking crying, Mom. What does it say?" I demanded.

She pulled her shit together. "It says, 'Congratulations! You have been admitted to the Fall 2009 Writing for Screen & Television MFA Program in the USC School of Cinematic Arts.' "

"Wow," I said. "That's unexpected."

The storm was over.

"God, I'm so proud of you. Wow. What an honor. What a fucking honor," she said, barely keeping it together.

My eyes welled up, and I started to weep. I was making an ass of myself in front of all the hipsters, but I didn't care. The acceptance, it wasn't much. It shouldn't have been that big of a deal. Millions of people go to millions of schools every year. But to me, it meant that I could officially start to rebuild. It meant that I had a way out of this situation. It meant that I was finally able to move on. Sure, it was going to still be a horrific battle to turn that education into a profession in such a batshit crazy industry, but at least I would get to try.

In an abstract way, this whole thing—this whole Lou Gehrig's mess—got me to my dream. Quitting my job, moving home, caring for my dad, feeding him, keeping him alive on a respirator, trying to make the end of his life as good as possible, dealing with my crazy mom, driving Chelsea around town—it all seemed worth it. I now had a chance to start my life over. And, fuck, it was about time I got some good news.

So there I was, with my cancer mom, stumbling around the USC campus. I knew I was going to go there. I didn't really have to look at it. The school could have been taught in a shed in the middle of a mudslide, and I still would have attended.

"Come on, they've stopped. We can catch them," I said, looking up at the group.

My mom winced in pain. Her leg was acting up again. "Shit, you okay, Mom?"

"Yeah, I'm fine," she said, sitting on a bench in the shade. I looked up at the group of students—their biggest worries being about which classes to take—then back to my mom. I was torn. Should I stay and help her? Or should I move on? Could I just leave her here? Would a little, weak woman be okay on this campus in the middle of South Central Los Angeles?

"Dan, go ahead. I'll be fine. I just need to rest," she said.

"I don't think I should leave my crippled mom in the middle of this neighborhood. You're liable to get raped," I said.

"Who's going to rape a little old lady with cancer?" she said, smiling.

"Good point," I said. I looked around. The campus was filled with students hustling about, chatting it up, planning the next party, working toward a career, trying to get laid, etc. A few campus police officers drove by. My mom was safe. It was time to move on.

"Okay, well, call me if, you know, you're about to get raped, or whatever," I said.

"I will," my loving mom said. I was thankful she came. She needed this, too. She needed to see that her kids were going to be okay. She needed to see that there was still hope for us all. She needed to see me go.

I started off. "Wait," she yelled. I turned back, expecting some horrible shit to have already happened. "Thanks for letting me come. Dad and I are very proud of you." She extended a shiny penny my way. "I found this. You take this one." I smiled as I grabbed the penny from her and dropped it into my pocket.

"Thanks, Mom," I said, and ran to catch up with the group, ready to start my new life.

ACKNOWLEDGMENTS

This book would not exist if it weren't for my family (for obvious reasons). It's hard to have some mean asshole write about you, and my family, for some reason, tolerated it and even encouraged me.

Thanks especially to my terrific mom, who has provided so much love and support in my life. She believed in me before anyone else did. Her fight with cancer is an inspiration. Before starting her latest round of chemo in the fall of 2014, she said, "I've got to keep on living so you little fuckers have someone to write about."

Thanks to Tiffany for being a great older sister full of Dad-like advice. Thanks to Greg for being my best friend and reading so many drafts of my work. Thanks to Jessica for putting up with all my shit and still loving me. Thanks to Chelsea for being so funny and not suing me, despite threatening to countless times.

Thanks to all the great people at Flatiron. Thanks to Colin Dickerman for taking a chance on a crude, unknown voice and being one hell of an editor. Thanks to Whitney Frick for reading the book countless times and taking the material to the next level. And to Marlena Bittner, publicist extraordinaire. Thank you, Bob Miller, Liz Keenan, James Melia, David Lott, Emily Walters, and copy editor Greg Villepique.

Thanks to my agent, Elisabeth Weed, for changing my life. The book file sat on a corner of my computer screen untouched for several years before she got her miracle-worker hands on it. Special thanks to Jenny Meyer for all her hard work. And thanks to Dana Murphy.

Thanks to those who read really early and really shitty drafts. (Can you believe there were even shittier versions than this?) Thanks to Charles Finch for being the first champion of the book. Thanks to Matteo Borghese, John O'Connor, Chuck MacLean, Dave Cowen, Giles Andrew, Katie O'Reilly, Gabriel Reilich, Bob Leavitt, Sarah Streicher, Mike Steffen, Ivy Pruss, Gary Neuenschwander, and Matt

Olson for their terrific notes, which helped shape and improve the book. Much thanks to Rob Turbovsky, John Phillips, Morgan Matson, and Sonia Kharkar for their support of the book.

Home Is Burning started out as notes I would post to Facebook. Writers are fueled by encouragement and the belief that they have something to say that people actually want to hear. So thanks to all those people who "liked" the stories and writing, even when they were poorly conceived Facebook notes full of typos and even filthier language.

Thanks to all my friends for listening to me bitch about life and laughing at all my stupid jokes. I don't want to name people here because if I left someone like Tigg Casper off the list, then he'd get all bitchy about it and we wouldn't be friends anymore. But friends, you know who you are. Thank you!

Thanks to all the additional family and friends who supported us during this difficult time. All the lasagnas, letters, visits, and love got us through it. Thanks to our neighbors. I shit on Mormons, but they really are some of the nicest people in the world.

And last, thanks to my dad for his brave battle with Lou Gehrig's disease. His courage taught me so much about life. Throughout his fight, he remained supportive of my dreams. One of the last things he told me was that I should pursue writing because it seemed like the career that would make me happiest. And it has. Even though I'm still pretty depressed all the time.

ALS ASSOCIATION DONATIONS

If you can't tell from the hundreds of pages you've just read, ALS is a horrible disease. Scientists, doctors, and researchers are working their asses off trying to find ways to prevent, treat, and cure it. But they need help. Thus, because I'm a hero (of sorts) in the same category as, say, Mother Teresa, I will be donating a portion of the proceeds from the sales of this book to the ALS Association. If you'd like to learn more about ALS than what I already poetically taught you, or if you'd like to make a donation, visit www.alsa.org. Thanks, and fuck Lou Gehrig's disease!